Clinical Updates on the Aortic Aneurysm and Aortic Dissection

Clinical Updates on the Aortic Aneurysm and Aortic Dissection

Guest Editors
Benedikt Reutersberg
Matthias Trenner

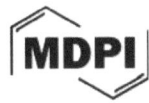

Basel • Beijing • Wuhan • Barcelona • Belgrade • Novi Sad • Cluj • Manchester

Guest Editors

Benedikt Reutersberg
Department of Vascular Surgery
University Hospital Zurich
Zurich
Switzerland

Matthias Trenner
Division of Vascular Medicine
St. Josefs-Hospital Wiesbaden
Wiesbaden
Germany

Editorial Office
MDPI AG
Grosspeteranlage 5
4052 Basel, Switzerland

This is a reprint of the Special Issue, published open access by the journal *Journal of Clinical Medicine* (ISSN 2077-0383), freely accessible at: https://www.mdpi.com/journal/jcm/special_issues/6PIKFCH743.

For citation purposes, cite each article independently as indicated on the article page online and as indicated below:

Lastname, A.A.; Lastname, B.B. Article Title. *Journal Name* **Year**, *Volume Number*, Page Range.

ISBN 978-3-7258-3103-6 (Hbk)
ISBN 978-3-7258-3104-3 (PDF)
https://doi.org/10.3390/books978-3-7258-3104-3

© 2025 by the authors. Articles in this book are Open Access and distributed under the Creative Commons Attribution (CC BY) license. The book as a whole is distributed by MDPI under the terms and conditions of the Creative Commons Attribution-NonCommercial-NoDerivs (CC BY-NC-ND) license (https://creativecommons.org/licenses/by-nc-nd/4.0/).

Contents

Jasmin Epple, Dittmar Böckler and Reinhart T. Grundmann
Sex Differences in Long-Term Survival and Cancer Incidence After Ruptured Abdominal Aortic Aneurysm Repair
Reprinted from: *J. Clin. Med.* **2024**, *13*, 6934, https://doi.org/10.3390/jcm13226934 1

Tamer Ghazy, Nesma Elzanaty, Helmut Karl Lackner, Marc Irqsusi, Ardawan J. Rastan, Christian-Alexander Behrendt and Adrian Mahlmann
Prevalence and Influence of Genetic Variants on Follow-Up Results in Patients Surviving Thoracic Aortic Therapy
Reprinted from: *J. Clin. Med.* **2024**, *13*, 5254, https://doi.org/10.3390/jcm13175254 11

Leonard Pitts, Michael C. Moon, Maximilian Luehr, Markus Kofler, Matteo Montagner, Simon Sündermann, et al.
The Ascyrus Medical Dissection Stent: A One-Fits-All Strategy for the Treatment of Acute Type A Aortic Dissection?
Reprinted from: *J. Clin. Med.* **2024**, *13*, 2593, https://doi.org/10.3390/jcm13092593 25

Roland Bozalka, Anna-Leonie Menges, Alexander Zimmermann and Lorenz Meuli
Hospital Incidence and Treatment Outcomes of Patients with Aneurysms and Dissections of the Iliac Artery in Switzerland—A Secondary Analysis of Swiss DRG Statistics Data
Reprinted from: *J. Clin. Med.* **2024**, *13*, 2267, https://doi.org/10.3390/jcm13082267 36

Frederike Meccanici, Carlijn G. E. Thijssen, Arjen L. Gökalp, Annemijn W. Bom, Guillaume S. C. Geuzebroek, Joost F. ter Woorst, et al.
Long-Term Health-Related Quality of Life following Acute Type A Aortic Dissection with a Focus on Male–Female Differences: A Cross Sectional Study
Reprinted from: *J. Clin. Med.* **2024**, *13*, 2265, https://doi.org/10.3390/jcm13082265 50

Cosmin M. Banceu, Diana M. Banceu, David S. Kauvar, Adrian Popentiu, Vladimir Voth, Markus Liebrich, et al.
Acute Aortic Syndromes from Diagnosis to Treatment—A Comprehensive Review
Reprinted from: *J. Clin. Med.* **2024**, *13*, 1231, https://doi.org/10.3390/jcm13051231 62

Panagiotis Doukas, Nicola Dalibor, András Keszei, Jelle Frankort, Julia Krabbe, Rachad Zayat, et al.
Factors Associated with Early Mortality in Acute Type A Aortic Dissection—A Single-Centre Experience
Reprinted from: *J. Clin. Med.* **2024**, *13*, 1023, https://doi.org/10.3390/jcm13041023 78

Joscha Mulorz, Agnesa Mazrekaj, Justus Sehl, Amir Arnautovic, Waseem Garabet, Kim-Jürgen Krott, et al.
Relative Thrombus Burden Ratio Reveals Overproportioned Intraluminal Thrombus Growth—Potential Implications for Abdominal Aortic Aneurysm
Reprinted from: *J. Clin. Med.* **2024**, *13*, 962, https://doi.org/10.3390/jcm13040962 89

Ilaria Puttini, Marvin Kapalla, Anja Braune, Enrico Michler, Joselyn Kröger, Brigitta Lutz, et al.
Aortic Vascular Graft and Endograft Infection–Patient Outcome Cannot Be Determined Based on Pre-Operative Characteristics
Reprinted from: *J. Clin. Med.* **2024**, *13*, 269, https://doi.org/10.3390/jcm13010269 101

Mohammed Al-Tawil, Mohamed Salem, Christine Friedrich, Shirin Diraz, Alexandra Broll, Najma Rezahie, et al.
Preoperative Imaging Signs of Cerebral Malperfusion in Acute Type A Aortic Dissection: Influence on Outcomes and Prognostic Implications—A 20-Year Experience
Reprinted from: *J. Clin. Med.* **2023**, *12*, 6659, https://doi.org/10.3390/jcm12206659 . . . . **117**

Hazem El Beyrouti, Mohamed Omar, Cristi-Teodor Calimanescu, Hendrik Treede and Nancy Halloum
Paracolic Gutter Routing: A Novel Retroperitoneal Extra-Anatomical Repair for Infected Aorto-Iliac Axis
Reprinted from: *J. Clin. Med.* **2023**, *12*, 5765, https://doi.org/10.3390/jcm12175765 . . . . **128**

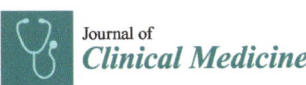

Article

Sex Differences in Long-Term Survival and Cancer Incidence After Ruptured Abdominal Aortic Aneurysm Repair

Jasmin Epple [1], Dittmar Böckler [1] and Reinhart T. Grundmann [2],*

[1] Department of Vascular and Endovascular Surgery, University Hospital Heidelberg, 69120 Heidelberg, Germany
[2] University Heart and Vascular Center Hamburg, Department for Vascular Medicine, University Hospital Hamburg-Eppendorf, 20251 Hamburg, Germany
* Correspondence: reinhart@prof-grundmann.de; Tel.: +49-8677-878483

Abstract: Background: Long-term gender-specific survival and cancer incidence in patients with ruptured abdominal aortic aneurysm (rAAA) were investigated after endovascular (EVAR) and open repair (OAR). **Methods**: Data from 2933 patients (EVAR n = 1187, OAR n = 1746) from a health insurance company in Germany (men n = 2391, women n = 542) were analyzed. All patients were cancer-free in their history. **Results:** Perioperative mortality was significantly higher after OAR (42.6%) than after EVAR (21.2%; $p < 0.001$). Women had significantly higher in-hospital mortality (41.5%) than men (32.2%). Notably, the 5-year survival was 36.9% after OAR and 40.8% after EVAR ($p < 0.001$), and 40.7% in men and 29.1% in women ($p < 0.001$). Overall, 17.2% of EVAR and 14.6% of OAR patients had cancer at 5 years ($p = 0.328$). Cancer incidence did not differ significantly between men and women. Patients with cancer had a significantly less favorable outcome compared to patients with no cancer ($p = 0.002$). Treatment of rAAA was also indicated in octogenarians, with survival rates of 19.9% after 5 years and even 38.4% with perioperative deaths excluded. **Conclusions**: Cancer represents a significant risk factor for survival in patients with rAAA. These patients should be monitored during follow-up, particularly regarding the development of lung cancer.

Keywords: ruptured abdominal aortic aneurysm; cancer incidence; gender; long-term outcome; octogenarians

Citation: Epple, J.; Böckler, D.; Grundmann, R.T. Sex Differences in Long-Term Survival and Cancer Incidence After Ruptured Abdominal Aortic Aneurysm Repair. *J. Clin. Med.* **2024**, *13*, 6934. https://doi.org/10.3390/jcm13226934

Academic Editor: Aaron S. Dumont

Received: 1 September 2024
Revised: 4 November 2024
Accepted: 12 November 2024
Published: 18 November 2024

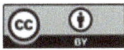

Copyright: © 2024 by the authors. Licensee MDPI, Basel, Switzerland. This article is an open access article distributed under the terms and conditions of the Creative Commons Attribution (CC BY) license (https://creativecommons.org/licenses/by/4.0/).

1. Introduction

This study focuses on the long-term gender-specific survival of patients with ruptured abdominal aortic aneurysm (rAAA) following endovascular (EVAR) and open repair (OAR). Our aim is to determine the expected tumor incidence during follow-up and to specifically assess the survival of patients over 80 years old with rAAA, for which relatively few data are available. In the randomized IMPROVE trial [1], after more than 3 years of follow-up, 179/316 (56.6%) deaths were observed following rAAA repair with EVAR, including 19/179 (10.6%) due to cancer. In the OAR group, there were 183/297 (61.6%) deaths, of which 13/183 (7.1%) were cancer-related. Specific gender-related data were not provided. Varkevisser et al. [2] reported a 5-year survival rate of 63% after EVAR and 52% after OAR for rAAA repair in a cohort from the SVS Vascular Quality Initiative (VQI) clinical registry (2013–2019), but did not provide information on tumor incidence or patient gender. Ettengruber et al. [3] examined a cohort of patients with intact abdominal aortic aneurysm (iAAA). They found that patients with cancer had a significantly worse outcome compared to those without cancer (HR 1.68; 95% CI 1.59–1.78, $p < 0.001$). After nine years, the estimated survival rates were 27.0% for patients with cancer and 55.4% for those without ($p < 0.001$). A comparable study on rAAA does not yet exist. Li et al. [4] reported a survival rate of 36.7% for women vs. 49.5% for men ($p = 0.02$) after endovascular and open AAA repair in a multicenter retrospective cohort study using prospectively collected VQI data, including 1160 women and 4148 men with rAAA, followed up for up to 8 years. Women had higher perioperative and long-term mortality. Data from the Dutch Surgical Aneurysm Audit (DSAA) were analyzed by Alberga et al. [5], including 2879 patients, of whom 1146 were treated with EVAR (382 octogenarians, 33%) and 1733 with OAR (410 octogenarians, 24%). The perioperative mortality rate for all octogenarians was 43.8% compared with 24.1% in all non-octogenarians. Although aneurysm repair was associated with high mortality in this patient category, especially after OAR, these authors noted that a substantial proportion of octogenarians (1/3 after EVAR and 1/5 after OAR) experienced an uneventful recovery after rAAA repair. Roosendaal et al. [6] reported a 2-year mortality rate of 66% (25/38) after EVAR and 62% (34/55) after OAR in 110 octogenarian patients with rAAA. They concluded that surgery for rAAA in active octogenarians should not be denied based on age alone. Gender-specific data or cancer incidence were not reported. Also, given the poor prognosis for patients undergoing rAAA repair, it remains uncertain whether a tumor would still play a significant role in long-term survival. This study aims to fill this gap by presenting long-term outcomes and cancer incidence after rAAA repair in men and women, as well as in patients under and over 80 years old, based on a large database from a German health insurance provider.

2. Materials and Methods

In this retrospective study, patient data from the nationwide health insurance company, AOK-Die Gesundheitskasse, were analyzed. The data were provided and anonymized by WIDO (Wissenschaftliches Institut der AOK). The analysis of the health insurance data involved an evaluation of the complete medical history of each patient. Therefore, this study is not limited to a specific hospital group or medical department. All diagnoses and procedures were coded using the International Classification of Diseases, Tenth Revision (ICD-10) and Operations and Procedures (OPS) codes.

This study includes data on all patients who underwent either endovascular (OPS code: 5-38a.1) or open repair (OPS code: 5-384.7) of a ruptured abdominal aortic aneurysm (rAAA) (ICD code: I71.3 abdominal aortic aneurysm, ruptured) between 1 January 2010 and 31 December 2016. A total of 3227 patients with rAAA were identified. A total of 294 patients with a history of cancer were excluded from the study. Cancer was identified if a cancer-specific ICD was found in the insurance database prior to aneurysm repair (ICD codes: C00–C97). The remaining 2933 rAAA patients were then divided into two groups according to gender. An analysis of comorbidities and perioperative and postoperative complications was performed using documented ICD and OPS codes. The AOK dataset is comprehensive, capturing standardized billing and diagnostic information from all healthcare facilities. As a result, missing data in this dataset are minimal and generally limited to clinical information not covered by ICD or OPS coding, such as specific lifestyle factors or laboratory results. Where such information was unavailable, no imputation was performed; analyses were strictly based on the coded data available. Since it was not possible to determine whether the deaths occurred in the treating hospital, after transfer, or during rehabilitation, perioperative mortality was defined as 60-day mortality. All patients were followed up until 31 December 2018.

Statistical Analysis

The analysis was performed with SPSS 27 (IBM Deutschland GmbH, Ehningen, Germany). To assess significant differences between the two genders, Chi-square tests were performed for non-metric variables. For metric variables, a Mann–Whitney U-test was used.

For estimating overall survival and cancer incidence in the follow-up, Kaplan–Meier tables were generated, and the log-rank test was used to test for significance between the two groups. A univariable Cox proportional model was implemented before a multivariable Cox proportional model to assess the impact of comorbidities, age, and gender on overall survival. All parameters demonstrating a statistically significant influence on survival in the univariable analysis ($p < 0.05$) were tested in the multivariable analysis.

Significance was assessed using log-rank tests. p-values less than 0.05 were considered statistically significant.

3. Results

3.1. Patients

Patient characteristics and comorbidities are shown in Table 1. In the rAAA cohort, 2391 patients were male (81.5%), and 542 were female (18.5%). A total of 40.8% of male patients underwent EVAR compared to 38.9% of female patients (p = 0.418). A total of 59.2% of male patients and 61.1% of female patients underwent OAR (p = 0.418). Women were significantly older than men with a mean age of 79.6 vs. 73.9 years (p < 0.001). Female patients had significantly more diabetes mellitus type 2 (male: 10.8%, female: 15.9%, p = 0.001) and arterial hypertension (male: 35.1%, female: 47.4%, p < 0.001). A history of myocardial infarction was significantly more common in men (men: 8.4%, women: 5.2%, p = 0.011).

Table 1. Baseline characteristics of male and female patients undergoing ruptured abdominal aortic aneurysm repair (all patients were cancer-free at time of repair).

Parameter	Male n = 2391	Female n = 542	p-Value
EVAR, n (%)	976 (40.8)	211 (38.9)	0.418
OAR, n (%)	1415 (59.2)	331 (61.1)	0.418
Age, mean ± SD in years, median (min–max)	73.9 ± 9.6, 75 (25–97)	79.6 ± 8.7, 81 (36–100)	<0.001
Patients ≥ 80 years, n (%)	719 (30.1)	314 (57.9)	<0.001
History of myocardial infarction, n (%)	201 (8.4)	28 (5.2)	0.011
History of stroke, n (%)	85 (3.6)	29 (5.4)	0.051
History of intracerebral bleeding, n (%)	9 (0.4)	1 (0.2)	0.700
History of TIA, n (%)	43 (1.8)	11 (2.0)	0.718
Arterial hypertension, n (%)	840 (35.1)	257 (47.4)	<0.001
Diabetes mellitus type 2, n (%)	258 (10.8)	86 (15.9)	0.001
COPD, n (%)	261 (10.9)	66 (12.2)	0.400
Left heart failure (NYHA 2–4 and unspecified), n (%)	220 (9.2)	159 (10.9)	0.227
Chronic kidney disease (stage 3–5), n (%)	201 (8.4)	56 (10.3)	0.152
-Stage 3, n (%)	−159 (6.6)	−45 (8.3)	0.172
-Stage 4, n (%)	−32 (1.3)	−10 (1.8)	0.370
-Stage 5, n (%)	−10 (0.4)	−1 (0.2)	0.701
PAD (Fontaine stage 3–4), n (%)	62 (2.6)	14 (2.6)	0.989
-Stage 3, n (%)	−26 (1.1)	−5 (0.9)	0.735
-Stage 4, n (%)	−36 (1.5)	−9 (1.7)	0.791

EVAR: endovascular aneurysm repair, OAR: open aneurysm repair, SD: standard deviation, min–max: minimum–maximum, TIA: transient ischemic attack, COPD: chronic obstructive pulmonary disease, NYHA: New York Heart Association, chronic kidney disease stage 3–5: glomerular filtration rate under 60 mL/min/1.73 m^2, PAD: peripheral artery disease.

3.2. Perioperative Outcome

Perioperative outcomes are shown in Table 2. Perioperative mortality was 32.2% for men and 41.5% for women (p < 0.001). In EVAR patients, 20.6% of men and 24.2% of women died perioperatively (p = 0.249). For OAR, the mortality rates were 40.2% for men and 52.6% for women (p < 0.001). Men aged ≥ 80 years had a mortality rate of 47.6% (EVAR 32.7%, OAR 60.6%) compared to 50.3% (EVAR 27.0%, OAR 65.1%) for women (p = 0.416). In comparison, perioperative mortality in patients < 80 years was lower with 25.6% (EVAR: 14.2%, OAR: 32.7%) in men and 29.4% (EVAR: 20.2%, OAR: 35.3%) in women (p = 0.222).

Table 2. Perioperative outcomes after ruptured abdominal aortic aneurysm repair.

Parameter	Male n = 2391	Female n = 542	p-Value
Perioperative mortality, n (%)	770 (32.2)	225 (41.5)	<0.001
Perioperative mortality EVAR, n (%)	201/976 (20.6)	51/211 (24.2)	0.249
Perioperative mortality OAR, n (%)	569/1415 (40.2)	174/331 (52.6)	<0.001
Perioperative mortality < 80 years, n (%)	428/1627 (25.6)	67/228 (29.4)	0.222
Perioperative mortality ≥ 80 years, n (%)	342/719 (47.6)	158/314 (50.3)	0.416
LOS, mean ± SD in days, median (min-max)	20.7 ± 22.3, 14 (0–281)	21.6 ± 24.1, 15 (0–226)	0.802
LOS of surviving patients, mean ± SD in days, median (min–max)	26.6 ± 23.7, 18 (1–281)	30.3 ± 26.3, 23 (1–226)	0.002
Blood transfusions, n (%)	1842 (77.0)	452 (83.4)	0.001
Intensive care treatment, n (%)	1541 (64.5)	345 (63.7)	0.727
Wound complications, n (%)	235 (9.8)	45 (8.3)	0.275
Myocardial infarction, n (%)	118 (4.9)	19 (3.5)	0.154
Stroke, intracerebral bleeding or TIA, n (%)	58 (2.4)	18 (3.3)	0.236
Dialysis, n (%)	462 (19.3)	86 (15.9)	0.062
Pneumonia, n (%)	432 (18.1)	84 (15.5)	0.156
Deep-vein thrombosis, n (%)	28 (1.2)	5 (0.9)	0.620
Major amputation, n (%)	20 (0.8)	3 (0.6)	0.500
Ileus, n (%)	153 (6.4)	26 (4.8)	0.160

EVAR: endovascular aneurysm repair, OAR: open aneurysm repair, SD: standard deviation, min–max: minimum–maximum, TIA: transient ischemic attack, LOS: length of stay.

Hospital stay did differ significantly between male (mean: 26.6 days) and female patients (mean: 30.3 days, $p = 0.002$) and was longer in patients ≥ 80 years (mean: 28.0 days) compared to patients < 80 years (mean: 26.9 days, $p = 0.040$) if the patients survived the operation.

Female patients were significantly more likely to require blood transfusions (83.4%) than male patients (77.0%) ($p = 0.001$). All other perioperative complications analyzed did not differ significantly between the two genders.

3.3. Long-Term Survival

The 5-year survival of male and female patients, differentiated by age and EVAR and OAR, is given in Table 3. In total, 40.8% of EVAR and 36.9% of OAR patients survived 5 years ($p < 0.001$). A total of 40.7% of male patients were still alive compared to 29.1% of female patients ($p < 0.001$, Figure 1). If the patients survived the initial repair (perioperative deaths excluded), 60.1% of male and 49.7% of female patients were still living after 5 years ($p < 0.001$).

Table 3. Survival 5 years after ruptured abdominal aortic aneurysm repair (all patients were cancer-free at time of repair). All percentages are Kaplan–Meier estimates.

Survival After 5 Years	Male n = 2391	Female n = 542	p-Value
Total cohort, n (%)	1025/2391 (40.7)	171/542 (29.1)	<0.001
EVAR, n (%)	453/976 (42.7)	81/211 (34.9)	0.001
OAR, n (%)	572/1415 (39.2)	90/331 (27.1)	<0.001
Patients < 80 years, n (%)	868/1672 (49.8)	101/228 (41.4)	0.003
Patients ≥ 80 years, n (%)	157/719 (19.7)	70/314 (20.3)	0.867
EVAR (perioperative deaths excluded), n (%)	453/775 (53.8)	77/160 (41.8)	0.001
OAR (perioperative deaths excluded), n (%)	572/846 (65.5)	94/157 (57.1)	0.004
Patients < 80 years (perioperative deaths excluded), n (%)	868/1244 (67.0)	101/161 (58.7)	0.003
Patients ≥ 80 years (perioperative deaths excluded), n (%)	157/377 (37.5)	70/156 (40.9)	0.556

EVAR: endovascular aneurysm repair, OAR: open aneurysm repair.

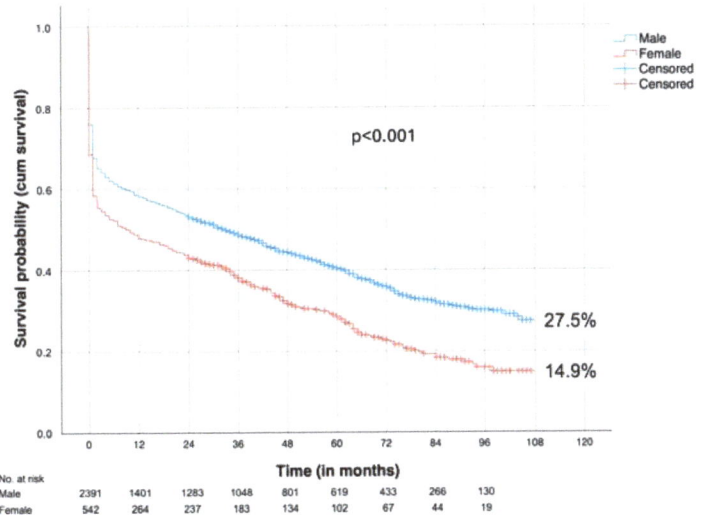

Figure 1. Survival (all patients were cancer-free at time of repair); male vs. female.

A total of 48.8% of patients < 80 years and 19.9% of patients ≥ 80 years survived 5 years ($p < 0.001$, Figure 2).

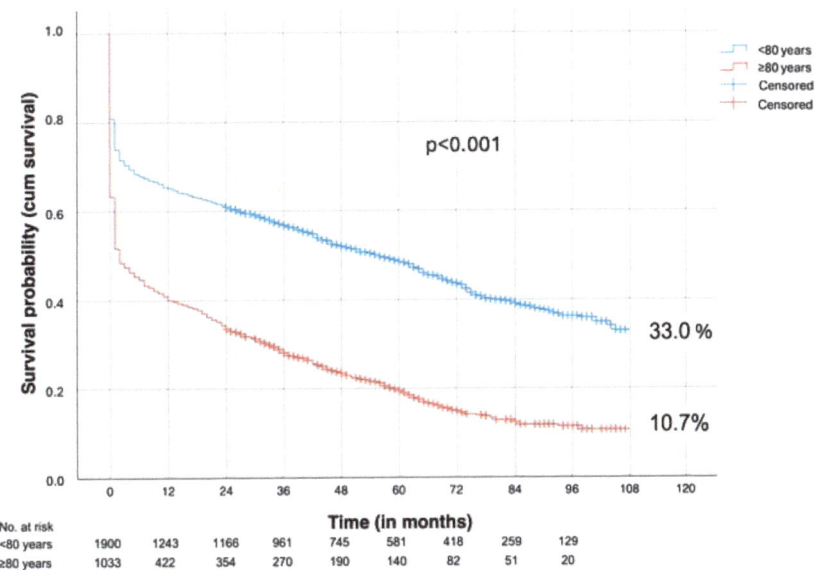

Figure 2. Survival (all patients were cancer-free at time of repair); <80 years vs. ≥80 years.

The factors influencing long-term outcomes were identified for patients who survived the initial rAAA repair (Table 4). Age ≥ 80 years (HR: 2.013, $p < 0.001$), COPD (HR: 1.602, $p < 0.001$), chronic kidney disease stage 3–5 (HR: 1.545, $p < 0.001$), cancer (HR: 1.318, $p = 0.002$), and left heart failure (NYHA 2–4) (HR: 1.269, $p = 0.043$) negatively influenced survival.

Table 4. Hazard ratio (HR) and proportional hazard model (multivariable analysis) for long-term mortality (all patients were cancer-free at time of repair). All patients included in the analysis survived the initial intervention.

	HR	95% CI	p-Value
Age ≥ 80 years	2.013	1.747–2.321	<0.001
COPD	1.602	1.303–1.970	<0.001
Chronic kidney disease (stage 3–5)	1.545	1.232–1.937	<0.001
Cancer	1.318	1.112–1.564	0.002
Left heart failure (NYHA 2–4 and unspecified)	1.269	1.008–1.599	0.043
OAR (vs. EVAR)	0.838	0.731–0.960	0.011
Women (vs. Men)	1.161	0.980–1.376	0.084
History of myocardial infarction	1.170	0.915–1.497	0.211
History of stroke, intracerebral bleeding, or TIA	1.050	0.779–1.415	0.749
Arterial hypertension	1.076	0.919–1.261	0.362
Diabetes mellitus type 2	1.112	0.898–1.377	0.331
PAD (Fontaine stage 3–4)	1.091	0.727–1.638	0.673

EVAR: endovascular aneurysm repair, OAR: open aneurysm repair, HR: hazard ratio, CI: confidence interval, TIA: transient ischemic attack, COPD: chronic obstructive pulmonary disease, chronic kidney disease stage 3–5: glomerular filtration rate under 60 mL/min/1.73 m^2, NYHA: New York Heart Association, PAD: peripheral artery disease.

Gender had no significant effect on survival (HR: 1.161, p = 0.084).

3.4. Cancer Incidence in the Follow-Up

In total, 17.2% of EVAR patients and 14.6% of OAR patients were diagnosed with cancer after five years (p = 0.328). Cancer incidence was not significantly higher in men (16.5%) compared to women (11.9%) (p = 0.153) (Table 5). This pattern was observed for both EVAR (men: 18.2%, women: 11.0%, p = 0.272) and OAR (men: 15.2%, women: 12.1%, p = 0.305). Lung cancer was the most common cancer during follow-up, affecting 4.4% of men and 2.7% of women (p = 0.288). The incidence of ureter and bladder cancer at five years (men: 2.8%, women: 1.0%, p = 0.098) and colon cancer (men: 2.0%, women: 1.4%, p = 0.598) did not differ significantly between the sexes. Prostate cancer affected 2.5% of men after five years of follow-up.

Table 5. Cancer incidence 5 years after abdominal aortic aneurysm repair (all patients were cancer-free at time of repair and survived the intervention). All percentages are Kaplan–Meier estimates.

	Male n = 1621	Female n = 317	p-Value
Cancer incidence	16.5%	11.9%	0.153
Cancer incidence EVAR	18.2%	11.0%	0.272
Cancer incidence OAR	15.2%	12.1%	0.354
Cancer incidence < 80 years	15.1%	9.5%	0.251
Cancer incidence ≥ 80 years	22.7%	14.5%	0.139
Lung cancer incidence	4.4%	2.7%	0.288
Prostate cancer incidence	2.5%	0.0%	0.016
Colon cancer incidence	2.0%	1.4%	0.598
Ureter and bladder cancer incidence	2.8%	1.0%	0.098

EVAR: endovascular aneurysm repair, OAR: open aneurysm repair.

Figure 3 shows the post-discharge survival of patients who survived rAAA repair (excluding in-hospital mortality), differentiated by whether they developed cancer during follow-up. After five years, 59.9% of cancer-free patients and 50.5% of cancer patients were still alive (p < 0.001).

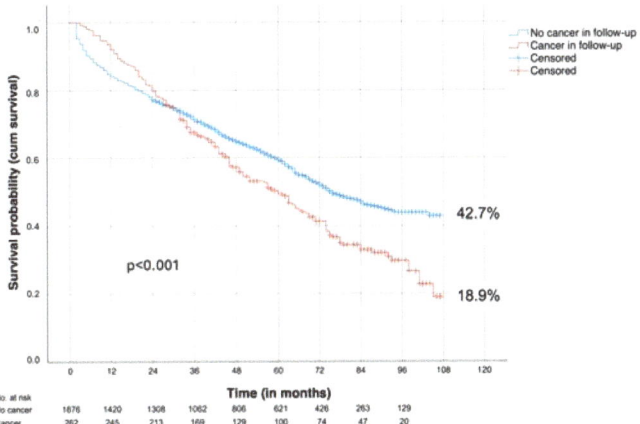

Figure 3. Survival of cancer-free patients and patients with cancer in the follow-up (all patients were cancer-free at time of repair. Perioperative deaths excluded).

4. Discussion

In our study, in-hospital mortality following rAAA repair was significantly higher after OAR at 42.6% compared to 21.2% after EVAR ($p < 0.001$). This finding aligns with the results of a comprehensive literature review and a meta-analysis of approximately 267,259 patients from 136 studies, which demonstrated that EVAR carries a lower perioperative mortality risk than open surgery (Kontopodis et al. [7]). Women had a significantly higher in-hospital mortality rate of 41.5% following rAAA repair compared to 32.2% in men, which was attributable solely to the higher mortality rate associated with OAR, as no significant gender differences were observed after EVAR (Table 2). Similarly, in the IMPROVE trial [8], women particularly benefited from the endovascular approach, with a 30-day mortality rate of 37% after EVAR versus 57% after OAR. A higher in-hospital mortality rate was also reported by Ho et al. [9] in the Vascular Quality Initiative (VQI) registry from 2013 to 2019 for rAAA patients. In this study, which included a total of 1775 patients (23.8% female), the in-hospital mortality rate after EVAR was 45.9% in women compared to 34.5% in men ($p < 0.01$).

In this study, the 5-year survival rate was 36.9% after OAR and 40.8% after EVAR ($p < 0.001$), which is less favorable than the survival rates reported by Varkevisser et al. [2] (63% after EVAR and 52% after OAR). However, Varkevisser et al. did not specify the percentage of patients over 80 years old, which in our study was 30.1% for men and 57.9% for women. Among patients who survived the initial AAA repair (excluding in-hospital mortality), better post-discharge survival was observed after OAR compared to EVAR, with 64.2% vs. 51.8% at 5 years ($p < 0.001$). This was also confirmed by multivariate regression analysis (HR: 0.838 [CI, 0.731–0.960]; $p = 0.011$).

In contrast, Salata et al. [10] found in a population-based study of 2692 rAAA patients (261 EVAR [10%] and 2431 OAR [90%]) that there were lower hazards for all-cause mortality and major adverse cardiovascular events (MACEs) within 30 days of surgery in favor of EVAR but no differences in mid- or long-term outcomes. Similarly, Kontopodis et al. [11] reported in a meta-analysis involving a total of 31,383 patients that there were no significant differences in the hazard of death after discharge from the hospital between the EVAR and open repair groups (HR, 1.10; 95% CI, 0.85–1.43; $p = 0.47$).

In our study, men exhibited a significantly better 5-year survival rate of 40.7% compared to 29.1% in women ($p < 0.001$) (Figure 1). This trend persisted even when excluding in-hospital mortality, with a 5-year survival rate of 60.1% for men and 49.7% for women, which can be attributed to the higher age of the female patients.

Li et al. [4] also found a less favorable long-term survival for women compared to men in an analysis of the Vascular Quality Initiative database, extending up to 8 years after rAAA repair, and similarly attributed this to the older age of the female patients. However, unlike the study by Li et al., no gender-specific differences were found in the proportion of patients with chronic kidney disease in the current study. The only significant differences observed were a higher prevalence of diabetes and arterial hypertension among women (Table 1).

Biancari et al. [12] reported on 200 patients aged 80 years or older who underwent emergency open repair for rAAA. They found a survival rate of 68% at three years and 45% at five years among the 82 patients who survived the procedure, concluding that an active approach is warranted even in this age group for hemodynamically stable patients. Roosendaal et al. [6] reached a similar conclusion in their analysis of outcomes in 110 octogenarian patients who underwent either endovascular or open repair of rAAA. In their study, half of the patients were still alive one year after the procedure, and more than 80% were living at home, comparable to the general population of 80-year-olds in the Netherlands, where approximately 14% reside in nursing homes. Thus, age alone should not be a criterion to question the feasibility of rAAA repair. This is further demonstrated by the present study, which observed a 5-year survival rate of 19.9% among patients over 80 years old (Figure 2) and an even higher survival when perioperative deaths were excluded (38.4%).

Pirinen et al. [13] analyzed 9464 patients with rAAA repair in Finland and Sweden. The mean survival after EVAR was 7.5 (95% CI 6.9–8.1 years) for patients younger than 65 years, 5.1 (5.4–5.3 years) for patients aged 65–79 years, and 3.1 (2.7–3.4 years) for patients aged >80 years. The results showed that the long-term survival of patients aged 80 years or older after successful AAA treatment is similar to that of the general population. It seems important, however, to consider not only the age but also the frailty of the patient when determining the indication for surgery. Yu et al. [14] identified 5806 patients (age, 72 ± 9 years; 77% male; EVAR, 65%) with rAAA in the VQI database, of whom 36% were frail and 10% were very frail. The overall observed 1-year mortality rate was 52.7%, with higher mortality in the OAR group compared to the EVAR group (55.8% vs. 51.1%; $p = 0.001$). Among very frail patients (n = 566), the 1-year mortality was 70% with EVAR vs. 69.9% with OAR, though patient age was not specifically analyzed. These authors concluded that very frail patients lack the resilience to withstand the stressors of aortic rupture, regardless of the repair technique.

In this study, all patients were cancer-free at the time of repair. After a follow-up period of 5 years, 16.5% of men and 11.9% of women developed cancer (Table 5). Patients who developed cancer had a significantly less favorable outcome compared to those without cancer (HR 1.318; 95% CI 1.112–1.564, $p = 0.002$). Ettengruber et al. [3] analyzed 18,802 iAAA patients. They concluded that patients with a history of cancer had worse long-term survival than those without (HR 1.68; 95% CI 1.59–1.78, $p < 0.001$). At the nine-year mark, the estimated survival rates were 27.0% for patients with cancer and 55.4% for those without ($p < 0.001$). They also analyzed tumor incidence after EVAR and OAR, and EVAR showed an increased risk in postoperative development of abdominal cancer (HR 1.20; 95% CI 1.07–1.35, $p = 0.002$). Markar et al. [15] also analyzed 14,150 patients who underwent EVAR and 24,645 patients who underwent open repair. EVAR was associated with an increased risk in postoperative abdominal cancer (hazard ratio [HR], 1.14; 95% confidence interval [CI], 1.03–1.27) and all cancers (HR, 1.09; 95% CI, 1.02–1.17). In this rAAA cohort, where 17.2% of EVAR patients and 14.6% of OAR patients were diagnosed with cancer at five years ($p = 0.328$), no significant difference was found between the two operation methods.

Comparative data on rAAA patients are scarce in the literature, with only Troisi et al. [16] reporting on 405 patients who underwent endovascular and open rAAA repair, among whom 58.2% survived after 5 years. In this cohort, cancer was the most common cause of death among the 135 fatalities (n = 25; 18.5%).

Based on the present data, it can be cautiously concluded that the development of cancer adversely affects patient survival as early as three years after rAAA repair (Figure 3). Therefore, patients who have undergone rAAA repair should not be excluded from routine cancer screening. Given the smoking history of many of these patients, lung cancer screening in particular should be considered, as it is the most frequently observed tumor in this population.

The present study has several evident limitations. The comprehensiveness of the datasets relies on the coding accuracy of individual hospitals and the documentation provided by the health insurance company, which leaves room for potential coding errors. The data reflect the patient demographics of a specific health insurance company, capturing its social structure, and may not necessarily represent the entire German population. However, it is worth noting that AOK is the largest health insurance company in Germany, with a market share of 37%. The anonymity of the datasets prevented analysis of the treated hospitals and their case volumes. Additionally, the causes of death and the exact dates of death remained indeterminable. The aortic diameter is not included in the health insurance data. Conversely, a notable strength of this study lies in its ability to document the long-term survival of all patients for up to nine years.

5. Conclusions

In summary, the perioperative mortality rate for rAAA repair was lower with EVAR compared to OAR, but OAR was associated with better long-term survival. Women had less favorable survival outcomes than men, which can be attributed to their higher age. Even in octogenarians, rAAA repair is indicated, with survival rates of 19.9% after 5 years and even higher when perioperative deaths are excluded (38.4%). Cancer remains a significant risk factor for survival in patients with rAAA, with a survival rate after five years of 59.9% in cancer-free patients versus 50.5% in those who developed cancer. Given the high risk of lung cancer development, these patients should be closely monitored during follow-up.

Author Contributions: Conceptualization, J.E., D.B. and R.T.G.; methodology, J.E. and R.T.G.; formal analysis, J.E.; investigation, J.E. and R.T.G.; resources, R.T.G.; data curation, J.E.; writing—original draft preparation, R.T.G.; writing—review and editing, J.E., D.B. and R.T.G.; visualization, J.E.; supervision, R.T.G. and D.B.; project administration, R.T.G. All authors have read and agreed to the published version of the manuscript.

Funding: This research received no external funding.

Institutional Review Board Statement: Ethical review and approval were waived for this study because this is health insurance data and analysis of this data does not require an ethical review and approval.

Informed Consent Statement: Patient consent was waived because this is health insurance data and analysis of this data does not require consent.

Data Availability Statement: The collected datasets can be requested in anonymized form from the corresponding author upon justified request.

Conflicts of Interest: The authors declare no conflicts of interest.

References

1. IMPROVE Trial Investigators. Comparative clinical effectiveness and cost effectiveness of endovascular strategy v open repair for ruptured abdominal aortic aneurysm: Three year results of the IMPROVE randomised trial. *BMJ* **2017**, *359*, j4859.
2. Varkevisser, R.R.B.; Swerdlow, N.J.; de Guerre, L.E.V.M.; Dansey, K.; Stangenberg, L.; Giles, K.A.; Verhagen, H.J.M.; Schermerhorn, M.L.; Society for Vascular Surgery Vascular Quality Initiative. Five-year survival following endovascular repair of ruptured abdominal aortic aneurysms is improving. *J. Vasc. Surg.* **2020**, *72*, 105–113.e4. [CrossRef] [PubMed]
3. Ettengruber, A.; Epple, J.; Schmitz-Rixen, T.; Böckler, D.; Grundmann, R.T.; DIGG gGmbH. Long-term outcome and cancer incidence after abdominal aortic aneurysm repair. *Langenbecks Arch. Surg.* **2022**, *407*, 3691–3699. [CrossRef] [PubMed]
4. Li, B.; Eisenberg, N.; Witheford, M.; Lindsay, T.F.; Forbes, T.L.; Roche-Nagle, G. Sex Differences in Outcomes Following Ruptured Abdominal Aortic Aneurysm Repair. *JAMA Netw. Open* **2022**, *5*, e2211336. [CrossRef]
5. Alberga, A.J.; de Bruin, J.L.; Gonçalves, F.B.; Karthaus, E.G.; Wilschut, J.A.; van Herwaarden, J.A.; Wever, J.J.; Verhagen, H.J.M.; Collaboration with the Dutch Society of Vascular Surgery, the Steering Committee of the Dutch Surgical Aneurysm Audit and the Dutch Institute for Clinical Auditing. Nationwide Outcomes of Octogenarians Following Open or Endovascular Management After Ruptured Abdominal Aortic Aneurysms. *J. Endovasc. Ther.* **2023**, *30*, 419–432. [CrossRef] [PubMed]

6. Roosendaal, L.C.; Wiersema, A.M.; Yeung, K.K.; Ünlü, Ç.; Metz, R.; Wisselink, W.; Jongkind, V. Survival and Living Situation After Ruptured Abdominal Aneurysm Repair in Octogenarians. *Eur. J. Vasc. Endovasc. Surg.* **2021**, *61*, 375–381. [CrossRef] [PubMed]
7. Kontopodis, N.; Galanakis, N.; Antoniou, S.A.; Tsetis, D.; Ioannou, C.V.; Veith, F.J.; Powell, J.T.; Antoniou, G.A. Meta-Analysis and Meta-Regression Analysis of Outcomes of Endovascular and Open Repair for Ruptured Abdominal Aortic Aneurysm. *Eur. J. Vasc. Endovasc. Surg.* **2020**, *59*, 399–410. [CrossRef] [PubMed]
8. IMPROVE Trial Investigators; Powell, J.T.; Sweeting, M.J.; Thompson, M.M.; Ashleigh, R.; Bell, R.; Gomes, M.; Greenhalgh, R.M.; Grieve, R.; Heatley, F.; et al. Endovascular or open repair strategy for ruptured abdominal aortic aneurysm: 30 day outcomes from IMPROVE randomised trial. *BMJ* **2014**, *348*, f7661.
9. Ho, V.T.; Rothenberg, K.A.; George, E.L.; Lee, J.T.; Stern, J.R. Female sex is independently associated with in-hospital mortality after endovascular aortic repair for ruptured aortic aneurysm. *Ann. Vasc. Surg.* **2022**, *81*, 148–153. [CrossRef] [PubMed]
10. Salata, K.; Hussain, M.A.; de Mestral, C.; Greco, E.; Awartani, H.; Aljabri, B.A.; Mamdani, M.; Forbes, T.L.; Bhatt, D.L.; Verma, S.; et al. Population-based long-term outcomes of open versus endovascular aortic repair of ruptured abdominal aortic aneurysms. *J. Vasc. Surg.* **2020**, *71*, 1867–1878.e8. [CrossRef] [PubMed]
11. Kontopodis, N.; Galanakis, N.; Ioannou, C.V.; Tsetis, D.; Becquemin, J.-P.; Antoniou, G.A. Time-to-event data meta-analysis of late outcomes of endovascular versus open repair for ruptured abdominal aortic aneurysms. *J. Vasc. Surg.* **2021**, *74*, 628–638.e4. [CrossRef] [PubMed]
12. Biancari, F.; Venermo, M.; Finnish Arterial Disease Investigators. Open repair of ruptured abdominal aortic aneurysm in patients aged 80 years and older. *Br. J. Surg.* **2011**, *98*, 1713–1718. [PubMed]
13. Pirinen, R.; Laine, M.T.; Mani, K.; Gunnarsson, K.; Wanhainen, A.; Sund, R.; Venermo, M. The Outcome after Endovascular and Open Repair of Abdominal Aortic Aneurysms—A Binational Study Conducted between 1998 and 2017. *J. Clin. Med.* **2024**, *13*, 4449. [CrossRef] [PubMed]
14. Yu, J.; Khamzina, Y.; Kennedy, J.; Liang, N.L.; Hall, D.E.; Arya, S.; Tzeng, E.; Reitz, K.M. The association between frailty and outcomes following ruptured abdominal aortic aneurysm repair. *J. Vasc. Surg.* **2024**, *80*, 379–388.e3. [CrossRef] [PubMed]
15. Markar, S.R.; Vidal-Diez, A.; Sounderajah, V.; Mackenzie, H.; Hanna, G.B.; Thompson, M.; Holt, P.; Lagergren, J.; Karthikesalingam, A. A population-based cohort study examining the risk of abdominal cancer after endovascular abdominal aortic aneurysm repair. *J. Vasc. Surg.* **2019**, *69*, 1776–1785.e2. [CrossRef] [PubMed]
16. Troisi, N.; Isernia, G.; Bertagna, G.; Adami, D.; Baccani, L.; Parlani, G.; Berchiolli, R.; Simonte, G. Preoperative factors affecting long-term mortality in patients survived to ruptured abdominal aortic aneurysm repair. *Int. Angiol.* **2023**, *42*, 318–326. [CrossRef] [PubMed]

Disclaimer/Publisher's Note: The statements, opinions and data contained in all publications are solely those of the individual author(s) and contributor(s) and not of MDPI and/or the editor(s). MDPI and/or the editor(s) disclaim responsibility for any injury to people or property resulting from any ideas, methods, instructions or products referred to in the content.

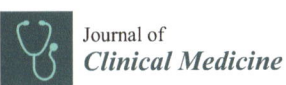

Article

Prevalence and Influence of Genetic Variants on Follow-Up Results in Patients Surviving Thoracic Aortic Therapy

Tamer Ghazy [1,*], Nesma Elzanaty [2], Helmut Karl Lackner [3], Marc Irqsusi [1], Ardawan J. Rastan [1], Christian-Alexander Behrendt [4,5] and Adrian Mahlmann [6,7]

1. Department of Cardiac and Thoracic-Vascular Surgery, University Hospital Giessen and Marburg, Philipps University of Marburg, 35043 Marburg, Germany; irqsusi@med.uni-marburg.de (M.I.); a.rastan@uk-gm.de (A.J.R.)
2. Department of Medical Physiology, Tanta Faculty of Medicine, Tanta University, Tanta 31527, Egypt; nesma.elzanaty@med.tanta.edu.eg
3. Division of Physiology, Otto Loewi Research Center for Vascular Biology, Immunology and Inflammation, Medical University of Graz, 8010 Graz, Austria; helmut.lackner@medunigraz.at
4. Department of Vascular and Endovascular Surgery, Asklepios Clinic Wandsbek, Asklepios Medical School, 20043 Hamburg, Germany; behrendt@hamburg.de
5. Brandenburg Medical School Theodor Fontane, 16816 Neuruppin, Germany
6. Centre for Vascular Medicine, Clinic of Angiology, St.-Josefs-Hospital, Katholische Krankenhaus Hagen gem. GmbH, 58099 Hagen, Germany; mahlmanna@kkh-hagen.de
7. Department of Internal Medicine III, University Hospital Carl Gustav Carus at Technische Universität Dresden, 01307 Dresden, Germany
* Correspondence: tamer.ghazy@uk-gm.de; Tel.: +49-6421-58-66223; Fax: +49-6421-58-68952

Citation: Ghazy, T.; Elzanaty, N.; Lackner, H.K.; Irqsusi, M.; Rastan, A.J.; Behrendt, C.-A.; Mahlmann, A. Prevalence and Influence of Genetic Variants on Follow-Up Results in Patients Surviving Thoracic Aortic Therapy. *J. Clin. Med.* **2024**, *13*, 5254. https://doi.org/10.3390/jcm13175254

Academic Editor: Maurizio Taramasso

Received: 16 July 2024
Revised: 18 August 2024
Accepted: 29 August 2024
Published: 5 September 2024

Correction Statement: This article has been republished with a minor change. The change does not affect the scientific content of the article and further details are available within the backmatter of the website version of this article.

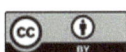

Copyright: © 2024 by the authors. Licensee MDPI, Basel, Switzerland. This article is an open access article distributed under the terms and conditions of the Creative Commons Attribution (CC BY) license (https://creativecommons.org/licenses/by/4.0/).

Abstract: Background/Objective: To investigate the prevalence and effects of genetic variants (GVs) in survivors of thoracic aortic dissection/aneurysm repair. **Methods:** Patients aged 18–80 years who survived follow-up after cardiosurgical or endovascular repair of thoracic aortic aneurysm or dissection at a single tertiary center between 2008 and 2019 and underwent genetic testing were enrolled. The exclusion criteria were age >60 years, no offspring, and inflammatory- or trauma-related pathogenesis. Follow-up entailed computed tomography-angiography at 3 and 9 months and annually thereafter. All patients underwent genetic analyses of nine genes using next-generation sequencing. In cases of specific suspicion, the analysis was expanded to include 32 genes. **Results:** The study included 95 patients. The follow-up period was 3 ± 2.5 years. GVs were detected in 40% of patients. Correlation analysis according to primary diagnosis showed no significant correlation in disease persistence, progression, or in reintervention rates in aneurysm patients and a correlation of disease persistence with genetic variants according to variant class in dissection patients ($p = 0.037$). Correlation analysis according to follow-up CD finding revealed that patients with detected dissection, irrespective of original pathology, showed a strong correlation with genetic variants regarding disease progression and reintervention rates ($p = 0.012$ and $p = 0.047$, respectively). **Conclusions:** The prevalence of VUS is high in patients with aortic pathology. In patients with dissected aorta in the follow-up, irrespective of original pathology, genetic variants correlate with higher reintervention rates, warranting extended-spectrum genetic testing. The role of VUS may be greater than is currently known.

Keywords: aortic surgery; aortic disease; genetic testing; heritable aortic disease

1. Introduction

Diseases of the thoracic aorta are often first diagnosed in the context of acute events, which frequently require urgent or emergent intervention. The disease course depends on the underlying aortic pathology and associated complications [1]. Known cardiovascular risk factors that predispose toward the development of thoracic aortic diseases over the course of life and increasing age contribute to the development of atherosclerosis, a potential pathophysiological cause of thoracic aortic pathologies. Moreover, traumatic or inflammatory influences can occasionally act as causative factors [2,3]. Conversely, diseases of the connective tissue of the aortic wall, such as Marfan syndrome or Ehlers-Danlos syndrome, which may be associated with thoracic aortic diseases, are more prevalent in younger patients [2]. Modern sequencing analyses allow for the targeted analysis of genetic loci associated with mutations linked to connective tissue diseases of the aortic wall, which can culminate in thoracic diseases of the aortic wall [2]. In addition to previously described and presumed disease-causing gene mutations, unclassified variants of unclear clinical significance (VUS) have been increasingly detected [4–10]. Furthermore, previous studies have focused on detecting and analyzing genetic changes that may be involved in the etiology of thoracic aortic diseases. However, the presence of VUS and their differential effects on the disease course, recurrence, and the type and number of subsequent surgical or endovascular interventions that may be needed based on these VUS have received very little attention. The primary aim of this study was to investigate the effect of genetic variants on the disease course in patients who underwent surgical or endovascular repair for thoracic aortic dissection or aneurysm. These findings are significant, not only for the patients themselves in structuring follow-up and selecting different therapeutic methods in the case of necessary reinterventions, but also potentially for future generations in the case of inheritable genetic aortic disease, enabling recommendations for screening examinations.

2. Materials and Method

The participating clinics/centers and collaborators included the University Vascular Center Dresden, Angiology Division, Medical Clinic and Polyclinic III, University Hospital Carl Gustav Carus, Dresden University of Technology; Heart Center, Dresden University Hospital, Department of Cardiac Surgery; and Community Practice for Human Genetics, Dresden, Germany (existing cooperation agreement with University Hospital Carl Gustav Carus).

The study was approved by the Ethics Committee of the Dresden University of Technology (EK317082014). Clinical data were obtained from the university aortic board, for which patient consent was waived. All participants provided written consent for inclusion in genetic testing.

2.1. Inclusion and Exclusion Criteria

All patients who underwent cardiosurgical or endovascular repair of thoracic aortic aneurysm (TAA) or thoracic aortic aneurysm and dissection (TAAD) at a single tertiary center between January 2008 and June 2019 were screened for eligibility. Screening was performed according to the primary diagnoses and treatments documented in the institutional database using the International Classification of Diseases codes.

The inclusion criteria were as follows:
- Patient age between 18 and 80 years;
- Survival during the procedure and follow-up period;
- Patient consent to undergo human genetic testing to clarify the pathogenesis of the underlying aortic wall disease.

The exclusion criteria were as follows:
- Confirmed inflammatory or trauma-related pathogenesis of thoracic aortic disease
- Missing follow-up data;
- Failure to provide consent.

In compliance with German health insurance regulations, patients aged above 60 years without any offspring were excluded from the study.

2.2. Recruited Patients/Sample Size

The primary diagnosis and treatment of the thoracic aortic pathology of 1334 patients were reviewed, and their primary data and patient records were screened. A total of

716 patients met the eligibility criteria. After contact, 118 patients consented to undergo genetic testing. Follow-up and human genetic data were missing for 23 patients; finally, 95 patients were enrolled in the study, as seen in Figure 1.

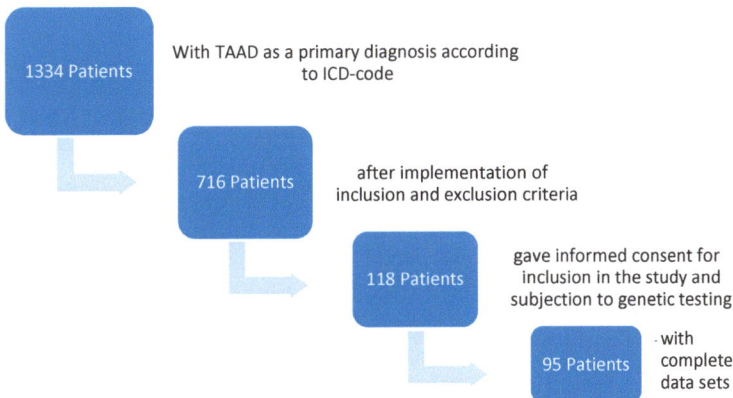

Figure 1. Selection criteria and patient recruitment.

2.3. Structured Follow-Up Examinations after Surgical or Endovascular Treatment of Aortic Pathology

Patients were subjected to the following structured clinical and image-based follow-up at the study institution after surgical treatment or thoracic endovascular aortic repair (TEVAR) for thoracic aortic pathology. During follow-up, the patient's medical history, current medication, cardiovascular risk factors, and comorbidities were recorded. Routine follow-up examinations were typically conducted 3 and 9 months after the primary intervention, and annually thereafter. Unscheduled assessments were performed earlier, if indicated, which was determined by the interdisciplinary vascular conference (aortic board) comprising experts from cardiothoracic surgery, vascular surgery, interventional radiology, angiology, and cardiology.

If there were no contraindications, such as severely impaired renal function, clinical hyperthyroidism, or iodine allergy, computed tomography (CT) angiography was preferred at the 3-month and 1-year follow-ups. In cases with a stable course of aortic disease without the need for treatment, magnetic resonance angiography was performed annually, alternating with transesophageal echocardiography combined with abdominal aortic ultrasonography.

2.4. Human Genetic Analysis to Clarify the Pathogenesis of Aortic Disease

Next-generation sequencing (NGS) was performed after DNA extraction from the blood samples collected from the patients. Initially, capture-based enrichment was performed, followed by analysis using the MiSeq Desktop Sequencer© (Illumina, San Diego, CA, USA). For the genes listed in Table 1, biometric data evaluation, including copy number variation (CNV) analysis, was conducted to identify larger deletions or duplications. Areas that could not be adequately assessed were further analyzed using conventional Sanger sequencing or multiplex ligation-dependent probe amplification. The identified polymorphisms, which are considered non-pathogenic according to current knowledge, have been reported separately. A five-tier classification was applied based on the methodology of Plon et al. and the Yale Aortic Institute Team [10,11]:

1. Class 1: Not disease-causing/nonpathogenic or of no clinical relevance;
2. Class 2: probably not disease-causing or of minor clinical relevance;
3. Class 3: VUS;
4. Class 4: likely disease-causing and pathogenic;
5. Class 5: disease-causing/pathogenic.

Table 1. Investigated gene loci associated with syndromic or non-syndromic thoracic aortic diseases with aneurysm and/or dissection.

Gene Name	Protein	Associated Aortic Disease/Syndrome
ACTA2 (NM_001613.2)	Smooth muscle α-actin	TAAD, AAT6 multisystem smooth muscle dysfunction, MYMY5
AEBP1 (NM_001129.4)	AE binding protein 1	BAA, EDS
BGN (NM_01711.5)	Biglycan	TAAD, Meester-Loeys Syndrome
COL1A1 (NM_000088.3)	Collagen type I α1 chain	TAAD, EDS
COL3A1 (NM_000090.3)	Collagen type III α1 chain	TAAD, EDS vascular Type (IV)
COL4A5 (NM_000495.3)	Collagen type IV α5 chain	TAAD, Alport Syndrome (Collagen type IV deficiency)
COL5A1 (NM_000093.4)	Collagen type V α1 chain	TAAD, EDS classical Type I
COL5A2 (NM_000393.4)	Collagen type V α2 chain	TAAD, EDS classical Type II
EFEMP2 (FBLN4)(NM_016938.4)	Fibulin-4	TAAD, other arterial aneurysms, Cutis laxa (autosomal recessive) Type Ib
ELN (NM_000501.3, NM_001278939.1)	Elastin	TAAD, Cutis laxa (autosomal dominant)
FBLN5 (NM_006329.3)	Fibulin 5	TAAD, Cutis laxa, Macular degeneration
FBN1 (NM_000138.4)	Fibrillin-1	TAAD, AAA, other arterial aneurysms, Marfan Syndrome
FBN2 (NM_001999.3)	Fibrillin-2	TAAD, Congenital Contractural Arachnodactyly
FLNA (NM_001110556.2)	Filamin A	TAAD, Periventricular nodular heterotopia, Otopalatodigital Syndromes
FOXE3 (NM_012186.2)	Forkhead box E3	TAAD, AAT11
GATA5 (NM_080473.4)	GATA binding protein 5	TAAD
LOX (NM_002317.6)	Lysyl oxidase	AAD, AAA, AAT10
MAT2A (NM_005911.5)	Methionine adenosyltransferase II α	TAA, FTAA
MFAP5 (NM_003480.3)	Microfibril-associated glycoprotein 2	TAAD, AAT9
MYH11 (NM_002474.2)	Smooth muscle myosin heavy chain	TAAD, AAT4
MYLK (NM_053025.3)	Myosin light chain kinase	TAAD, AAT7
NOTCH1 (NM_017617.4)	Notch receptor 1	TAAD, AOVD
NOTCH3 (NM_000435)	Notch receptor 3	TAAD
PLOD1 (NM_000302.3)	Procollagen-lysine,2-oxoglutarate 5-dioxygenase 1	TAAD, EDS
PRKG1 (NM_006258.3)	Type I cGMP-dependent protein kinase	TAAD, AAA, AAT8
RLP26 (NM_000987.4)	Receptor-like protein 26	TAAD
SKI (NM_003036.3)	Sloan Kettering proto-oncoprotein	TAA, Shprintzen-Goldberg Syndrome
SLC2A10 (NM_030777.3)	Glucose transporter 10	TAA, other arterial aneurysm

AAT (n): familial thoracic aortic aneurysms (1–11) TAA: thoracic aortic aneurysm, TAAD: thoracic aortic aneurysm and dissection, EDS: Ehlers-Danlos syndrome, BAA: abdominal artery aneurysm; AOVD: aortic valve disease.

Table 1 shows the gene loci studied in the cohort, which were classified into classes 4 and 5 based on Plon et al.'s [11] study.

Initially, the nine genes assumed to most commonly harbor disease-causing variants were examined. In cases of specific suspicion, such as familial aggregation, the analysis was expanded to a total of 32 genes, covering the currently known genetic causes of non-syndromic TAAD to a large extent, after obtaining consent again from the patient. If indications of a syndromic form were present, additional investigations such as chromosome analysis for suspected Turner Syndrome were initiated.

2.5. Applied Statistical Methods

Continuous variables were presented as the mean ± standard deviation and binary data as a percentage of the population. Pearson's chi-squared and F-tests were used to examine the correlation between distinct binary traits. As cardiovascular risk factors were not metrically scaled, Kendall's tau was used for the calculation. Statistical significance was set at $p < 0.5$ (two-sided). SPSS Statistics software (version 27, IBM, New York, NY, USA) was used for the statistical analysis.

3. Results

3.1. Demographic and Preoperative Data

The study population included 95 patients with a preponderance of males (71% men vs. 29% women). There was no significant difference in the age distribution at initial diagnosis, during human genetic examination, and on the cutoff date of 30 June 2019 (defined as the end of data collection) (Tables 2 and 3).

Table 2. Age distribution of the patient population.

Patients	Women (n = 28)	Men (n = 67)	p (t-Test)
Age at diagnosis	52.4 ± 12.4	51.3 ± 12.2	0.696
Age at genetic testing	55.3 ± 12.6	53.8 ± 12.5	0.596
Age as of 30 June 2019	55.8 ± 12.2 years	54.5 ± 12.0 years	0.612

Table 3. Primary treatment for the main diagnosis of thoracic aortic dissection/aneurysm based on age and sex.

Patients	Primarily Treated with Endovascular Therapy (n = 30)	Primarily Treated with Open Cardiosurgery (n = 65)	p-Value
Age (in years) at genetic testing	59.4 ± 12.0	48.0 ± 10.5	<0.001 (t-test)
Age as of 30 June 2019	63.7 ± 11.5	50.8 ± 10.0	<0.001 (t-test)
Sex (n) (women/men)	13/17	15/50	0.044 (Chi-Squared Test)

Patients who underwent surgical treatment were older than those who underwent endovascular therapy (59.4 ± 12.0 vs. 48.0 ± 10.5 years, respectively, $p < 0.001$); the frequency of men was higher in the surgical treatment group ($p = 0.044$).

Irrespective of sex, arterial hypertension was the dominant preexisting cardiovascular risk factor, as seen in 83% of patients, followed by a history of smoking and hypercholesterolemia (34 and 33%, respectively) and coronary heart disease (14%). Carotid stenosis/stroke, peripheral arterial occlusive disease, chronic obstructive pulmonary disease, or renal insufficiency were present in <10% of patients (Table 4).

Nearly all the patients were on long-term medication; 95% of patients were receiving beta-blocker therapy, and 83% were on angiotensin-converting enzyme inhibitors or angiotensin II type 1 receptor antagonists. Other antihypertensive agents were used in 21% of patients. Statin therapy was documented in 33% of patients. Antiplatelet therapy was administered to 43% of patients. Oral anticoagulants were administered to 37% of the study cohort (Table 5); the indications for therapeutic anticoagulation included mechanical heart valve replacement, atrial fibrillation/flutter, or past history of venous thromboembolism (Table 5).

Table 4. Comorbidities and cardiovascular risk factors in the patient population.

Cardiovascular Risk Factors	n	Percentage
Arterial Hypertension	79	83%
(Ex) Smoking	32	34%
Hypercholesterolemia	31	33%
Diabetes Mellitus	8	8%
Coronary Heart Disease	13	14%
Comorbidities		
Renal Insufficiency	9	9%
Carotid Stenosis/Stroke	5	5%
Peripheral Arterial Occlusive Disease (PAOD)	4	4%
COPD	2	2%

COPD: chronic obstructive pulmonary disease.

Table 5. Long-term medication of the patient population.

Medication	n	Percentage
Beta-Blockers	90	95%
ACE Inhibitors/AT1 Receptor Antagonists	79	83%
Platelet Aggregation Inhibitors	40	42%
Calcium Antagonists	39	41%
Oral Anticoagulants	35	37%
Statins	31	33%
Other Antihypertensives	20	21%

ACE: angiotensin-converting enzyme, AT1: angiotensin II type 1.

Overall, 57% of patients had thoracic aortic dissection, and 41% of patients had thoracic aneurysm. At the time of the initial diagnosis, 2% of patients exhibited a concomitance of both conditions. Contained rupture of the aortic aneurysm was confirmed radiologically in 6.3% of patients. Intramural hematoma and penetrating aortic ulcer were observed in 8.4% and 2.1% of patients, respectively.

3.2. Operative Data

Surgery constituted the primary treatment for thoracic aortic pathologies in 68% of this patient population, while an endovascular interventional approach was employed in the remaining 32%. The main aortic diagnosis (thoracic aortic dissection vs. aneurysm) and the type of treatment implemented (surgical vs. endovascular) did not differ significantly in this cohort (Pearson Chi-Square, $\chi^2 = 0.278$, $p = 0.598$). The aortic procedures are summarized in Table 6.

Table 6. Management of the primary diagnosis.

Procedure	Frequency
Isolated replacement of the ascending aorta	22%
Aortic root replacement with/out valve sparing, with hemiarch replacement	32%
Aortic arch replacement	3%
(Frozen) Elephant trunk operation (FET)	7%
TEVAR (all)	25%

Table 6. *Cont.*

Procedure	Frequency
TEVAR with complete stenting of left subclavian artery	11%
TEVAR with partial stenting of left subclavian artery	8%
With creation of carotid-carotid bypass	2%
With creation of carotid-subclavian bypass	0%
TEVAR octopus debranching and EVAR	1%

EVAR: endovascular aortic aneurysm repair, TEVAR: thoracic endovascular aortic aneurysm repair.

3.3. Follow-Up Data

3.3.1. Data Analysis According to Primary Diagnosis

General Results

The average follow-up duration was about 3 ± 2.5 years. Imaging studies showed complete resolution of the existing aortic pathology after the primary procedure in 31% of patients. The distribution of residual pathology is shown in Table 7.

Table 7. Distribution of residual aortic pathology.

	Type of Persistent Pathology			Total
	Resolved Pathology	Residual Aneurysm	Residual Dissection	
Resolved Pathology	28	0	0	28
Residual pathology	1	9	57	67
Total	29	9	57	95

The correlation analysis showed no significant correlation of genetic variants to the persistence of pathology ($p = 0.414$), diameter expansion, development of new aneurysms ($p = 0.369$), or reinterventional rate ($p = 0.742$). The analysis showed a significant correlation with the development of new dissections or the expansion of dissection to previously non-dissected segments ($p = 0.042$).

During follow-up, 38% of patients required one or more reinterventions; a maximum of four additional surgical or endovascular procedures were performed during follow-up. There was no significant correlation with genetic variant detection ($p = 0.742$).

Aortic Aneurysm Patients

Secondary expansion of the aortic diameter or de novo development of aortic ectasia/aneurysm occurred in 23 patients. Six patients with an initial aortic aneurysm subsequently developed aortic dissection in non-treated segments during follow-up. No retrograde aortic dissection was observed after TEVAR.

In patients who were primarily treated for aortic aneurysm and developed new dissections in the subsequent follow-up, the prevalence of genetic variants was 80%, and that of VUS was 60%. In patients who developed a de novo aneurysm or further expansion of an existing aneurysm in distant segments, the prevalence of genetic variants was 50%, and that of VUS was 37.5%. However, there were no statistically significant differences in the prevalence compared to the stable cohort ($p = 0.405$ and $p = 0.633$ respectively). Supplementary Table S1 lists the detected genetic variants in aneurysm patients and the state of disease progression in each patient with a genetic variant. The analysis of reintervention rates showed no significant correlation with genetic variant detection ($p = 0.248$).

Aortic Dissection Patients

Table 8 presents the trends in thrombosis of the false lumen over time after the primary procedure for all treated dissections. Overall, 65.6% of the cohort retained a completely or partially perfused false lumen after aortic dissection during follow-up, whereas 32.3% showed complete thrombosis immediately after the primary procedure or during follow-up imaging.

Table 8. Aortic dissections: Dynamics of false lumen thrombosis at follow-up.

Trend in False Lumen	Frequency
Not perfused/resolved immediately postoperatively	26.9%
Completely thrombosed at follow-up	54%
Partial thrombosis stable	18.3%
Progressive thrombosis	9.7%
Completely perfused	37.6%

The correlation analysis of persistent pathology with genetic variants shows a borderline significance ($p = 0.05$, Table 9) when all variants are evaluated as one pool.

Table 9. Correlation of persistence of dissection to genetic variants.

	Presence of Genetic Variants			
	Non-Present	Present		
Resolution of aortic pathology	2	4	6	
Residual dissection	35	13	48	
	37	17	54	$p = 0.05$

The correlation analysis of persistent pathology with genetic variants according to variant class shows a significant correlation ($p = 0.037$, Table 10).

Table 10. Correlation of persistence of dissection to genetic variant classes.

	Presence of Genetic Variant Class				
	Non-Present	Class 4 or 5	Lower Classes		
Resolution of aortic pathology	2	0	4	6	
Residual dissection	35	2	11	48	
	37	2	15	54	$p = 0.037$

In the event of residual aortic dissection after the primary dissection procedure, 85% of patients followed a stable course during subsequent follow-ups. In 15% of patients with residual dissections, progression with extension into the initially unaffected vessel sections was detected. The prevalence of genetic variants was 24%, and that of VUS was 22% in patients with a stable disease course. The prevalence of genetic variants was 42% in patients with disease progression, all of which were VUS. There was no significant correlation between disease progression and genetic variants ($p = 0.426$). Supplementary Table S2 enumerates the genetic variants detected in patients with dissection progression. The analysis of reintervention rates showed no significant correlation with genetic variant detection ($p = 0.250$).

3.3.2. Data Analysis According to Follow-Up CT-Finding

The evaluation of all patients with detected aortic dissection at follow-up (i.e., aneurysm patients who show a new dissection in the follow-up and dissection patients who show a persistent dissection in follow-up) showed a strong correlation with the presence of genetic variants (Spearman $R^2 = 0.321$, $p = 0.012$; Kendall Tau $R^2 = 0.321$, $p = 0.019$).

The analysis of reintervention rates showed a positive correlation in reintervention rates in patients with detected variants (Spearman $R^2 = 0.256$, $p = 0.046$; Kendall Tau $R^2 = 0.243$, $p = 0.047$).

3.4. Human Genetic Analysis: Gene Variants Distribution in the Studied Cohort

Human genetic analysis revealed variants in the target candidate genes with a known connection to connective tissue diseases involving the aortic vessel wall in 40.7% of patients (n = 38, Table 11). Seven patients (7.4% of the total cohort, 18.4% of all variants) harbored a class 5 variant with an established association with connective tissue diseases [8].

Table 11. Overview of the results of variant analysis.

Affected Gene	Variant Class 4 or 5	Absolute Number of Patients	Percentage of Cohort
FBN1	yes	3	7.9%
	no	10	26%
COL3A1	yes	1	2.6%
SMAD3	no	1	2.6%
TGFB2	yes	1	2.6%
	no	3	7.9%
TGFBR1	no	2	5.3%
MYLK	no	2	5.3%
MYH11	no	8	21%
PRKG1	no	1	2.6%
NOTCH1	no	3	7.9%
NOTCH3	yes	1	2.1%
TGRBR2	no	1	2.1%
ACTA2	no	2	5.3%
SMAD6	yes	1	2.6%

Upon strict segregation of cases with a singular occurrence of a class 5 pathological variant, a lower-class variant, or a combination thereof, the following frequencies emerged: Thirty-one patients harbored a lower-class variant, accounting for 81.6% of all detected variants; four patients (10.5%) exclusively harbored a pathological class 5 variant; in three patients (7.9%), both a pathological variant and a lower-class variant were found. Table 11 details the affected genes and variant classes. The analysis discovered no difference in the detected variants with respect to sex (Pearson's Chi-Square: $\chi^2 = 0.684$; $p = 0.408$).

4. Discussion

Aortic aneurysms or dissections can remain asymptomatic for a long time but can emerge suddenly, causing acute life-threatening events. Despite intensive research and the accumulation of extensive data, definitive identification of the individual pathophysiological causes of aortic vascular wall pathologies is not often possible. In addition to a likely combination of various cardiovascular risk factors such as arterial hypertension, hyperlipoproteinemia, diabetes mellitus, or smoking, the familial form, including connective tissue diseases, is the second most common cause [6,7]. In syndromic connective tissue diseases such as Marfan syndrome or Ehlers-Danlos syndrome, screening for aortic manifestations using imaging techniques has been established because of the known association with aortic involvement [12,13].

Rapid advancements in the field of genetic diagnostics have fundamentally altered the diagnosis and investigation of many disease patterns. The ability to completely analyze the human genome is particularly significant for identifying the causes of familial clustering. Specific deviations from the norm, i.e., the wild-type, can be clinically and pathophysiologically correlated with the pathological findings and can be classified as pathological, allowing screening and early diagnostics to be offered to the relatives of affected individuals. The frequency of detection of previously unclassified mutation variants is on the rise, which must be evaluated in terms of their clinical significance and the pathogenesis of aortic diseases.

In recent years, numerous scientific studies have undertaken a search for genetic triggers of thoracic aortic diseases such as aneurysms or dissections [5,7,10,11,14]. In addition to the importance of known mutations, such as changes in the fibrillin 1 gene (FBN1) in Marfan syndrome, which have already been described in association with connective tissue diseases [8,15], other genes have also been recognized as relevant to the disease-causing process and investigated in greater depth, expanding knowledge about the variety of possible genetic triggers [4,9,16–19].

In the presence of genetic aortopathy, depending on the type and severity of the aortic connective tissue disease, treatable secondary aortic pathologies may develop over time, even after surgical or endovascular treatment of the thoracic aneurysm or dissection, with varying dynamics. Currently, data are insufficient on the influence of genetic variants on the development of these secondary aortic manifestations, with potential indications for re-treatment/reintervention in patients with gene mutations/mutation variants related to aortic connective tissue diseases.

Many studies have focused on the prevalence of changes in the genotype as the pathogenic basis for TAAD, yielding results similar to those of the current study. Poninska et al. analyzed 10 known disease-associated genes in 51 patients with TAAD and found mutations in 41.2% of participants, with 35.3% being classified as LP or pathogenic disease-causing variants. The inclusion of patients was primarily but not exclusively based on the presence of familial clustering, early age of onset, and suspected connective tissue disease [14]. Fang et al. investigated 11 causal genes in 70 patients with TAAD from southern China using NGS and found deviations from the wild-type in 51.4% of patients. Of these, 7.5% were definitively pathological, 25% were likely pathological variants, and 32.5% were potentially disease-causing mutations that closely matched the results of the present study. Familial clustering was not a prerequisite for inclusion, but if present, the variant detection rate was 92.3% compared to 45.6% in participants without familial clustering [20]. Ziganshin et al. included 102 patients with TAAD, familial clustering, and early age of onset, who were examined using whole-exome sequencing for 21 genes. Here, variants were described in 27.5% of all tested patients, with 21.6% in the VUS category [21]. In a study conducted in northwest China by Li et al., 51.4% of 212 patients with TAAD tested positive for mutations using NGS. A total of 31.6% fell into the LP and definitely pathological variant group and 19.8% into VUS. The working group tested 15 genes associated with TAAD [22]. An even larger genetic sample was studied by Li et al. in southern China, who searched for mutations in 129 genes in 151 patients with sporadic or familial TAAD and described abnormalities in 62.3% of all cases. The majority of these genotypic changes fell into the VUS group, and 22.5% included likely and definitely pathological deviations [23].

Nonetheless, the Yale Aortic Institute team examined a cohort of 967 participants with and without familial clustering using NGS for 15 TAAD-associated genes and described VUS, LP, and pathogenic variants in only 12% of the participants. Forty-nine cases of pathological or likely pathological variants were identified, accounting for 4.9%. It is noteworthy that approximately half of these participants had no relevant family history [10].

All the above-mentioned studies, as well as the present one, concur that disease-associated changes occurred most frequently in the FBN1 gene. The frequencies of variants in MYH11, MYLK, NOTCH1, ACTA2, COL1A1/2, COL3A1, and COL5A1/2 were not entirely uniform [5,10,20,21,23,24]. Further investigation of other gene loci and their pathogenic associations with TAAD is required, especially in non-syndromic diseases with familial clustering [24,25].

To date, mutations in 37 gene loci with a pathophysiological association with thoracic aortic aneurysms and dissections have been detected [5]. Li et al. clearly showed that research on other causal genes (with 129 detected gene loci) is rapidly progressing and will continue to do so [23]. The frequency of detected variants varies greatly among studies, ranging from 12% to 62.3% without further selection or from 4.9% to 35.3% when considering only likely and definite pathological variants. The large variation in prevalence in these studies can be attributed to different study designs with a narrower/broader selection of patients and expansion of the gene loci under examination [5,10,14,20,21,23,24]. Apropos of the variant prevalence in the current study, especially considering the sample size and the number of analyzed gene loci, the results align with existing evidence. Nevertheless, closer examination of these studies may pave the way for more refined indications for genetic testing. At this juncture, we believe that genetic testing should continue to expand, as further examination of gene loci, specific mutations, and their prevalence and clinical relevance is needed to determine clearer pathways for future decision-making.

Regarding a possible connection/influence of a confirmed genetic variant and the rate of required reinterventions during follow-up, the present study found no significant correlation with the primary diagnosis. Interestingly, there was a statistically significant increase in the risk of reintervention for patients with detected aortic dissection in the follow-up with a genetic variant. This is consistent with the results of Poninska et al., who described a shorter event-free interval for patients with pathological and likely pathological mutations in their study [14]. This may indicate a closer, more meticulous follow-up in this cohort, which may lead in the future to a lower threshold for intervention/reintervention.

Nevertheless, these consequences are dependent on the confirmation/exclusion of genetic variants in patients with dissection, which is not always logistically possible as genetic-variant analysis using NGS is currently only approved for TAAD with familial clustering or conspicuous age or phenotype. This strategy should be parsed critically from an economic perspective. Performing human genetic-variant testing to clarify the pathogenesis of aortic disease is valuable, as it may have clinical relevance for the patient, such as admission to a structured follow-up in specialized centers to ensure timely detection of dynamic aortic changes and reinterventions (if required), or for his/her offspring to facilitate early detection of potentially at-risk offspring and offer genetic testing, imaging screening, and follow-up. These benefits also offer sound economic arguments for prophylactic medicine, and the economic advantages should be studied and included in the decision-making processes. Currently, from an economic perspective, the question of a possible age limit or cutoff value from which genetic testing is no longer meaningful arises, especially since at an older age, the first manifestation of aortic diseases is more likely to be caused by atherosclerosis than by a connective tissue disease based on genetic variants. Although the data from our study show that patients with the first manifestation of a thoracic aortic dissection or aneurysm disease and a confirmed genetic variant were, on average, about six years younger, this trend did not attain significance in the analysis by age group, and the prevalence of genetic variants did not significantly differ according to the age group, indicating that genetic testing can be beneficial to older patients.

The first step in this pathway was recommended by Caruana et al., who recommended genetic analysis irrespective of age in the absence of risk factors and pre-existing conditions, but with an absolute cutoff of 70 years [26]. Even though a cutoff to determine the age limit of human genetic testing would be desirable, it cannot yet be conclusively determined owing to the current paucity of data. Our results do not show a clinical benefit for patients with aortic aneurysm, but based on the significantly higher percentage of reintervention in patients with detected dissection in the follow-up with genetic variants in our study, we suggest the following flowchart for decision-making regarding genetic testing in TAAD patients according to our results (Figure 2).

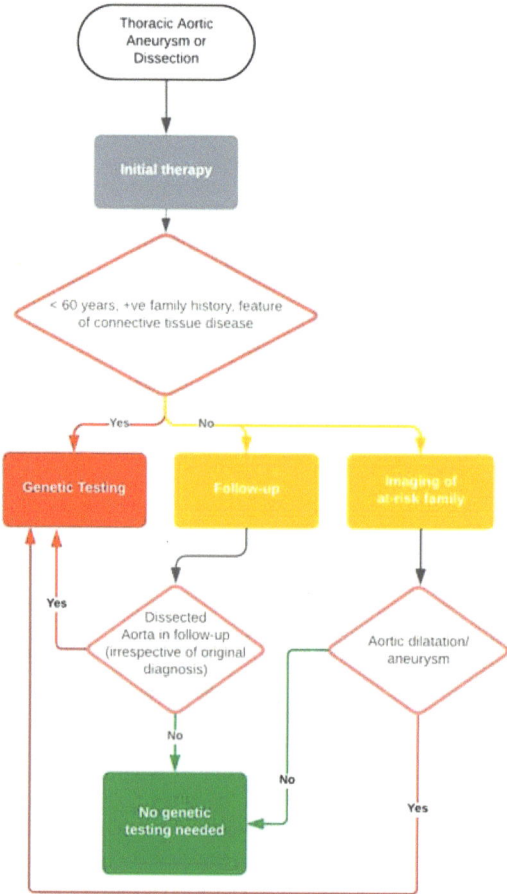

Figure 2. Decision-making flowchart for genetic testing of patients with TAAD.

Our data and suggestions might be a step on a long way to gathering evidence on a topic that lacks supporting data. This is confirmed in the last guidelines of the European Association of Cardiothoracic Surgery for diagnosing and treating acute and chronic syndromes of the aortic organ [27], which confirm the lack of evidence-based standardized follow-up protocol specific to each disease and treatment modality. Although variants of specific genes are now included in the guidelines, with a lower threshold for indicating therapy, large nationwide or multinational cohort studies are urgently needed to expand the knowledge on genetic variants affecting the aortic disease and its course.

Limitations

The study limitations include retrospective enrolment of patients with a subsequent inevitable lower recruitment percentage, which would have affected the generalizability of the study results. However, our group eliminated selection bias in an earlier publication with the same patient cohort [28]. Furthermore, the results concur with those of most previous studies. The genetic analysis included a specific group of genes as approved by the German health authorities. Expanding the spectrum of genetic testing might provide further insights, which our study group intends to perform in future research. Furthermore, it should be noted that mosaicism or other functionally significant genetic alterations in the examined genes or influencing regions cannot be entirely excluded. The study was performed at a single center, which might have influenced or limited the geographical area from which the patient sample was drawn. The influence of surgeons/surgery type on reintervention was not investigated.

5. Conclusions

The prevalence of genetic variants is high in patients with aortic pathology, a large percentage of which are currently classified as VUS. In patients with dissected aorta in the follow-up, irrespective of original pathology, the detected genetic variants correlated with higher reintervention rates, which indicates that VUS may, in fact, play a larger role than is currently known. Studies with larger cohorts are needed to further examine the detected variants to confirm their correlation and change their class to pathological or probably pathological.

Supplementary Materials: The following supporting information can be downloaded at: https://www.mdpi.com/article/10.3390/jcm13175254/s1, Table S1: Genetic Variants Detected in Patients with Aneurysm and Their Correlation with Disease Progression; Table S2: Genetic Variants Detected in Patients with Dissection and Their Correlation with Disease Progression.

Author Contributions: Conceptualization: A.M. and T.G.; Methodology, investigation, and data curation: A.M.; Formal analysis: H.K.L.; Writing: T.G. and N.E.; Editing: M.I. and C.-A.B.; Resources: A.J.R.; Project administration: A.M. and T.G. All authors have read and agreed to the published version of the manuscript.

Funding: Open Access funding was provided by the Open Access Publishing Fund of the Philipps University of Marburg.

Institutional Review Board Statement: The study was conducted in accordance with the tenets of the Declaration of Helsinki and approved by the Institutional Review Board of the Dresden University of Technology (File number: EK317082014, 13 August 2014).

Informed Consent Statement: Clinical data were obtained from the university aortic board, for which patient consent was waived. All participants provided written consent for inclusion in genetic testing. Informed consent was obtained from all patients involved in the study.

Data Availability Statement: The data supporting the findings of this study are available from the corresponding author upon reasonable request. The data will be available for five years after publication.

Conflicts of Interest: The authors declare no conflict of interest.

References

1. Liu, B.; David, X.; Granville, J.; Golledge, J.; Kassiri, Z. Pathogenic mechanisms and the potential of drug therapies for aortic aneurysm. *Am. J. Physiol. Heart Circ. Physiol.* **2020**, *318*, 652–670. [CrossRef]
2. Saeyeldin, A.A.; Velasquez, C.A.; Mahmood, S.U.B.; Brownstein, A.J.; Zafar, M.A.; Ziganshin, B.A.; Elefteriades, J.A. Thoracic aortic aneurysm: Unlocking the "silent killer" secrets. *Gen. Thorac. Cardiovasc. Surg.* **2019**, *67*, 1–11. [CrossRef] [PubMed]
3. Stone, J.R.; Bruneval, P.; Angelini, A.; Bartoloni, G.; Basso, C.; Batoroeva, L.; Buja, L.M.; Butany, J.; D'Amati, G.; Fallon, J.T.; et al. Consensus statement on surgical pathology of the aorta from the Society for Cardiovascular Pathology and the Association for European Cardiovascular Pathology: I. Inflammatory diseases. *Cardiovasc. Pathol.* **2015**, *24*, 267–278. [CrossRef]
4. Chesneau, B.; Edouard, T.; Dulac, Y.; Colineaux, H.; Langeois, M.; Hanna, N.; Boileau, C.; Arnaud, P.; Chassaing, N.; Julia, S.; et al. Clinical and genetic data of 22 new patients with SMAD3 pathogenic variants and review of the literature. *Mol. Genet. Genom. Med.* **2020**, *8*, e1132. [CrossRef] [PubMed]
5. Vinholo, T.F.; Brownstein, A.J.; Ziganshin, B.A.; Zafar, M.A.; Kuivaniemi, H.; Body, S.C.; Bale, A.E.; Elefteriades, J.A. Genes Associated with Thoracic Aortic Aneurysm and Dissection: 2019 Update and Clinical Implications. *Aorta* **2019**, *7*, 99–107. [CrossRef]
6. Pinard, A.; Jones, G.T.; Milewicz, D.M. Genetics of thoracic and abdominal aortic diseases. *Circ. Res.* **2019**, *124*, 588–606. [CrossRef] [PubMed]

7. Renner, S.; Schüler, H.; Alawi, M.; Kolbe, V.; Rybczynski, M.; Woitschach, R.; Sheikhzadeh, S.; Stark, V.C.; Olfe, J.; Roser, E.; et al. Next-generation sequencing of 32 genes associated with hereditary aortopathies and related disorders of connective tissue in a cohort of 199 patients. *Genet. Med.* **2019**, *21*, 1832–1841. [CrossRef]
8. Syx, D.; De Wandele, I.; Symoens, S.; De Rycke, R.; Hougrand, O.; Voermans, N.; De Paepe, A.; Malfait, F. Bi-allelic AEBP1 mutations in two patients with Ehlers–Danlos syndrome. *Hum. Mol. Genet.* **2019**, *28*, 1853–1864. [CrossRef]
9. Takeda, N.; Hara, H.; Fujiwara, T.; Kanaya, T.; Maemura, S.; Komuro, I. TGF-β Signaling-Related Genes and Thoracic Aortic Aneurysms and Dissections. *Int. J. Mol. Sci.* **2018**, *19*, 2125. [CrossRef]
10. Weerakkody, R.; Ross, D.; Parry, D.A.; Ziganshin, B.; Vandrovcova, J.; Gampawar, P.; Abdullah, A.; Biggs, J.; Dumfarth, J.; Ibrahim, Y.; et al. Targeted genetic analysis in a large cohort of familial and sporadic cases of aneurysm or dissection of the thoracic aorta. *Genet. Med.* **2018**, *20*, 1414–1422. [CrossRef]
11. Plon, S.E.; Eccles, D.M.; Easton, D.; Foulkes, W.D.; Genuardi, M.; Greenblatt, M.S.; Hogervorst, F.B.L.; Hoogerbrugge, N.; Spurdle, A.B.; Tavtigian, S.V. Sequence variant classification and reporting: Recommendations for improving the interpretation of cancer susceptibility genetic test results. *Hum. Mutat.* **2008**, *29*, 1282–1291. [CrossRef]
12. Wozniak-Mielczarek, L.; Sabiniewicz, R.; Nowak, R.; Gilis-Malinowska, N.; Osowicka, M.; Mielczarek, M. New Screening Tool for Aortic Root Dilation in Children with Marfan Syndrome and Marfan-Like Disorders. *Pediatr. Cardiol.* **2020**, *41*, 632–641. [CrossRef]
13. Cikach, F.; Desai, M.Y.; Roselli, E.E.; Kalahasti, V. Thoracic aortic aneurysm: How to counsel, when to refer. *Clevel. Clin. J. Med.* **2018**, *85*, 481–492. [CrossRef] [PubMed]
14. Poninska, J.K.; Bilinska, Z.T.; Franaszczyk, M.; Michalak, E.; Rydzanicz, M.; Szpakowski, E.; Pollak, A.; Milanowska, B.; Truszkowska, G.; Chmielewski, P.; et al. Next-generation sequencing for diagnosis of thoracic aortic aneurysms and dissections: Diagnostic yield, novel mutations and genotype phenotype correlations. *J. Transl. Med.* **2016**, *14*, 115. [CrossRef] [PubMed]
15. Schoenhoff, F.S.; Carrel, T.P. Re-interventions on the thoracic and thoracoabdominal aorta in patients with Marfan syndrome. *Ann. Cardiothorac. Surg.* **2017**, *6*, 662–671. [CrossRef] [PubMed]
16. Guo, D.-C.; Gong, L.; Regalado, E.S.; Santos-Cortez, R.L.; Zhao, R.; Cai, B.; Veeraraghavan, S.; Prakash, S.K.; Johnson, R.J.; Muilenburg, A.; et al. MAT2A mutations predispose individuals to thoracic aortic aneurysms. *Am. J. Hum. Genet.* **2015**, *96*, 170–177. [CrossRef]
17. Hu, X.; Jiang, W.; Wang, Z.; Li, L.; Hu, Z. Nox1 negatively modulates fibulin-5 in vascular smooth muscle cells to affect aortic dissection. *Biol. Pharm. Bull.* **2019**, *42*, 1464–1470. [CrossRef]
18. Li, M.; Dong, X.; Chen, S.; Wang, W.; Yang, C.; Li, B.; Liang, D.; Yang, W.; Liu, X.; Yang, X. Genetic polymorphisms and transcription profiles associated with intracranial aneurysm: A key role for NOTCH3. *Aging* **2019**, *11*, 5173–5191. [CrossRef] [PubMed]
19. Regalado, E.S.; Guo, D.-C.; Prakash, S.; Bensend, T.A.; Flynn, K.; Estrera, A.; Safi, H.; Liang, D.; Hyland, J.; Child, A.; et al. Aortic disease presentation and outcome associated with ACTA2 mutations. *Circ. Cardiovasc. Genet.* **2015**, *8*, 457–464. [CrossRef]
20. Fang, M.; Yu, C.; Chen, S.; Xiong, W.; Li, X.; Zeng, R.; Zhuang, J.; Fan, R. Identification of Novel Clinically Relevant Variants in 70 Southern Chinese patients with Thoracic Aortic Aneurysm and Dissection by Next-generation Sequencing. *Sci. Rep.* **2017**, *7*, 10035. [CrossRef]
21. Ziganshin, B.A.; Bailey, A.E.; Coons, C.; Dykas, D.; Charilaou, P.; Tanriverdi, L.H.; Liu, L.; Tranquilli, M.; Bale, A.E.; Elefteriades, J.A. Routine genetic testing for thoracic aortic aneurysm and dissection in a clinical setting. *Ann. Thorac. Surg.* **2015**, *100*, 1604–1611. [CrossRef] [PubMed]
22. Li, J.; Yang, L.; Diao, Y.; Zhou, L.; Xin, Y.; Jiang, L.; Li, R.; Wang, J.; Duan, W.; Liu, J. Genetic testing and clinical relevance of patients with thoracic aortic aneurysm and dissection in northwestern China. *Mol. Genet. Genom. Med.* **2021**, *9*, e1800. [CrossRef]
23. Li, Y.; Fang, M.; Yang, J.; Yu, C.; Kuang, J.; Sun, T.; Fan, R. Analysis of the contribution of 129 candidate genes to thoracic aortic aneurysm or dissection of a mixed cohort of sporadic and familial cases in South China. *Am. J. Transl. Res.* **2021**, *13*, 4281–4295. [PubMed]
24. Ostberg, N.; Zafar, M.; Ziganshin, B.; Elefteriades, J. The Genetics of Thoracic aortic aneurysms and Dissection: A Clinical perspective. *Biomolecules* **2020**, *10*, 182. [CrossRef] [PubMed]
25. Brownstein, A.; Kostiuk, V.; Ziganshin, B.; Zafar, M.; Kuivaniemi, H.; Body, S.; Bale, A.; Elefteriades, J. Genes Associated with Thoracic Aortic Aneurysm and Dissection: 2018 Update and Clinical Implications. *Aorta* **2018**, *6*, 13–20. [CrossRef]
26. Caruana, M.; Baars, M.J.; Bashiardes, E.; Benke, K.; Björck, E.; Codreanu, A.; De Moya Rubio, E.; Dumfarth, J.; Evangelista, A.; Groenink, M.; et al. HTAD patient pathway: Strategy for diagnostic work-up of patients and families with (suspected) heritable thoracic aortic diseases (HTAD). A statement from the HTAD working group of VASCERN. *Eur. J. Med. Genet.* **2023**, *66*, 104673. [CrossRef] [PubMed]
27. Czerny, M.; Grabenwöger, M.; Berger, T.; Aboyans, V.; Della Corte, A.; Chen, E.P.; Desai, N.D.; Dumfarth, J.; Elefteriades, J.A.; Etz, C.D.; et al. EACTS/STS Guidelines for Diagnosing and Treating Acute and Chronic Syndromes of the Aortic Organ. *Eur. J. Cardio-Thorac. Surg.* **2024**, *65*, ezad426. [CrossRef]
28. Mahlmann, A.; Elzanaty, N.; Saleh, M.; Irqsusi, M.; Rastan, A.; Leip, J.L.; Behrendt, C.-A.; Ghazy, T. Prevalence of Genetic Variants and Deep Phenotyping in Patients with Thoracic Aortic Aneurysm and Dissection: A Cross-Sectional Single-Centre Cohort Study. *J. Clin. Med.* **2024**, *13*, 461. [CrossRef]

Disclaimer/Publisher's Note: The statements, opinions and data contained in all publications are solely those of the individual author(s) and contributor(s) and not of MDPI and/or the editor(s). MDPI and/or the editor(s) disclaim responsibility for any injury to people or property resulting from any ideas, methods, instructions or products referred to in the content.

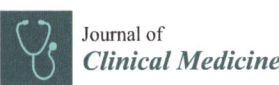

Review

The Ascyrus Medical Dissection Stent: A One-Fits-All Strategy for the Treatment of Acute Type A Aortic Dissection?

Leonard Pitts [1,2,*,†], Michael C. Moon [3,†], Maximilian Luehr [4], Markus Kofler [1,2,5], Matteo Montagner [1,2], Simon Sündermann [1,2,5], Semih Buz [1,2,5], Christoph Starck [1,2,5], Volkmar Falk [1,2,5,6] and Jörg Kempfert [1,2,5]

1 Deutsches Herzzentrum der Charité (DHZC), Department of Cardiothoracic and Vascular Surgery, Augustenburger Platz 1, 13353 Berlin, Germany; markus.kofler@dhzc-charite.de (M.K.); matteo.montagner@dhzc-charite.de (M.M.); simon.suendermann@dhzc-charite.de (S.S.); semih.buz@dhzc-charite.de (S.B.); christoph.starck@dhzc-charite.de (C.S.); volkmar.falk@dhzc-charite.de (V.F.); joerg.kempfert@dhzc-charite.de (J.K.)
2 Charité—Universitätsmedizin Berlin, Corporate Member of Freie Universität Berlin and Humboldt-Universität zu Berlin, Charitéplatz 1, 10117 Berlin, Germany
3 Division of Cardiac Surgery, University of Alberta, Edmonton, AB T6G 1H9, Canada; mmoon@ualberta.ca
4 Department of Cardiothoracic Surgery, Heart Centre, University of Cologne, 50923 Cologne, Germany; maximilian.luehr@uk-koeln.de
5 DZHK (German Centre for Cardiovascular Research), Partner Site Berlin, 10785 Berlin, Germany
6 Translational Cardiovascular Technologies, Institute of Translational Medicine, Department of Health Sciences and Technology, Swiss Federal Institute of Technology (ETH), 8092 Zurich, Switzerland
* Correspondence: leonard.pitts@dhzc-charite.de; Tel.: +49-30-4593-2059
† These authors contributed equally to this work.

Abstract: The treatment of DeBakey type I aortic dissection remains a major challenge in the field of aortic surgery. To upgrade the standard of care hemiarch replacement, a novel device called an "Ascyrus Medical Dissection Stent" (AMDS) is now available. This hybrid device composed of a proximal polytetrafluoroethylene cuff and a distal non-covered nitinol stent is inserted into the aortic arch and the descending thoracic aorta during hypothermic circulatory arrest in addition to hemiarch replacement. Due to its specific design, it may result in a reduced risk for distal anastomotic new entries, the effective restoration of branch vessel malperfusion and positive aortic remodeling. In this narrative review, we provide an overview about the indications and the technical use of the AMDS. Additionally, we summarize the current available literature and discuss potential pitfalls in the application of the AMDS regarding device failure and aortic re-intervention.

Keywords: acute type A aortic dissection; aorta; Ascyrus Medical Dissection Stent; endovascular; malperfusion; frozen elephant trunk; thoracic endovascular aortic repair

1. Introduction

Acute type A aortic dissection (ATAAD) is associated with poor outcomes [1]. Although there has been great progress in terms of surgical and perioperative technologies over the last decades, morbidity and mortality are still high [2]. Advanced age and preoperative malperfusion contribute significantly to a higher surgical risk, considering that open surgery remains the therapy of choice in the treatment of ATAAD [3,4]. The resection of the entry tear in combination with an open distal anastomosis under adequate cerebral protection is recommended to prevent aortic rupture, reestablish antegrade flow in the true lumen and resolve malperfusion [5,6]. According to the current guidelines, this includes the resection of the ascending aorta at least in terms of a hemiarch replacement [7,8]. Though this strategy effectively treats the ascending aorta, the aortic arch and descending aorta remain untouched in the case of DeBakey type I dissection. Especially in the case of supraaortic vessel involvement or consecutive aortic branch vessel malperfusion, more extensive repair may be advantageous [9]. For this scenario, the Ascyrus Medical Dissection Stent

(AMDS; Artivion®, Atlanta, GA, USA) was developed to upgrade the standard of care hemiarch procedure, aiming to reduce complications deriving from true lumen collapse and false lumen patency [10,11].

2. Device Description and Surgical Procedure

The AMDS is a hybrid prosthesis consisting of a proximal cuff composed of polytetrafluorethylene and an uncovered superhelical nitinol stent (Figure 1).

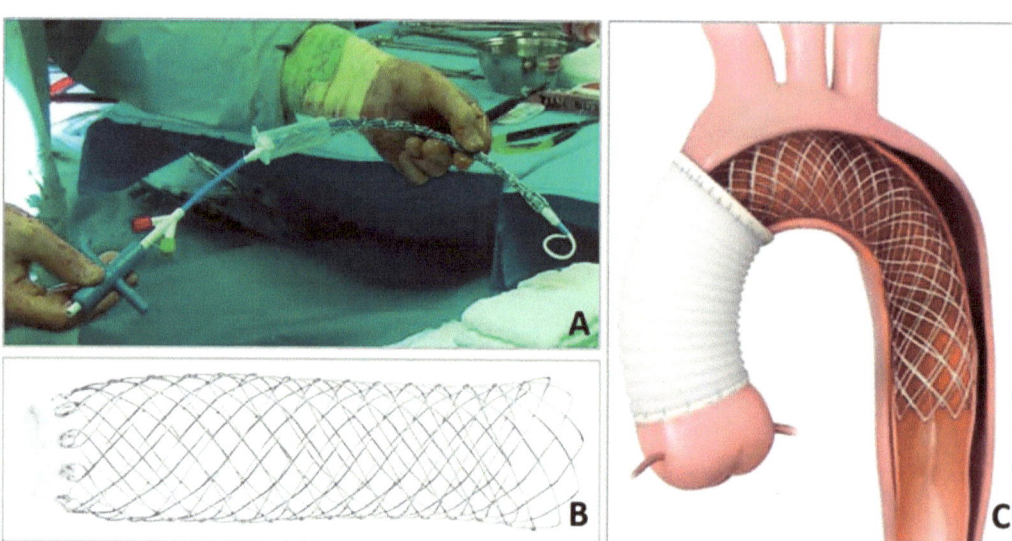

Figure 1. Graphical example of the AMDS device (used with the permission of Artivion®, Atlanta, GA, USA). (**A**) AMDS, including the delivery system before implantation. (**B**) Fully unfolded AMDS. (**C**) Hemiarch replacement and AMDS implantation at zone 0.

The aim of the cuff is to effectively seal the distal anastomosis and prevent false lumen flow as well as to lower the risk for distal anastomotic new entries (DANEs) [12]. Currently, two cuff sizes are available: 24 and 32 mm. The stent frame was designed for true lumen stabilization and consecutive positive aortic remodeling in the aortic arch and the downstream aorta. Flexibility is allowed to adapt to the curvature of the aortic arch, enabling insertion in zone 0. Two different shapes of the nitinol stent are currently available (straight and tapered) and four different sizes. The choice for the adequate size is made through an evaluation of a preoperative computed tomography scan and pragmatic measurement of the diameter at two aortic landmarks: zone 1 (aortic arch) and zone 4 (tracheal bifurcation). The appropriate stent can then be selected according to the sizing charts provided by the manufacturer. The device is simple to handle and does not significantly prolong the surgical procedure [13]. A corresponding video demonstrating the step-by-step implantation and providing surgical tips and tricks was recently published by our group [10]. A schematic of the procedure for implantation is shown in Figure 2.

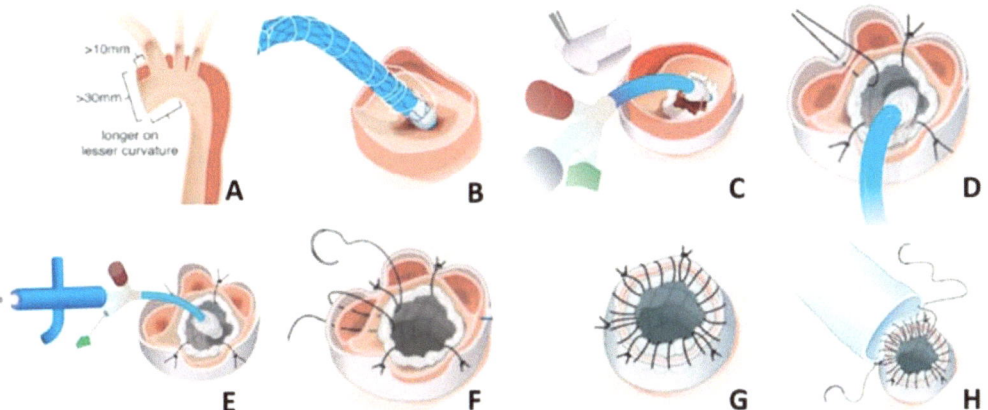

Figure 2. Schematic of the step-by-step implantation of the AMDS (used with the permission of Artivion®, Atlanta, GA, USA). In summary, the steps are as follows: (**A**) Leave > 10 mm distance to the innominate artery and longer on the lesser curvature when transecting the ascending aorta (the diameter at the distal anastomosis should be >30 mm). Store the AMDS in saline solution until implantation; (**B**) Insert the AMDS into the true lumen until the cuff reaches the plane of the transected aorta (if a guidewire is used, remove it before stent expansion); (**C**) Remove the plastic sheath to expose the polytetrafluoroethylene felt; (**D**) Place an external polytetrafluoroethylene felt strip around the aorta, and then place four single non-interrupting polypropylene sutures beginning at 6 o'clock, followed by 12, 3 and 9 o'clock to stabilize the cuff. This sandwich technique is highly recommended to avoid tearing the dissected aortic tissue; (**E**) While stabilizing the felt, unscrew the green cap counterclockwise to remove it completely. Pull back the sutures to expand the stent portion; (**F**) The delivery system can be removed once the stent is fully expanded and the tip of the delivery system is free from the stent. If tension appears, a stiff guidewire may be used to straighten the tip of the delivery system; (**G**) Perform a running suture in terms of a sandwich technique, consisting of the inner stent cuff, the aortic tissue and the outer felt. Avoid the enfolding of the inner cuff; (**H**) Finish the distal anastomosis by performing a running suture between the dacron graft and the sandwich cuff while ensuring to take all layers of the "felt–aortic–felt" complex with every stitch for the maximum seal of the distal anastomosis.

3. When to Use AMDS—And When to Avoid It

As already mentioned, the AMDS was conducted to upgrade the standard of care hemiarch procedure. Rylski et al. showed that the incidence for DANEs after hemiarch replacement in the setting of ATAAD may occur in up to 70% of cases [14]. False lumen perfusion ($p < 0.001$) and DANEs ($p < 0.001$) were strongly associated with the increased growth of the residual dissected aorta, which is a well-studied risk factor for further aortic-related interventions and death [14,15]. This is consistent with other studies, showing that a patent false lumen caused by DANEs after ATAAD repair shows greater aortic growth rate of the descending aorta and is one of the leading risk factors for distal aortic events [16]. The first try to address false lumen patency was the so-called Djumbodis Dissection System, a non-self-expanding bare metal stent, which was deployed into the aortic arch in addition to hemiarch replacement [17]. However, most of the patients had continuing antegrade perfusion of the false lumen, and the authors concluded that under these circumstances, no additive value as an adjunct to hemiarch replacement exists, most likely due to the non-self-expanding capability of the device. The main differences between the Djumbodis Dissection System and AMDS may be the non-availability of the proximal cuff to avoid the formation of DANEs and stent migration, as well as the non-self-expanding stent capability, which favors false lumen patency. Besides the low numbers of implantations, available data on the long-term outcome of patients who received an additional implantation of the Djumbodis Dissection Stent are limited to a minimum. Vendramin et al. summarized the long-term follow up and late complications of patients treated with the Djumbodis Dissection Stent and discovered high rates of late complications associated with the device, among them were stent fracture and stent migration [18]. The authors not only determined the insufficiency of this device, but also advised that patients with a Djumbodis Dissection Stent undergo regular monitoring to mitigate the risk of potential catastrophic incidents stemming from device failure.

This highlights the urgent need for an appropriate tool to address the challenges of the residual dissected aorta. However, there are a few key points (Table 1) that should be considered to identify potential candidates who benefit from additional AMDS implantations.

Table 1. Indications and contraindications for AMDS implantation.

Indications	Contraindications
DeBakey Type I dissection Primary entry in the ascending aorta or the aortic root	Aneurysm of the aortic arch or descending aorta Entries in the aortic arch or descending aorta including supra-aortic vessels Connective tissue disorder (e.g., Marfan syndrome) Nickel (nitinol) allergy

There is an ongoing debate on whether to perform hybrid arch repair using a frozen elephant trunk (FET) or the AMDS [19]. It must be stated clearly that these prostheses are two different kinds of animals, and therefore, their indications are also different. Indeed, the FET represents an excellent treatment option in case of DeBakey type I dissection with consecutive malperfusion. Outstanding results have been published in the past, bearing in mind that these data were derived from specialized aortic centers with corresponding expertise in the use of FET for total arch replacement [20,21]. Though representing the gold standard for definite and complete arch repair, it requires a professional aortic team with experienced aortic surgeons to achieve satisfactory results and low perioperative mortality rates because of its high complexity [22]. Performing a FET procedure in the setting of ATAAD may not be feasible for every surgeon on-call without advanced aortic surgery training and experience. Especially for this scenario, additional AMDS implantations and hemiarch replacements represent valid alternatives in case of a life-saving operation for DeBakey type I dissection. However, if contraindications exist, no compromises should be made, and total arch replacement, preferably using a FET, should be performed [23]. According to our expertise, entries not only in the aortic arch or descending aorta, but also in the supra-aortic vessels may contribute to a perfused false lumen after AMDS implantation, leading to aortic growth and a high risk for complex redo surgery. This highlights the importance of preoperative planning including multiplanar computed tomography reconstructions to assess the individual dissection patterns precisely and offer adequate aortic repair [1]. In a nutshell, the AMDS does not replace the FET, but offers a valid alternative in the case of DeBakey type I dissection and the absence of specific contraindications while upgrading the hemiarch procedure. In the case of chronic aortic dissection, no evidence is currently available in terms of AMDS implantation, and therefore, no reliable recommendations can be provided so far. According to our experience, AMDS implantation should not be considered for the treatment of chronic aortic dissection, e.g., of the aortic arch.

4. Current Clinical Results

The first results following AMDS implantation for the treatment of ATAAD were published by Boszo et al. in the "Dissected Aorta Repair Through Stent Implantation" (DARTS) trial [24]. In this safety and feasibility multicenter study, 16 patients with DeBakey type I dissection were enrolled, of whom 50% had evidence of preoperative malperfusion. The thirty-day mortality was 6.3%, and complete or partial thrombosis, including the remodeling of the aortic arch and descending aorta, was detected in 91.7% of cases (n = 11/12 with complete follow-up). Though the median follow-up time was only 130 ± 94 days, the results were promising and paved the way for further investigation. The DARTS trial expanded, and more centers participated, enrolling a total of 47 patients between 2017 and 2019 with a median follow-up time of 631 days [15]. Preoperative malperfusion was present in 56.5% of patients, including three cases of spinal malperfusion with consecutive paraplegia. The thirty-day mortality was 13%, and there were no device-related complications. The complete obliteration or thrombosis of the false lumen was observed in 74% in the aortic arch and in 53% in the descending aorta. Spinal malperfusion resolved in all cases. The AMDS promoted false lumen closure at the distal anastomosis in 90% of patients. A further sub-analysis of this cohort revealed excellent results for the restoration of malperfusion: 95.5% (n = 63) of branch vessel malperfusion cases resolved without an additional procedure [25]. New perioperative stroke, defined by the absence of preoperative cerebral malperfusion, occurred in 7.7% (n = 2) of patients. Preoperative cerebral malperfusion caused by the dissection of supra-aortic vessels is especially crucial and significantly increases the risk of perioperative stroke [5]. Current evidence is limited, but in a series of 16 patients, we were able to demonstrate satisfactory results in terms of supra-aortic vessel restoration and reached 100% regression of the totally occluded supra-aortic branches after the AMDS was implanted [26]. Later on, we published the currently largest available series of AMDS implantations for the treatment of DeBakey type I dissection, which includes 100 patients [6]. The thirty-day mortality and the rate of new postoperative stroke were 18% and 8%, respectively. Technical success was achieved in 76%, defined as the induced thrombosis of the false lumen in the medial segment of the descending aorta. Unfortunately, results for the long-term follow-up of aortic remodeling and false lumen patency are still missing. Recently, the three-year outcomes of the DARTS trial were published: the false lumen was completely or partially thrombosed in 90.5% in zone 0, 60.0% in zone 1, 68.2% in zone 2 and 89% in zone 5 [27]. Though AMDS was designed for zone 0 insertion, the partial replacement of the aortic arch and more distal implantation may be necessary in selected scenarios. Mehdiani et al. investigated the outcomes of eight patients receiving AMDS implantation beyond zone 0 [28]. No malperfusion was present in the survivors (7/8 patients), and true lumen was open in all patients, while the true lumen area was significantly higher in zone III ($p = 0.016$) and at the level of T11 ($p = 0.009$). The authors concluded that additional AMDS implantation beyond zone 0 can be safely performed and that it potentially avoids the risk for spinal cord injury, which is a rare but serious complication in the case of FETs [29]. Another series with 57 patients was published by Luehr et al., demonstrating an in-hospital mortality of 16% and a new postoperative stroke rate of 4%, which are in line with previous results [30]. Justified criticism has been raised about the additional use of an AMDS, questioning its potential benefit against standard hemiarch replacement, considering that the AMDS is way more expensive than a single dacron graft [31]. The first study comparing outcomes between single hemiarch replacement and additional AMDS implantation was recently published, investigating the impacts on aortic remodeling and risk for DANEs [12]. In this retrospective dual-center trial, 114 patients met the inclusion criteria and underwent hemiarch replacement in case of DeBakey type I dissection, whereas 37 patients received additional AMDS implantation. Despite no difference in mortality ($p = 0.768$) or other in-hospital adverse events, the incidence for DANEs was significantly lower with 11.8% (n = 4) in the AMDS group compared to 43.3% (n = 26) in the isolated hemiarch group ($p = 0.002$). Additionally, positive aortic remodeling in terms of false lumen thrombosis was superior in the AMDS group at the level of the aortic arch ($p = 0.029$), the proximal descending aorta ($p = 0.031$) and the level of pulmonary artery bifurcation ($p = 0.044$). These preliminary results are promising and suggest a broader application of the AMDS, considering that long-term follow-up data are still missing. The latest results of the DARTS trial and currently available studies (except case reports or case series) investigating outcomes after AMDS implantation are summarized in Table 2.

Table 2. Current study results investigating outcomes after AMDS implantation in DeBakey type I dissection.

Author and Year	Number of Patients	Preoperative Malperfusion, n (%)	Thirty-Day Mortality, n (%)	(New *) Postoperative Stroke, n (%)	Device Failure, n (%)	DANE, n (%)	False lumen Thrombosis (Complete or Partial), n (%)
Bozso, 2022 [27]	n = 47	26 (56.5%)	6 (13%)	1 (4.8%) *	0 (0%)	0 (0%)	Zone 0: 19 (91%) Zone 1: 12 (60%) Zone 2: 15 (68%) Zone 3: 16 (68%) Zone 5: 16 (89%)
Montagner, 2022 [6]	n = 100	46 (46%)	18 (18%)	8 (8%) *	3 (3%)	n.a.	Zone 4: 67 (76%)
Luehr, 2022 [30]	n = 57	41 (72%)	9 (16%)	2 (4%) *	5 (8%)	n.a.	n.a.
White, 2023 [12]	n = 37	13 (35%)	5 (14%)	8 (21.6%)	n.a.	4 (12%)	Zone A: 24 (73%) Zone B1: 24 (73%) Zone B2: 26 (81%) Zone B3: 25 (81%) Zone C: 21 (68%)

Zone A = aortic arch; Zone B1 = proximal descending; Zone B2: mid-descending; Zone B3: distal descending; Zone C: infradiaphragmatic. "*" defines "new" postoperative stroke. This is why it is stated in brackets and is separated from the general postoperative stroke rate without "*". This difference is often made in the aortic community.

5. Potential Risk for Device Failure

Due to the small number of implantations, current experience about potential device failure is limited. In their series of 57 AMDS implantations, Luehr et al. discovered that in 5 patients (8%), the proximal and distal AMDS portions were inflated while a complete central stent collapse was evident [30]. An example of AMDS collapse identified via postoperative computed tomography in one of our patients is shown in Figure 3.

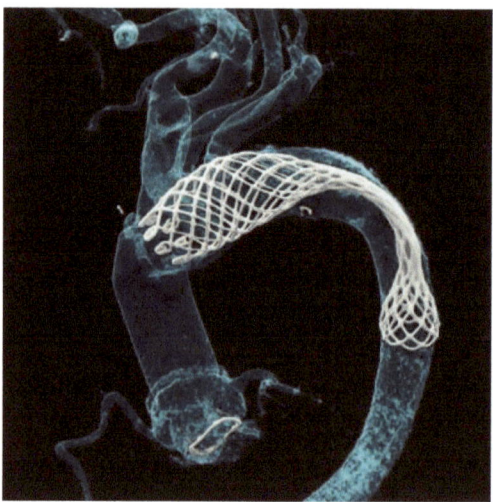

Figure 3. Postoperative computed tomography-based 3D reconstruction showing central AMDS collapse.

When comparing the inner ascending aortic graft length, patients without collapse showed significantly shorter lengths than patients with AMDS collapse (30.0 ± 5.9 vs. 39.6 ± 10.9 mm; $p = 0.029$). However, the proximal and distal stent portions remained inflated and did not seem to be affected by the central collapse. The increased stretching of the stent portion may result in a decrease in AMDS diameter favoring stent collapse as demonstrated by the authors. In standard hemiarch replacement, the proximal part of the aortic arch is resected transversely toward the inner arch's curvature, and the ascending aortic graft is shortened and resected with a corresponding shorter portion at the inner arch curvature. This approach aims to avoid the potential kinking of an elongated ascending graft. However, it may increase the tension of the AMDS toward the sinotubular junction, leading to a higher risk of stent collapse. Another potential risk factor may be the configuration of a gothic aortic arch or prominent aortic kinking of the arch and/or the descending aorta. Though no official contraindications exist for this scenario, AMDS implantation might be reconsidered under these circumstances to avoid stent collapse. Finally, aortic reshaping after the establishment of a pulsatile blood flow may lead to slight aortic elongation favoring stent collapse. On this basis, the authors proposed three key factors that might increase the risk for central stent collapse (Table 3). In our series of 100 AMDS implantations, we recognized the same phenomenon in three patients [6]. One of them was most likely caused due to the high tortuosity of the proximal descending aorta, which confirms the points mentioned by Luehr et al. [30]. One of three patients underwent successful endovascular dilatation of the collapsed stent. In the other two patients, endovascular dilatation was not a feasible option, but due to the uncovered stent design, no complications were observed in the further course and in-stent thrombosis was not evident during follow-up for these patients. However, we do recommend that in the case of AMDS collapse, medical anticoagulation therapy may be considered to avoid in-stent thrombosis [6,30].

Table 3. Potential risk factors for central AMDS collapse according to Luehr et al. [30].

Potential Risk Factors for Central AMDS Collapse		
Unfavorable anatomy	Device application	Aortic elongation
• Gothic aortic arch • Aortic kinking	• AMDS oversizing • Suboptimal aortic transection • Increased proximal tension	• During reperfusion

6. Aortic Re-Intervention after AMDS Implantation

Early re-intervention due to malperfusion after surgery for DeBakey type I dissection is not uncommon and was also observed after AMDS implantation [6,15]. Most of these cases caused by branch vessel related malperfusion can successfully be treated using an endovascular approach. Current evidence is limited to a minimum regarding the further treatment of the downstream aorta in case of DeBakey type I dissection using thoracic endovascular aortic repair (TEVAR) after AMDS implantation [32]. While the FET serves as an excellent landing zone for the treatment of residual aortic dissection, the suitability of the AMDS for this concept is unknown [33,34]. In a case series with three patients, El-Andari et al. demonstrated excellent results for TEVAR following AMDS implantation [35]. The time from initial AMDS implantation to TEVAR ranged from three months to two years. Two patients presented with a progression of thoracic distal aortic aneurysm and one patient with a patent entry tear in the distal aortic arch causing dissection expansion in the absence of DANEs. All patients underwent TEVAR, and one required additional carotid-subclavian bypass. However, more information is needed for the treatment of chronic residual dissection using TEVAR after AMDS implantation.

No data in terms of aortic redo surgery after AMDS implantation are currently available. In our opinion, aortic redo surgery after AMDS implantation can be crucial and should only be performed in specialized aortic centers with corresponding expertise in endovascular and aortic arch surgery. Indications may be the dissection progression of the aortic arch, anastomotic leakage or aortic graft infection, including AMDS cuff infection, which might be a vulnerable spot in the case of graft infection. According to our experience, complete AMDS removal may only be feasible in the case of early redo surgery after AMDS implantation. During the later course, the stent portion is stuck in the aortic arch and descending aorta, carrying the risk of aortic damage if manual extraction is forced. In this case, the only possibility may be FET implantation into the AMDS combined with a debranching of the supra-aortic vessels. Due to the radial force of the AMDS, cutting the stent portion should not be performed to avoid an uncontrolled expansion of the stent. Though this might be of interest for extended arch surgery and the graft replacement of the aortic arch, we do not recommend cutting the stent. If urgently needed, a possible strategy could be applying several polypropylene sutures through the aortic wall to stabilize the stent frame and adapt it to the aortic wall tightly. This may avoid the uncontrolled expansion of the stent frame and allow for cuff removal and graft replacement beyond zone 0. An example is shown in Figure 4, where we performed cuff removal in one of our patients. No data are currently available regarding the incidence or impact of arch entries after AMDS implantation or on the risk of stent-induced new entries. These topics may be of upmost importance for the surgical community to identify patients at risk. Corresponding data are urgently needed.

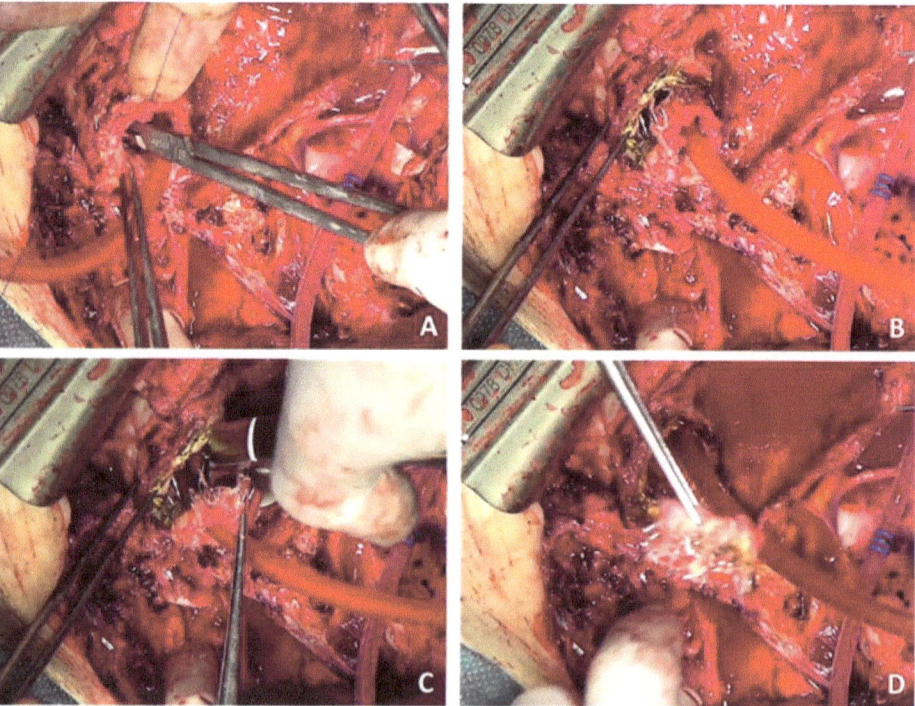

Figure 4. Example of AMDS shortening, including cuff removal. (**A**) Application of multiple single non-interrupting polypropylene sutures to stabilize the stent frame. (**B**) Careful dissection of the felt cuff. (**C**) Cutting the stent frame. (**D**) Complete removal of the cuff without an uncontrolled expansion of the stent.

7. Conclusions

Though experience and numbers are currently limited, the AMDS provides a promising and useful upgrade for standard hemiarch repair in the treatment of DeBakey type I dissection. Its use may be associated with a reduced risk for DANEs, positive aortic remodeling and the effective treatment of malperfusion. Preliminary studies show satisfactory short- and mid-term outcomes, considering that long-term data are urgently needed. Additionally, more data about standard hemiarch replacement compared to additional

AMDS implantation are needed. Compared to total arch replacement using a FET, the AMDS may represent a valid alternative in the setting of acute DeBakey type I dissection—if no contraindications are present. This highlights the importance of careful preoperative planning including multiplanar computed tomography reconstructions to offer adequate aortic repair. Further information in terms of device failure and re-intervention after AMDS implantation is highly needed to identify patients at risk.

Author Contributions: Conceptualization: all authors; methodology: L.P., M.C.M., M.L. and J.K.; validation: all authors; investigation: L.P., M.C.M., M.L. and J.K.; resources: M.C.M., M.L., V.F., J.K.; original draft preparation: L.P. and M.C.M.; writing—review and editing: all authors; visualization: L.P. and M.M.; supervision: all authors; project administration: L.P., M.C.M., M.L. and J.K.; funding acquisition: not required. All authors have read and agreed to the published version of the manuscript.

Funding: This research received no external funding.

Institutional Review Board Statement: Ethical review and approval were waived for this study due to the nature of a narrative review, involving no clinical data of our own or animals.

Informed Consent Statement: Patient consent was waived due to the nature of a narrative review with no active enrollment of patients.

Data Availability Statement: The original contributions presented in the study are included in the article. Further inquiries can be directed to the corresponding author.

Conflicts of Interest: M.C.M., M.L., V.F. and J.K. have received educational grants, including travel support, fees for lectures and speeches, and for professional consultation and research, along with study funds from Artivion® (Hechingen, Germany/Atlanta, GA, USA). M. Montagner has received speaker fees and travel grants from Artivion® (Hechingen, Germany). The remaining authors declare that the research was conducted in the absence of any commercial or financial relationships that could be construed as a potential conflict of interest.

Abbreviations

AMDS	Ascyrus Medical Dissection Stent
ATAAD	Acute type A aortic dissection
DANE	Distal anastomotic new entry
DARTS	Dissected aorta repair through stent implantation
FET	Frozen elephant trunk
TEVAR	Thoracic endovascular aortic repair

References

1. Pitts, L.; Montagner, M.; Kofler, M.; Van Praet, K.M.; Heck, R.; Buz, S.; Kurz, S.D.; Sündermann, S.; Hommel, M.; Falk, V.; et al. State of the Art Review: Surgical Treatment of Acute Type A Aortic Dissection. *Surg. Technol. Int.* **2021**, *38*, 279–288. [PubMed]
2. Montagner, M.; Kofler, M.; Pitts, L.; Heck, R.; Buz, S.; Kurz, S.; Falk, V.; Kempfert, J. Matched comparison of 3 cerebral perfusion strategies in open zone-0 anastomosis for acute type A aortic dissection. *Eur. J. Cardiothorac. Surg.* **2022**, *62*, ezac214. [CrossRef] [PubMed]
3. Pitts, L.; Kofler, M.; Montagner, M.; Heck, R.; Kurz, S.D.; Buz, S.; Falk, V.; Kempfert, J. The Impact of Malperfusion Patterns in Elderly Patients undergoing Surgery for Acute Type A Aortic Dissection. *Eur. J. Cardiothorac. Surg.* **2023**, *64*, ezad288. [CrossRef] [PubMed]
4. Pitts, L.; Heck, R.; Montagner, M.; Penkalla, A.; Kofler, M.; Falk, V.; Kempfert, J.; Buz, S. Case Report: Successful endovascular treatment of acute type A aortic dissection. *Front. Cardiovasc. Med.* **2023**, *10*, 1299192. [CrossRef] [PubMed]
5. Pitts, L.; Kofler, M.; Montagner, M.; Heck, R.; Iske, J.; Buz, S.; Kurz, S.D.; Starck, C.; Falk, V.; Kempfert, J. Cerebral Protection Strategies and Stroke in Surgery for Acute Type A Aortic Dissection. *J. Clin. Med.* **2023**, *12*, 2271. [CrossRef] [PubMed]
6. Montagner, M.; Kofler, M.; Seeber, F.; Pitts, L.; Starck, C.; Sundermann, S.H.; Kurz, S.; Grubitzsch, H.; Falk, V.; Kempfert, J. The arch remodelling stent for DeBakey I acute aortic dissection: Experience with 100 implantations. *Eur. J. Cardio-Thorac. Surg.* **2022**, *62*, ezac384. [CrossRef] [PubMed]

7. Isselbacher, E.M.; Preventza, O.; Black, J.H.; Augoustides, J.G.; Beck, A.W.; Bolen, M.A.; Braverman, A.C.; Bray, B.E.; Brown-Zimmerman, M.M.; Chen, E.P.; et al. 2022 ACC/AHA Guideline for the Diagnosis and Management of Aortic Disease: A Report of the American Heart Association/American College of Cardiology Joint Committee on Clinical Practice Guidelines. *Circulation* **2022**, *80*, e223–e393. [CrossRef] [PubMed]
8. Czerny, M.; Grabenwöger, M.; Berger, T.; Aboyans, V.; Della Corte, A.; Chen, E.P.; Desai, N.D.; Dumfarth, J.; Elefteriades, J.A.; Etz, C.D.; et al. EACTS/STS Guidelines for diagnosing and treating acute and chronic syndromes of the aortic organ. *Eur. J. Cardio-Thorac. Surg.* **2024**, *65*, ezad426. [CrossRef] [PubMed]
9. Wang, C.; Zhang, L.; Li, T.; Xi, Z.; Wu, H.; Li, D. Surgical treatment of type A acute aortic dissection with cerebral malperfusion: A systematic review. *J. Cardiothorac. Surg.* **2022**, *17*, 140. [CrossRef]
10. Montagner, M.; Kofler, M.; Buz, S.; Kempfert, J. Hybrid arch repair for acute type A aortic dissection: A new concept and step-by-step procedure. *Interact. Cardiovasc. Thorac. Surg.* **2021**, *32*, 837. [CrossRef]
11. Montagner, M.; Heck, R.; Kofler, M.; Buz, S.; Starck, C.; Sündermann, S.; Kurz, S.; Falk, V. New Hybrid Prosthesis for Acute Type A Aortic Dissection. *Surg. Technol. Int.* **2020**, *36*, 95–97.
12. White, A.; Elfaki, L.; O'Brien, D.; Manikala, V.; Bozso, S.; Ouzounian, M.; Moon, M.C. The use of the Ascyrus Medical Dissection Stent in acute type A aortic dissection repair reduces distal anastomotic new entry tear. *Can. J. Cardiol.* **2024**, *40*, 470–475. [CrossRef]
13. Elbatarny, M.; Youssef, A.; Bozso, S.J.; Moon, M.C.; Chung, J.; El-Hamamsy, I.; Dagenais, F.; Chu, M.W.A.; Ouzounian, M. Repair of acute type A dissection with distal malperfusion using a novel hybrid arch device. *Multimed. Man. Cardiothorac. Surg.* **2020**, *2020*.
14. Rylski, B.; Hahn, N.; Beyersdorf, F.; Kondov, S.; Wolkewitz, M.; Blanke, P.; Plonek, T.; Czerny, M.; Siepe, M. Fate of the dissected aortic arch after ascending replacement in type A aortic dissection†. *Eur. J. Cardio-Thorac. Surg.* **2017**, *51*, 1127–1134. [CrossRef]
15. Bozso, S.J.; Nagendran, J.; Chu, M.W.A.; Kiaii, B.; El-Hamamsy, I.; Ouzounian, M.; Kempfert, J.; Starck, C.; Moon, M.C. Midterm Outcomes of the Dissected Aorta Repair through Stent Implantation Trial. *Ann. Thorac. Surg.* **2020**, *111*, 463–470. [CrossRef]
16. Tamura, K.; Chikazawa, G.; Hiraoka, A.; Totsugawa, T.; Sakaguchi, T.; Yoshitaka, H. The prognostic impact of distal anastomotic new entry after acute type I aortic dissection repair. *Eur. J. Cardio-Thorac. Surg.* **2017**, *52*, 867–873. [CrossRef]
17. Czerny, M.; Stöhr, S.; Aymard, T.; Sodeck, G.H.; Ehrlich, M.; Dziodzio, T.; Juraszek, A.; Carrel, T. Effect on false-lumen status of a combined vascular and endovascular approach for the treatment of acute type A aortic dissection. *Eur. J. Cardio-Thorac. Surg.* **2012**, *41*, 409–413. [CrossRef]
18. Vendramin, I.; Piani, D.; Lechiancole, A.; Sponga, S.; Sponza, M.; Puppato, M.; Bortolotti, U.; Livi, U. Late complications of the Djumbodis system in patients with type A acute aortic dissection. *Interact. Cardiovasc. Thorac. Surg.* **2020**, *31*, 704–707. [CrossRef]
19. Al-Tawil, M.; Jubouri, M.; Tan, S.Z.; Bailey, D.M.; Williams, I.M.; Mariscalco, G.; Piffaretti, G.; Chen, E.P.; Velayudhan, B.; Mohammed, I.; et al. Thoraflex Hybrid vs. AMDS: To replace the arch or to stent it in type A aortic dissection? *Asian Cardiovasc. Thorac. Ann.* **2023**, *31*, 596–603. [CrossRef]
20. Shrestha, M.; Fleissner, F.; Ius, F.; Koigeldiyev, N.; Kaufeld, T.; Beckmann, E.; Martens, A.; Haverich, A. Total aortic arch replacement with frozen elephant trunk in acute type A aortic dissections: Are we pushing the limits too far? *Eur. J. Cardiothorac. Surg.* **2015**, *47*, 361–366; discussion 366. [CrossRef] [PubMed]
21. Benk, J.; Berger, T.; Kondov, S.; D'Inka, M.; Bork, M.; Walter, T.; Discher, P.; Rylski, B.; Czerny, M.; Kreibich, M. Comparative Study of Male and Female Patients Undergoing Frozen Elephant Trunk Total Arch Replacement. *J. Clin. Med.* **2023**, *12*, 6327. [CrossRef] [PubMed]
22. Dinato, F.J.; Dias, R.R.; Duncan, J.A.; Fernandes, F.; Ramires, F.J.A.; Mady, C.; Jatene, F.B. The learning curve effect on outcomes with frozen elephant trunk technique for extensive thoracic aorta disease. *J. Card. Surg.* **2019**, *34*, 796–802. [CrossRef] [PubMed]
23. Acharya, M.; Sherzad, H.; Bashir, M.; Mariscalco, G. The frozen elephant trunk procedure: Indications, outcomes and future directions. *Cardiovasc. Diagn. Ther.* **2022**, *12*, 708–721. [CrossRef] [PubMed]
24. Bozso, S.J.; Nagendran, J.; MacArthur, R.G.G.; Chu, M.W.A.; Kiaii, B.; El-Hamamsy, I.; Cartier, R.; Shahriari, A.; Moon, M.C. Dissected Aorta Repair through Stent Implantation trial: Canadian results. *J. Thorac. Cardiovasc. Surg.* **2019**, *157*, 1763–1771. [CrossRef] [PubMed]
25. Bozso, S.J.; Nagendran, J.; Chu, M.W.A.; Kiaii, B.; El-Hamamsy, I.; Ouzounian, M.; Kempfert, J.; Starck, C.; Shahriari, A.; Moon, M.C. Single-Stage Management of Dynamic Malperfusion Using a Novel Arch Remodeling Hybrid Graft. *Ann. Thorac. Surg.* **2019**, *108*, 1768–1775. [CrossRef] [PubMed]
26. Montagner, M.; Kofler, M.; Heck, R.; Buz, S.; Starck, C.; Kurz, S.; Falk, V.; Kempfert, J. Initial experience with the new type A arch dissection stent: Restoration of supra-aortic vessel perfusion. *Interact. Cardiovasc. Thorac. Surg.* **2021**, *33*, 276–283. [CrossRef] [PubMed]
27. Bozso, S.J.; Nagendran, J.; Chu, M.W.A.; Kiaii, B.; El-Hamamsy, I.; Ouzounian, M.; Forcillo, J.; Kempfert, J.; Starck, C.; Moon, M.C. Three-year outcomes of the Dissected Aorta Repair through Stent Implantation trial. *J. Thorac. Cardiovasc. Surg.* **2022**, *167*, 1661–1669.e3. [CrossRef] [PubMed]
28. Mehdiani, A.; Sugimura, Y.; Wollgarten, L.; Immohr, M.B.; Bauer, S.; Schelzig, H.; Wagenhäuser, M.U.; Antoch, G.; Lichtenberg, A.; Akhyari, P. Early Results of a Novel Hybrid Prosthesis for Treatment of Acute Aortic Dissection Type A with Distal Anastomosis Line Beyond Aortic Arch Zone Zero. *Front. Cardiovasc. Med.* **2022**, *9*, 892516. [CrossRef] [PubMed]
29. Chakos, A.; Jbara, D.; Yan, T.D.; Tian, D.H. Long-term survival and related outcomes for hybrid versus traditional arch repair-a meta-analysis. *Ann. Cardiothorac. Surg.* **2018**, *7*, 319–327. [CrossRef]

30. Luehr, M.; Gaisendrees, C.; Yilmaz, A.K.; Winderl, L.; Schlachtenberger, G.; Van Linden, A.; Wahlers, T.; Walther, T.; Holubec, T. Treatment of acute type A aortic dissection with the Ascyrus Medical Dissection Stent in a consecutive series of 57 cases. *Eur. J. Cardio-Thorac. Surg.* **2022**, *63*, ezac581. [CrossRef]
31. Pacini, D.; Murana, G. Novel hybrid graft for acute type A repair: Advance mastering of dissection stenting. *Eur. J. Cardio-Thorac. Surg.* **2022**, *62*, ezac408. [CrossRef] [PubMed]
32. O'Brien, D.J.; White, A.; Bozso, S.J.; Ferguson, D.; Moon, M.C.; Pozeg, Z. Thoracic Endovascular Aortic Repair Stent Deployed in the Ascyrus Medical Dissection Stent. *Ann. Thorac. Surg.* **2022**, *114*, e441–e442. [CrossRef] [PubMed]
33. Kreibich, M.; Berger, T.; Rylski, B.; Chen, Z.; Beyersdorf, F.; Siepe, M.; Czerny, M. Aortic reinterventions after the frozen elephant trunk procedure. *J. Thorac. Cardiovasc. Surg.* **2020**, *159*, 392–399.e1. [CrossRef] [PubMed]
34. Hostalrich, A.; Porterie, J.; Boisroux, T.; Marcheix, B.; Ricco, J.B.; Chaufour, X. Outcomes of Secondary Endovascular Aortic Repair after Frozen Elephant Trunk. *J. Endovasc. Ther.* **2023**, 15266028231169172. [CrossRef]
35. El-Andari, R.; Bozso, S.J.; O'Brien, D.; Chung, J.; Ouzounian, M.; Moon, M.C. Thoracic Endovascular Aortic Repair for Descending Thoracic Aortic Enlargement following Repair with the Ascyrus Medical Dissection Stent. *Can. J. Cardiol.* **2023**, *39*, 1698–1700. [CrossRef]

Disclaimer/Publisher's Note: The statements, opinions and data contained in all publications are solely those of the individual author(s) and contributor(s) and not of MDPI and/or the editor(s). MDPI and/or the editor(s) disclaim responsibility for any injury to people or property resulting from any ideas, methods, instructions or products referred to in the content.

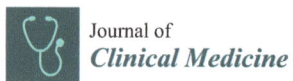

Article

Hospital Incidence and Treatment Outcomes of Patients with Aneurysms and Dissections of the Iliac Artery in Switzerland—A Secondary Analysis of Swiss DRG Statistics Data

Roland Bozalka [1], Anna-Leonie Menges [1], Alexander Zimmermann [1,*] and Lorenz Meuli [1,2]

1 Department of Vascular Surgery, University Hospital Zurich (USZ), University of Zurich (UZH), CH-8091 Zurich, Switzerland
2 Copenhagen Aortic Centre, Department of Vascular Surgery, Copenhagen University Hospital, 2100 Copenhagen Ø, Denmark
* Correspondence: alexander.zimmermann@usz.ch; Tel.: +41-44-255-2039

Citation: Bozalka, R.; Menges, A.-L.; Zimmermann, A.; Meuli, L. Hospital Incidence and Treatment Outcomes of Patients with Aneurysms and Dissections of the Iliac Artery in Switzerland—A Secondary Analysis of Swiss DRG Statistics Data. *J. Clin. Med.* **2024**, *13*, 2267. https://doi.org/10.3390/jcm13082267

Academic Editor: Ralf Kolvenbach

Received: 7 March 2024
Revised: 11 April 2024
Accepted: 12 April 2024
Published: 14 April 2024

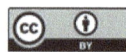

Copyright: © 2024 by the authors. Licensee MDPI, Basel, Switzerland. This article is an open access article distributed under the terms and conditions of the Creative Commons Attribution (CC BY) license (https://creativecommons.org/licenses/by/4.0/).

Abstract: **Background/Objectives:** Aneurysms and dissections of the iliac artery (ADIAs) are significant vascular conditions often associated with aortic pathologies. Despite their importance, reports on isolated iliac artery pathologies are rare. This study aimed to investigate the epidemiology of ADIA in Switzerland including treatment incidence and hospital outcomes. **Methods:** A retrospective analysis of diagnosis-related group (DRG) statistics from 2011 to 2018 in Switzerland was conducted, identifying all cases of ADIA while excluding those with concomitant treatment of aortic pathologies. Age-standardized incidence rates and treatment outcomes were assessed, with multivariable logistic regression performed to identify factors associated with hospital mortality. **Results:** From 2011 to 2018, 1037 ADIA cases were hospitalized in Switzerland. Incidence rates for elective treatment were significantly higher in men than women, increasing in men from 1.5 to 2.4 cases per 100,000 men ($p = 0.007$), while remaining stable in women at around 0.2 cases per 100,000 women. Acute treatment incidence rates were lower but still higher in men, at 0.9 cases per 100,000 men and 0.2 cases per 100,000 women. Crude hospital mortality rates were lower for endovascular repair than open surgical repair in both elective (0.8% vs. 3.1%, $p = 0.023$) and emergency treatment (6.7% vs. 18.4%, $p = 0.045$). Multivariable analysis showed that endovascular repair was associated with significantly reduced hospital mortality compared to open repair (OR 0.27, 95%-CI: 0.10 to 0.66, $p = 0.006$). **Conclusions:** This nationwide study of iliac artery pathologies shows that the treatment incidence was about 10 times higher in men than in women for elective procedures, but only about five times higher for emergency treatment. Endovascular procedures were associated with significantly lower hospital mortality than open procedures, while hospital mortality rates were comparable for men and women.

Keywords: aneurysm; iliac; artery; iliac; dissection; iliac; secondary data analysis; DRG

1. Introduction

An iliac artery aneurysm (IAA) is the dilation of the common iliac artery (CIA), the internal iliac artery (IIA), or the external iliac artery (EIA) by more than 1.5 times the normal diameter [1]. Different classification systems exist for IAA. Historical Swedish autopsy data on aortic and iliac aneurysms from the 1970s to 1980s show that about 17% of all abdominal aortic aneurysms (AAA) are accompanied by IAA [2]. These pathologies are generally referred to as aorto-iliac aneurysms. In clinical practice, the treatment of AAA often requires simultaneous treatment of the CIA, as these vessels are frequently ectatic or aneurysmal and do not allow either endovascular sealing or durable surgical suturing. Isolated IAAs were found in only 0.7% of all patients with aorto-iliac aneurysms. Thus, the treatment of isolated IAA pathologies remains rare and there is no solid and up-to-date data on the epidemiology of isolated IAAs. For isolated IAAs, Reber's classification according to anatomical extent has become established [3]. It comprises four types, with type I comprising isolated CIA aneurysms, type II isolated IIA aneurysms, type III a combination of CIA and IIA aneurysms, and type IV aneurysms in which all iliac vessels are dilated. The CIA is most affected, whereas the EIA is rarely affected by aneurysmal degeneration, possibly due to its different embryological origin [3].

The pathogenesis of IAA is similar to that of AAA and generally includes atherosclerotic degeneration of the medial wall [1]. Other etiologies include post-dissection aneurysms, infected native aneurysms, traumatic aneurysms, or pseudoaneurysms [1]. As with AAA, most patients with isolated degenerative IAA are male (90%) and usually over 70 years old at diagnosis [1].

IAA are generally asymptomatic but might cause symptoms due to compression of surrounding structures such as the ureter, sacral plexus, or iliac vein [4,5]. As with aortic aneurysms, the risk of a life-threatening rupture increases with increasing diameter [1,6,7]. However, the natural history of IAA is less well established than for AAA. The diameter threshold where elective IAA treatment should be considered has recently been increased to ≥ 4.0 cm (class of recommendation IIa, level of evidence C) by the European Society of Vascular Surgery (ESVS) [1]. In contrast, limited data exist on isolated dissections of the iliac arteries. Most often, case reports describe iatrogenic dissections. Reports on spontaneous dissections of the iliac arteries often involve underlying pathologies such as fibromuscular dysplasia or connective tissue diseases [8,9]. As for aortic dissections, emergent surgical treatment is generally indicated when there is evidence of rupture, or malperfusion (i.e., limb ischemia). For chronic dissections treatment is generally recommended if there is a concomitant IAA ≥ 4.0 cm [1], or can be considered in patients with clinically relevant malperfusion of the limb [10]. Treatment options encompass both endovascular and open procedures. While open therapy was the standard until the 1990s, the rapid advancement of endovascular techniques has shifted the trend towards endovascular approaches. As with AAA, endovascular procedures are associated with lower complication rates and shorter hospital stays [11]. The current ESVS guidelines recommend that the choice of surgical technique for IAA should be based on individual patient and lesion characteristics (Class IIa, Level B) [1].

This study aimed to describe the epidemiology of isolated IAA and iliac artery dissections through a secondary data analysis of Diagnosis Related Group (DRG) statistics in Switzerland.

2. Materials and Methods

2.1. Data Source

This is a secondary data analysis of case-related hospital discharge data from the Swiss Federal Statistical Office (SFSO). Every medical institution in Switzerland, including hospitals, birthing centres, and medical specialty institutions, is bound to report all hospitalizations to the SFSO annually. The SFSO collects baseline characteristics like age, sex, and insurance class, as well as a primary diagnosis and up to 49 secondary diagnoses. Diagnoses are recorded using the 10th revision of the International Classification of Diseases (ICD-10). Further, general information like the type of admission (planned or emergent), the total length of stay in days, length of stay in the intensive care unit (ICU) in hours, and discharge information, including hospital mortality, are recorded. Finally, up to 100 procedure codes are captured for each hospital stay using the Swiss classification of surgical interventions (CHOP). The full CHOP code is available online: http://tinyurl.com/mwzux9xb (accessed on 13 April 2024). The main CHOP code for endovascular implantation of a stent graft in the iliac artery, "39.79.12", was only available since 2011. Before 2011, only unspecific coding for endovascular therapy without anatomical location was available. In addition, there are codes for endovascular coil embolization or occlusion of abdominal vessels "39.79.26" and for other extracranial vessels ("x.20 and x.29") available. Since 2014, the additional codes "39.78.11, x.12, x.13, x.19" were added to differentiate between iliac stent grafts without a side branch ("x.11"), iliac stent grafts with a side branch ("x.12"), iliac stent graft with fenestration ("x.13"), and other stent graft ("x.19"). The CHOP codes for open surgical treatment were "38.36.17", "39.25.11, x.12, x.19, x.21, x.22, x.99", and "39.57.48". These codes did not change during the observed period. Further details on ICD and CHOP codes are available in the Supplementary Material.

Data are fully anonymized due to personal data protection regulations. Thereby, each patient receives a new unique identifier for each admission. This obscures the identification of readmissions of the same patient. Further, the institution number is encoded and grouped into five levels of care, with level one indicating university hospitals, level two indicating larger non-university hospitals ("major hospitals"), and levels three to five indicating smaller hospitals for secondary care ("regional hospitals") [12]. The analysis of this fully anonymized dataset did not require ethical approval (waived by the local ethics board: BASEC-Nr. Req-2021-01010). This study is reported in accordance with the STROBE statement [13].

2.2. Inclusion and Exclusion Criteria

All cases with "I72.3" as a primary or secondary diagnosis (ICD-10: aneurysm or dissection of the iliac artery; ADIA) were identified during the reporting years 2011–2018. Several additional filters were applied to identify cases that were truly admitted for this diagnosis. The Supplementary Table S1 provided an overview on the patient identification process. In short, cases with ADIA as a secondary diagnosis only and without a CHOP code for surgical treatment were excluded. Likewise, all elective admissions with ADIA as primary diagnosis but without a CHOP code for surgical treatment were excluded. Further, all cases with a primary diagnosis of any aortic aneurysm (ICD I71.3–I71.6) or any aortic dissection (ICD I71.00–I70.07), as well as all cases with both endovascular and open surgical treatment codes were excluded. Finally, all acute admissions without a surgical treatment code and with discharge to another acute care hospital were excluded to avoid duplicates.

2.3. Statistical Analysis

Factor variables were summarized with counts and percentages and compared using the Chi-squared test. Continuous variables were summarized with the median and quartiles 25 and 75 and compared using the Kruskal–Wallis rank test. Comorbidities were summarized using a sum score of weighted Elixhauser ICD-10 diagnosis groups according to van Walraven [14]. This involves evaluating the presence of ICD-10 codes within each comorbidity category for every case, and then aggregating them using a weighting system using the "comorbidity" R package version 0.5.3 by Gasparini [15]. The used ICD-10 codes are available in the Supplementary Tables S2 and S3. Hospital incidence rates were age-standardized using the 2013 European standard population and for the Swiss population data from the SFSO as previously described [16–18].

A multivariable logistic regression model was built to analyze the association between treatment modality and hospital mortality. The continuous variables of age and the van Walraven comorbidity score, as well as the factor variables of sex, type of admission, type of treatment, insurance class, hospital level, and period of treatment (2011–2014 vs. 2015–2018) were included in this model to adjust for potential confounding. Cases without surgical treatment were excluded. Regression coefficients were presented using odds ratios (OR) and the corresponding 95% confidence intervals (95%-CI). Hospital levels from 3 to 5 were merged to obtain a reasonable number of patients in this group. The data structure does not allow for missing data. All analyses were performed using R version 4.2.3 on macOS 12.5.1 [19]. All *p*-values were two-sided with an alpha-level of 5%.

3. Results

From 01.01.2011 to 31.12.2018, 8808 cases were hospitalized with ADIA as a primary or secondary diagnosis. After excluding 7664 cases, a total of 1144 cases were included in this study. Figure 1 details the patient flow with reasons for exclusion. In total, 787 (68.8%) were electively treated for ADIA, 164 (14.3%) received urgent or emergent treatment for

ADIA, and the remaining 193 (16.9%) received conservative treatment for ADIA. Data were complete for the published variables.

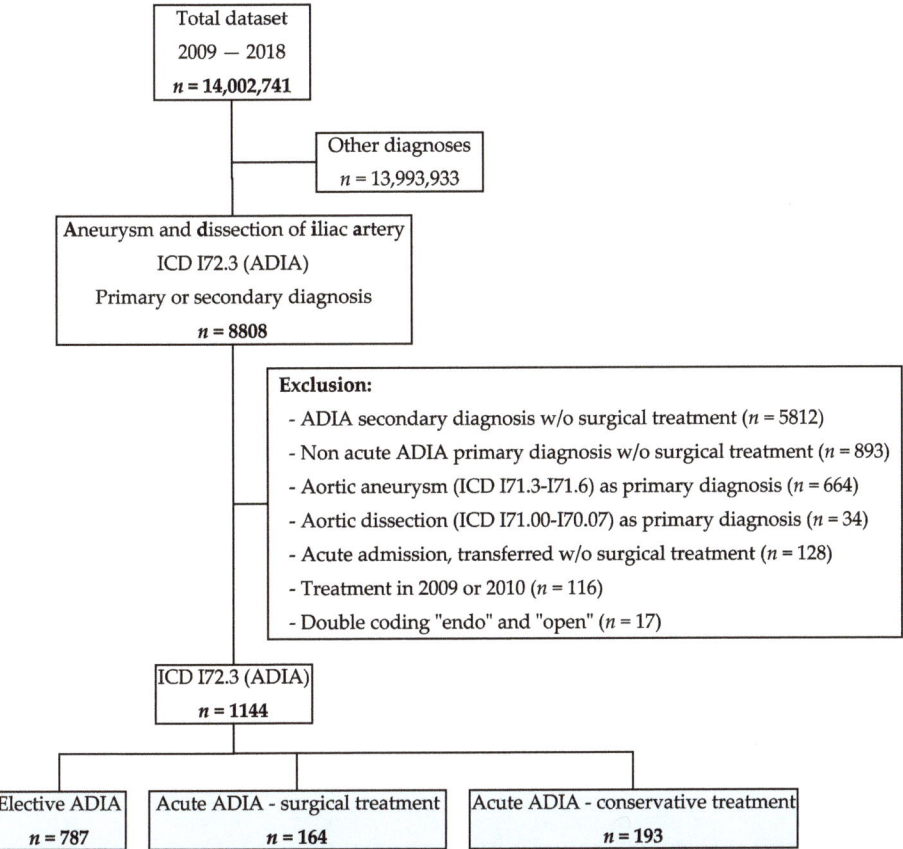

Figure 1. The total dataset contained all hospitalizations in the Swiss population in the years from 2009 to 2018. ICD = International Classification of Diseases (version 10); ADIA = aneurysm and dissection of iliac artery. w/o = without.

Tables 1 and 2 show the baseline characteristics of electively treated cases and surgically treated emergencies, each stratified by treatment modality. Cases receiving endovascular therapy were significantly older compared to cases that received open surgical repair: 74 versus 69 years in the elective cases, $p < 0.001$, and 75 versus 72.5 years in emergency cases, $p = 0.02$. In the elective setting, the proportion of endovascular treatment was significantly higher in the later treatment period (2015 to 2018) compared to the more historic period (2011 to 2014), $p < 0.001$. The same tendency was seen in the emergency setting but did not reach statistical significance. The change in treatment modality is illustrated by the Supplementary Figure S1. The overall proportion of endovascular repair steadily increased from 20.4% in 2011 to 58.7% in 2018, whereas the proportion of open repair (46.6% to 24.5%) and conservative management (33.0% to 16.8%) decreased during the same period. Characteristics and hospital mortality of the acute cases with ADIA without surgical therapy are summarized in the Supplementary Table S4.

Table 1. Baseline characteristics of elective cases.

Variable	Endovascular Repair (n = 492)	Open Repair (n = 295)	Total (n = 787)	p Value
Male sex	455 (92)	269 (91)	724 (92)	0.518
Age, years	75 (68, 80)	69 (63, 75)	73 (66, 79)	<0.001
van Walraven score	2 (0, 6)	3 (0.5, 10)	2 (0, 8)	<0.001
Coronary artery disease	114 (23)	78 (26)	192 (24)	0.301
Chronic heart failure	19 (3.9)	15 (5.1)	34 (4.3)	0.414
Cerebrovascular disease	30 (6.1)	18 (6.1)	48 (6.1)	0.998
Arterial hypertension	246 (50)	144 (49)	390 (50)	0.747
Chronic pulmonary disease	41 (8.3)	29 (9.8)	70 (8.9)	0.475
Diabetes mellitus	61 (12)	32 (11)	93 (12)	0.514
Chronic kidney disease	85 (17)	50 (17)	135 (17)	0.906
Cancer	7 (1.4)	7 (2.4)	14 (1.8)	0.329
Obesity	16 (3.3)	8 (2.7)	24 (3.0)	0.670
Type of hospital				0.045
University hospital (Level 1)	181 (37)	135 (45.8)	316 (40)	
Major hospital (Level 2)	267 (54)	138 (46.8)	405 (51)	
Other (Level 3 to 5)	44 (8.9)	22 (7.5)	66 (8.4)	
Location before admission				0.182
Home	455 (92)	272 (92)	727 (92)	
Acute care hospital	34 (6.9)	19 (6.4)	53 (6.7)	
Nursing home	2 (0.4)	0 (0.0)	2 (0.3)	
Other	1 (0.2)	4 (1.4)	5 (0.6)	
Treatment period				<0.001
2011–2014	115 (29.3)	162 (54.9)	277 (40.3)	
2015–2018	278 (70.7)	133 (45.1)	411 (59.7)	

Data are complete. Counts are presented with percentages and compared using Chi2 tests. Continuous variables are summarized with median and percentiles 25 and 75 and compared using Kruskal–Wallis rank tests. ICD-10 codes to identify comorbidities are available in the supplement.

Table 2. Baseline characteristics of surgically treated emergent cases.

Variable	Endovascular Repair (n = 91)	Open Repair (n = 73)	Total (n = 164)	p Value
Male sex	74 (81)	66 (90)	140 (85)	0.102
Age, years	74 (65, 81)	73 (60, 78)	73 (62, 80)	0.154
van Walraven score	10 (2, 19)	10 (3, 17)	10 (3, 18)	0.984
Coronary artery disease	22 (24)	17 (23)	39 (24)	0.894
Chronic heart failure	10 (11)	6 (8.2)	16 (9.8)	0.552
Cerebrovascular disease	5 (5.5)	1 (1.4)	6 (3.7)	0.227
Arterial hypertension	35 (38)	27 (37)	62 (38)	0.846
Chronic pulmonary disease	14 (15)	12 (16)	26 (16)	0.854
Diabetes mellitus	7 (7.7)	9 (12)	16 (9.8)	0.320
Chronic kidney disease	26 (29)	20 (27)	46 (28)	0.868
Cancer	3 (3.3)	0 (0)	3 (1.8)	0.254
Obesity	1 (1.1)	1 (1.4)	2 (1.2)	0.999
Type of hospital				0.668
University hospital (Level 1)	42 (46)	28 (38)	70 (43)	
Major hospital (Level 2)	45 (49)	41 (56)	86 (52)	
Other (Level 3 to 5)	4 (4.4)	4 (5.5)	8 (4.9)	
Location before admission				0.196
Home	69 (76)	59 (81)	128 (78)	
Acute care hospital	16 (18)	14 (19)	30 (18)	
Nursing home	2 (2.2)	0 (0)	2 (1.2)	
Other	4 (4.4)	0 (0)	4 (2.4)	
Treatment period				0.487
2011–2014	35 (38)	32 (44)	67 (41)	
2015–2018	56 (62)	41 (56)	97 (59)	

Data are complete. Counts are presented with percentages and compared using Chi2 tests. Continuous variables are summarized with median and percentiles 25 and 75 and compared using Kruskal–Wallis rank tests. ICD-10 codes to identify comorbidities are available in the supplement.

3.1. Epidemiology

The age-standardized incidence rates for elective surgical treatment of ADIA in Switzerland are plotted in Figure 2. The incidence rates were about 10 times higher in men than in women. They significantly increased in men from 1.75 (95%-CI: 1.4 to 2.2) to 2.7 (2.2 to 3.2) cases per 100,000 men, $p = 0.012$, and were stable in women at around 0.2 (0.1 to 0.4) per 100,000 women, $p = 0.674$.

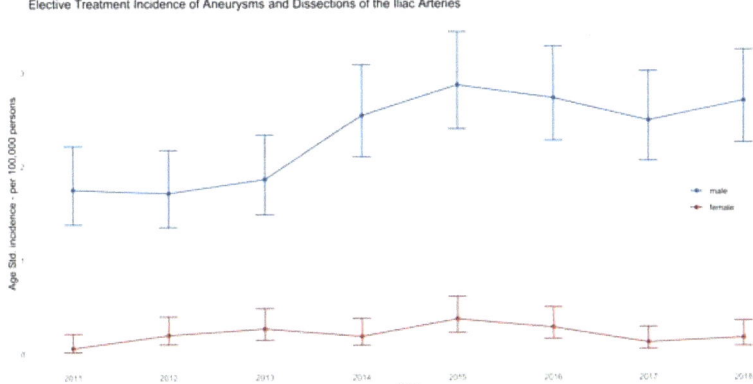

Figure 2. Age-standardized incidence rates of elective treatment of iliac artery aneurysms or dissections in Switzerland between 2011 and 2018 with 95% confidence intervals stratified by sex. The incidence significantly increased in males ($p = 0.012$) and was stable in females ($p = 0.674$) in the observed eight years.

The age-standardized incidence rates for emergent hospital admission for ADIA in Switzerland are plotted for 2011 to 2018 in Figure 3. These figures included both surgically treated cases and cases with conservative management. The incidence rates were about five times higher in men than in women. They were stable in both sexes in the observed period at around 0.9 (95%-CI: 0.7 to 1.3) cases per 100,000 men and around 0.2 (0.1 to 0.4) cases per 100,000 women.

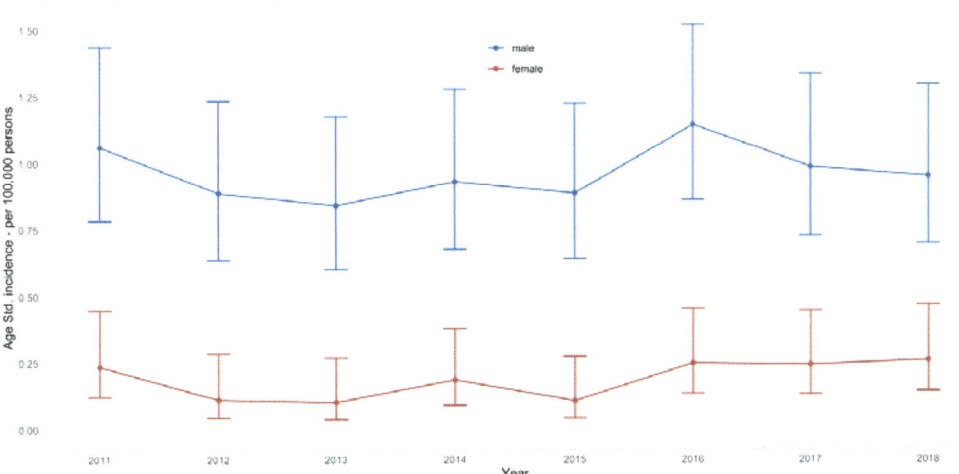

Figure 3. Age-standardized incidence rates of all emergent admissions for iliac artery aneurysms or dissections in Switzerland between 2011 and 2018 with 95% confidence intervals stratified by sex (both surgically treated and conservatively managed). The incidence rates were stable in the observed eight years in both males ($p = 0.688$) and females ($p = 0.212$).

3.2. Treatment Modality

There was a steady increase in endovascular therapy in the observed period. In 2011, only 27% of the cases were treated using an endovascular approach, where it was 63.3% in 2018. On the other hand, the proportion of conservatively managed cases and cases managed with open surgical treatment decreased in the period from 29.7% to 14.2%, and from 43.2 to 22.5%, respectively. A figure detailing these proportions is available in the Supplementary Material. Figure 4 shows an overall Venn diagram of the type of endovascular therapy including elective and emergency treatments. Subcodes for tube, branched, or fenestrated grafts were only available for the years from 2014 to 2018. Three cases were coded with a fenestrated graft, and these were excluded to increase readability. Most cases were coded with tube stent graft implantation (40.3%), the second largest group was coded with an isolated vessel occlusion (24.4%), and an additional 16.9% were coded to have a branched device implanted without additional vessel occlusion. A total of 47 cases (13.1%) were coded with endovascular occlusion and tube graft implantation. All other combinations were relatively seldom.

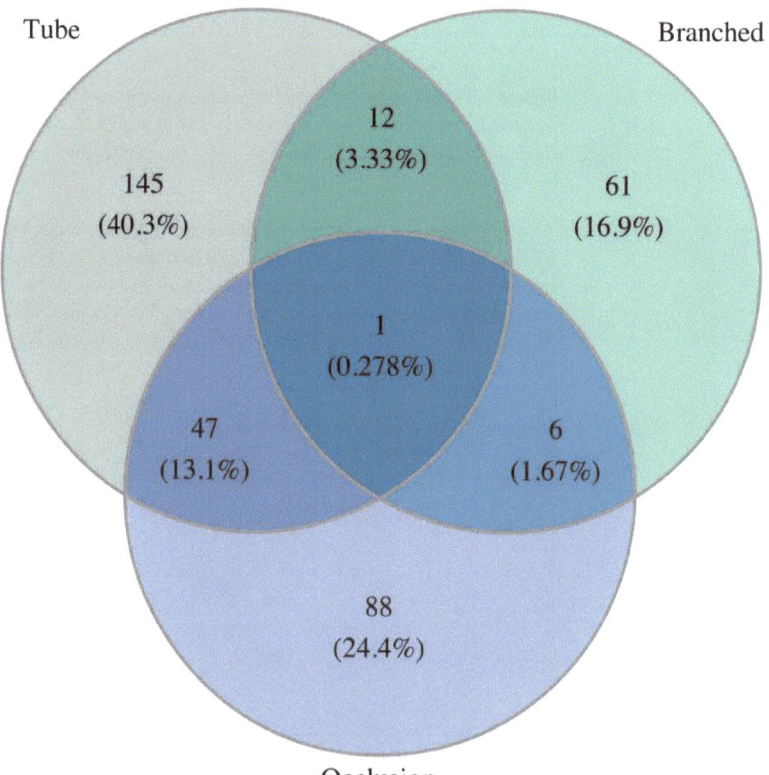

Figure 4. Venn diagram showing coding of endovascular therapy for elective or acute treatment of ADIA for the years from 2014 to 2018, excluding 3 cases coded with a fenestrated graft.

3.3. Treatment Outcomes—Elective

Table 3 summarizes the procedural details and treatment outcomes of cases with elective treatment for ADIA. There were significant differences in both the length of intensive care unit admission and length of hospital stay in favor of endovascular therapy, both $p < 0.001$. Likewise, the proportion of cases needing packed red blood cell transfusion was significantly higher after open surgical repair than endovascular repair, $p < 0.001$. In general, the number of reported complications was low for both endovascular and open repair, except for lower limb ischemia, with 6.5% of cases after endovascular repair and 14.2% after open repair, $p < 0.001$. Despite the high rate of lower limb ischemia, crural fasciotomy was only coded in 0.6%, and major amputation was never coded.

Table 3. Treatment details and outcomes of elective cases.

Variable	Endovascular Repair (n = 492)	Open Repair (n = 295)	Total (n = 787)	p Value
Length of stay ICU, hours	0 (0, 0)	16 (0, 26)	0 (0, 19)	<0.001
Length of hospital stay, days	4 (3, 6)	9 (7, 14)	6 (3, 10)	<0.001
Packed red blood cells				<0.001
0	430 (87)	201 (68.1)	631 (80)	
1–5	46 (9.3)	66 (22.4)	112 (14)	
>5	16 (3.3)	28 (9.5)	44 (5.6)	
Fresh frozen plasma				0.010
0	487 (99)	283 (95.9)	770 (98)	
1–5	4 (0.8)	10 (3.4)	14 (1.8)	
>5	1 (0.2)	2 (0.7)	3 (0.4)	
Platelet transfusion				0.609
0	491 (100)	294 (99.7)	785 (100)	
1–5	1 (0.2)	0 (0.0)	1 (0.1)	
>5	0 (0)	1 (0.3)	1 (0.1)	
Myocardial infarction	2 (0.4)	1 (0.3)	3 (0.4)	0.999
Acute mesenteric ischemia	3 (0.6)	8 (2.7)	11 (1.4)	0.024
Large intestine resection	1 (0.2)	7 (2.4)	8 (1.0)	0.005
Small intestine resection	2 (0.4)	3 (1.0)	5 (0.6)	0.369
Acute lower limb ischemia	32 (6.5)	42 (14.2)	74 (9.4)	<0.001
Crural fasciotomy	1 (0.2)	4 (1.4)	5 (0.6)	0.068
Major amputation	0 (0)	0 (0.0)	0 (0)	NA
Destination after discharge				<0.001
Home	443 (90)	240 (81.4)	683 (87)	
Rehabilitation	21 (4.3)	37 (12.5)	58 (7.4)	
Acute care hospital	14 (2.8)	8 (2.7)	22 (2.8)	
Nursing home	8 (1.6)	0 (0.0)	8 (1.0)	
Other	2 (0.4)	1 (0.3)	3 (0.4)	
Hospital mortality	4 (0.8)	9 (3.1)	13 (1.7)	0.022

Data are complete. Counts are presented with percentages and compared using Chi2 tests. Continuous variables are summarized with median and percentiles 25 and 75 and compared using Kruskal–Wallis rank tests. ICD-10 codes to identify comorbidities are available in the supplement. ICU = intensive care unit. Destination after discharge also includes mortality; this level is not shown as it is redundant with the hospital mortality variable. NA = not applicable (no events in both groups).

3.4. Treatment Outcomes—Emergency

Table 4 summarizes the procedural details and treatment outcomes of cases with emergency surgical treatment for ADIA. Like the elective setting, the length of intensive care stay, and the total length of hospital stay were significantly lower after endovascular repair. On the other hand, the need for transfusion was similar in both groups. Complication rates were dramatically higher than in the elective setting, with an overall rate of myocardial infarction of 4.9% compared to 0.4% in the elective setting. Notably, mesenteric ischemia was coded significantly more often after open surgical repair than after endovascular therapy, 12% versus 2.2%, $p = 0.012$. Likewise, small- and large-bowel resection was coded more often after open surgery than after endovascular treatment, without reaching statistical significance. Lower limb ischemia and major amputation were quite common and seen after both endovascular- and open-surgical repair without statistically significant differences.

Table 4. Treatment details and outcomes for surgically treated emergent cases.

Variable	Endovascular Repair (n = 91)	Open Repair (n = 73)	Total (n = 164)	p Value
Length of stay ICU, hours	0 (0, 43)	46 (15, 109)	23 (0, 83)	<0.001
Length of hospital stay, days	11 (6, 19)	16 (10, 28)	13 (7, 21)	0.003
Packed red blood cells				0.171
0	43 (47)	26 (36)	69 (42)	
1–5	30 (33)	24 (33)	54 (33)	
>5	18 (20)	23 (32)	41 (25)	
Fresh frozen plasma				0.799
0	85 (93)	67 (92)	152 (93)	
1–5	4 (4.4)	5 (6.8)	9 (5.5)	
>5	2 (2.2)	1 (1.4)	3 (1.8)	
Platelet transfusion				0.254
0	88 (97)	73 (100)	161 (98)	
1–5	3 (3.3)	0 (0)	3 (1.8)	
>5	0 (0)	0 (0)	0 (0)	
Myocardial infarction	2 (2.2)	6 (8.2)	8 (4.9)	0.141
Acute mesenteric ischemia	2 (2.2)	9 (12)	11 (6.7)	0.012
Large intestine resection	2 (2.2)	6 (8.2)	8 (4.9)	0.141
Small intestine resection	1 (1.1)	4 (5.5)	5 (3.0)	0.173
Acute lower limb ischemia	9 (9.9)	14 (19)	23 (14)	0.089
Crural fasciotomy	2 (2.2)	4 (5.5)	6 (3.7)	0.408
Major amputation	2 (2.2)	2 (2.7)	4 (2.4)	>0.999
Destination after discharge				0.201
Home	54 (59)	37 (51)	91 (55)	
Rehabilitation	13 (14)	15 (21)	28 (17)	
Acute care hospital	11 (12)	4 (5.5)	15 (9.1)	
Nursing home	3 (3.3)	1 (1.4)	4 (2.4)	
Other	1 (1.1)	2 (2.7)	3 (1.8)	
Hospital mortality	9 (9.9)	14 (19)	23 (14)	0.089

Data are complete. Counts are presented with percentages and compared using Chi2 tests. Continuous variables are summarized with median and percentiles 25 and 75 and compared using Kruskal–Wallis rank tests. ICD-10 codes to identify comorbidities are available in the supplement. ICU = intensive care unit. Destination after discharge also includes mortality; this level is not shown as it is redundant with the hospital mortality variable.

3.5. Hospital Mortality

The crude hospital mortality rates for elective treatment of ADIA were 0.8% after endovascular repair and 3.1% after open surgical repair, $p = 0.022$. For surgical emergency treatment, the crude hospital mortality rates were 9.9% after endovascular repair and 19% after open repair, $p = 0.089$. The hospital mortality rate in the conservatively treated cohort was 27%; see Supplementary Table S4.

The differences in treatment outcomes between open and endovascular repair cases were analyzed in a multivariable logistic regression analysis; see Figure 5. Endovascular repair was associated with a significantly reduced hospital mortality compared to open repair, OR 0.35 (0.16 to 0.73, $p = 0.006$). The adjusted mortality rate was significantly higher in the acute setting compared to elective treatment, OR 7.03 (3.38 to 15.14, $p < 0.001$). Further, increasing age at the time of treatment, OR 1.04 (1.01 to 1.09) per year, $p = 0.023$, and an increasing van Walraven score, OR 1.05 (1.02 to 1.09) per point, $p = 0.001$, were associated with higher hospital mortality. Sex, hospital level, insurance class, and period of treatment were not significantly associated with hospital mortality.

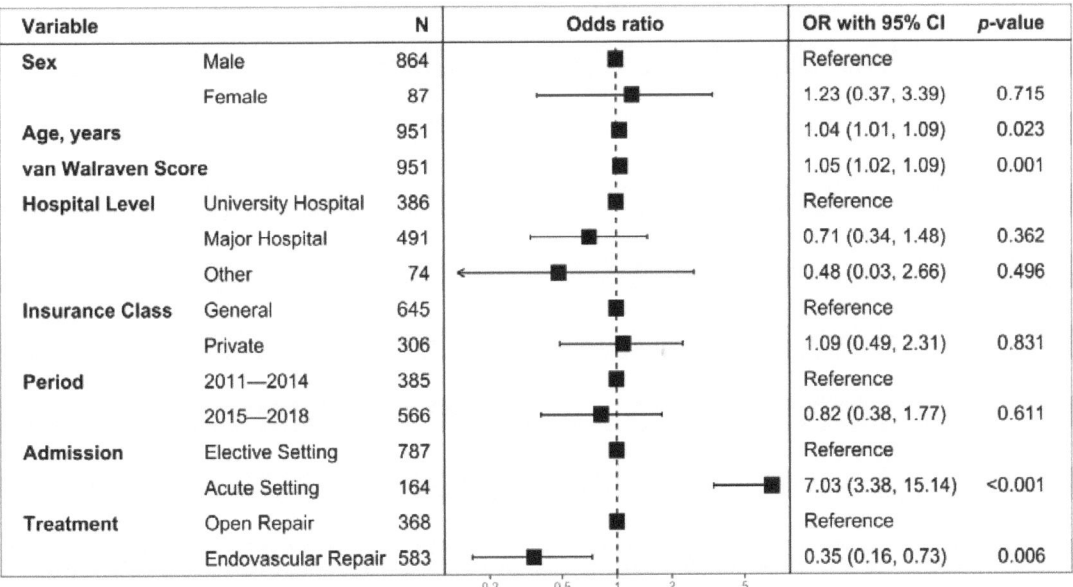

Figure 5. Multivariable logistic regression model on hospital survival. Data are complete. Analysis of 951 cases with 36 events (= hospital deaths). OR = odds ratio; 95% CI = 95% confidence interval of odds ratio.

4. Discussion

This is the first study to show comprehensive nationwide epidemiological data on the surgical treatment of iliac artery pathologies. The study shows several remarkable findings. First, the treatment incidence rate for men was roughly 10 times higher in the elective setting compared to women but only roughly five times higher for emergency treatments. Second, the data show favorable hospital outcomes for endovascular procedures compared to open surgical treatments. And third, there was no statistically significant difference in hospital treatment outcomes between men and women.

An important note is required when interpreting these findings; in contrast to aortic pathologies, the current ICD coding for diseases of the iliac arteries does not differentiate between dissections and aneurysms. Therefore, there is also no classification between asymptomatic, symptomatic, or ruptured aneurysms of the iliac artery. The grouping into elective and acute cases was determined in this study by coding the hospitalization as either elective or emergency. An indirect verification of this grouping by the coding of hemorrhagic or hypovolemic shock (ICD R57.1) did not provide any additional information, as it is not clear whether the condition was present on admission or occurred during treatment as a complication of an originally elective treatment. Therefore, the specific mortality rate for the conservative treatment of iliac artery dissections as well as the specific mortality rate for symptomatic or ruptured iliac artery aneurysms remain unknown as these pathologies cannot be distinguished. The comparatively low hospital mortality in the "conservative management cohort" for acute ADIA of only 27% indicates that there might be a substantial proportion of dissections captured that were treated with the best medical therapy only. This hypothesis is also supported by the fact that another investigation for ruptured AAA (rAAA) has shown a hospital mortality rate in the palliative cohort of 95.7%. It seems very likely that the hospital mortality rate for palliative cases in patients with ruptured IAA might be at a comparable level [20].

4.1. Epidemiology

There is currently no comprehensive epidemiological data available to put our findings in an international context. The incidence of ADIA was roughly 10% of the incidence rates for AAA in the same period in Switzerland (2009–2018 for AAA versus 2011–2018 for ADIA) [16]. Comparison with historic data from a single institution in Switzerland (1972–1988) reported 7% of isolated IAA within all aorto-iliac aneurysms [21]. Both rates are substantially higher than the historic Swedish autopsy data that observed a prevalence of isolated IAA of only 0.7% of all aorto-iliac aneurysms [2]. The comparison is however difficult since this study describes treatment incidence, whereas the Swedish data described aneurysm prevalence in autopsies with a definition of ≥ 1.5 cm diameter.

While the treatment incidence rates for AAA were stable in the last decade in Switzerland, there was a significant increase in elective treatment incidence in men for ADIA. On the other hand, the incidence rates for acute ADIA remained stable in both sexes. A possible and very likely explanation for the significant increase in the frequency of treatment in men is the increasing use of less invasive endovascular therapies, which led to the rise in the number of patients eligible for elective IAA repairs [22,23]. This is emphasized by the fact that the endovascularly treated cases were six years older than open repair cases. However, this argument would also apply to women, but the absolute number of cases may need to be bigger to capture any trends in females.

Another remarkable finding is that the proportion of females was substantially higher in emergency cases (15%) compared to elective cases (8%). A possible explanation could be a higher proportion of dissections in the emergency cohort, in which the proportion of women could also be higher. It is well-established for aortic diseases that, the proportion of females is higher in dissections compared to aneurysms [16,24].

The epidemiological data also show a decrease in the proportion of conservatively managed patients (Supplementary Figure S1). Reasons for this finding might be an increase in surgical treatment for dissections of the iliac arteries. Advances in diagnostics allow for better visualization of dynamic obstructions due to intimal flaps that might cause intermittent claudication [10]. On the other hand, there is emerging evidence that the risk for rupture of IAA might be lower than previously assumed [6,7]. Therefore, the recently published ESVS guidelines on this subject increased the diameter indication threshold from 3.5 cm to 4.0 cm [1]. It will be interesting to see whether these changes also have an impact on the number of ruptures or only reduce the number of elective procedures performed. Again, comprehensive clinical data from registries rather than administrative data are needed to answer this question.

4.2. Treatment Outcomes

The multivariable-adjusted analysis showed an approximate three times lower hospital mortality after endovascular repair than open surgical repair (OR 0.35, 95% CI: 0.16 to 0.73, $p = 0.006$). On the other hand, emergency procedures were associated with a seven times higher hospital mortality rate (OR 7.03, 95%-CI: 3.38 to 15.14, $p < 0.001$). This is not surprising, as higher hospital mortality rates for ruptured IAA must be expected. In line with previously published analyses on DRG data for different aortic pathologies in Switzerland, higher age, and an increase in the van Walraven score were significantly associated with hospital mortality [16,20]. In contrast to these earlier analyses, however, there were no differences between men and women in treating ADIA in Switzerland.

Interestingly, we observed an unexpectedly high rate of mesenteric complications following elective open surgery for ADIA. Acute mesenteric ischemia was diagnosed in 2.7% of cases undergoing open repair, compared to only 0.6% following endovascular therapy ($p = 0.024$). Large bowel resection was performed in 2.4% of cases after open repair, as opposed to only 0.2% after endovascular repair ($p = 0.005$). Additionally, small intestine resection occurred in 1% of cases after open repair, while it was only 0.4% after endovascular repair ($p = 0.369$). These complications are all serious; unfortunately, the dataset does not allow us to definitively establish their etiology. Mesenteric ischemia following treatment of the iliac arteries is presumably most often related to an insufficient collateral network in situations where the IIA is occluded intentionally or as a bailout in complicated situations [11]. The importance of IIA patency is underlined by the clear recommendation (Class I, Level C) that blood flow to at least one IIA should be preserved during either open or endovascular repair of IAA [1]. Besides the potential risk for colonic ischemia, other complications associated with IIA occlusion are buttock claudication, erectile dysfunction, and spinal cord ischemia [25]. Knowledge on an impaired collateral network due to occlusion of the contralateral IAA or the inferior mesenteric artery is essential when planning ADIA treatment but also when comparing treatment outcomes. This information is not available in our data and thus hinders us from drawing any conclusions on the risk of a specific treatment with these dramatic complications. Of note, acute mesenteric ischemia was coded in one of the 178 cases (0.6%) treated with coiling and in another two of the 314 cases (0.6%) that had endovascular therapy coded without coiling. Alternative explanations for mesenteric ischemia may also be intestinal hypoperfusion due to reduced perioperative arterial blood flow, especially in cases of hemorrhagic shock, so-called non-occlusive mesenteric ischemia (NOMI) [26]. Furthermore, concomitant acute mesenteric ischemia can also occur unrelated to the procedure itself during the hospital stay in patients with arteriosclerotic disease [27].

Within its limitations, this study provides a comprehensive picture of the epidemiology and periprocedural outcomes of patients treated for iliac artery pathology. As with many less invasive endovascular treatment alternatives, this study shows lower hospital mortality. However, this study lacks important information on the follow-up of these patients. Endovascular treatment of isolated IAA has been associated with higher rates of re-intervention than open surgical repair in cohort studies [28]. Further studies should focus on long-term outcomes and evaluate the burden of possible re-interventions and late complications to obtain a complete picture of the treatment for iliac artery pathologies. An individualized treatment decision must consider patient characteristics including anatomical parameters and patient preferences. In this shared decision, all perioperative benefits must be weighed against a higher rate of potential re-interventions.

4.3. Limitations

There are several limitations to this analysis. First, the reported cohort is heterogeneous and includes both aneurysms and dissections. The ICD coding does not allow for the differentiation between aneurysms and dissections. Further, there is no specific ICD code for ruptured IAA. Identification of the cases with acute pathologies was indirectly achieved via a variable for admission. Thus, treatment-specific outcomes are reported rather than disease-specific outcomes.

Secondly, these administrative data do not include the cardiovascular risk profile, the functional capacity of the treated individuals, the hemodynamic situation in dissections or ruptures, or anatomical characteristics of the pathology. Hence, adjustments were only possible for age, sex, the van Walraven comorbidity score, and the insurance state. Such unmeasured factors could explain the observed differences in survival rates to some extent and could theoretically explain the differences.

Thirdly, the data allow non-independent observations of patients treated twice for the same ICD code. It must be assumed that some individuals were treated for both sides at different hospital admissions. The data structure does not allow for the identification of these cases; thus, it is likely that some non-independent observations are present in this cohort.

Fourthly, we present epidemiological data on hospital admissions and treatments in Switzerland. Incidence rates depend not only on the disease itself, but also on less generalizable factors such as the organization and reimbursement of costs in the Swiss healthcare system.

Lastly, coding errors cannot be excluded, and the anonymized data structure does not allow for data validation. Nevertheless, the data provide almost complete coverage of the Swiss population since reimbursement depends on reporting the cases to the Swiss authorities. Selection bias and the risk of information bias in hard outcomes such as hospital mortality is therefore low [29].

5. Conclusions

This nationwide study of iliac artery pathologies shows that the treatment incidence was about 10 times higher in men than in women for elective procedures, but only about five times higher for emergency treatment. Hospital mortality rates were dramatically higher in emergency procedures compared to elective procedures. Endovascular procedures were associated with significantly lower hospital mortality than open procedures, while hospital mortality rates were comparable for men and women.

Supplementary Materials: The following supporting information can be downloaded at: https://www.mdpi.com/article/10.3390/jcm13082267/s1, Supplementary Figure S1: Management of ADIA; Supplementary Table S1: Patient Identification; Supplementary Table S2: CHOP codes, Supplementary Table S3: ICD-codes for ComplicaTons; Supplementary Table S4: Characteristics and outcomes of conservative management for ADIA.

Author Contributions: Conceptualization, R.B., A.-L.M., A.Z. and L.M.; methodology, L.M. and A.Z.; formal analysis, L.M.; resources, A.Z.; data curation, L.M.; writing—original draft preparation, R.B.; writing—review and editing, A.-L.M., A.Z. and L.M.; visualization, L.M.; supervision, A.Z. and L.M.; project administration, A.Z.; funding acquisition, L.M. and A.Z. All authors have read and agreed to the published version of the manuscript.

Funding: This research has partly been funded by the Swiss National Science Foundation (SNSF), grant P500PM_217674 / 1.

Institutional Review Board Statement: Ethical review and approval were waived for this study due to the nature of the analyzed data (fully anonymized administrative data, BASEC-Nr. Req-2021-01010).

Informed Consent Statement: Patient consent was waived due to fully anonymised data (BASEC-Nr. Req-2021-01010).

Data Availability Statement: Data can be requested at the Swiss Federal Statistical Office: https://www.bfs.admin.ch/bfs/en/home/services/contact.html (accessed on 11 April 2024).

Acknowledgments: We thank Klaus Steigmiller for his contribution to the statistical analysis of the dataset.

Conflicts of Interest: The authors declare no conflicts of interest. The funders had no role in the design of the study; in the collection, analyses, or interpretation of data; in the writing of the manuscript; or in the decision to publish the results.

References

1. Wanhainen, A.; Van Herzeele, I.; Bastos Goncalves, F.; Bellmunt Montoya, S.; Berard, X.; Boyle, J.R.; D'Oria, M.; Prendes, C.F.; Karkos, C.D.; Kazimierczak, A.; et al. Editor's Choice--European Society for Vascular Surgery (ESVS) 2024 Clinical Practice Guidelines on the Management of Abdominal Aorto-Iliac Artery Aneurysms. *Eur. J. Vasc. Endovasc. Surg.* **2024**, *67*, 192–331. [CrossRef]
2. Brunkwall, J.; Hauksson, H.; Bengtsson, H.; Bergqvist, D.; Takolander, R.; Bergentz, S.-E. Solitary Aneurysms of the Iliac Arterial System: An Estimate of Their Frequency of Occurrence. *J. Vasc. Surg.* **1989**, *10*, a13733. [CrossRef]
3. Reber, P.U.; Brunner, K.; Hakki, H.; Stirnemann, P.; Kniemeyer, H.W. Häufigkeit, Klassifikation Und Therapie Der Isolierten Beckenarterienaneurysmen. *Der Chir.* **2001**, *72*, 419–424. [CrossRef]
4. Perini, P.; Mariani, E.; Fanelli, M.; Ucci, A.; Rossi, G.; Massoni, C.B.; Freyrie, A. Surgical and Endovascular Management of Isolated Internal Iliac Artery Aneurysms: A Systematic Review and Meta-Analysis. *Vasc. Endovasc. Surg.* **2021**, *55*, 254–264. [CrossRef]
5. Sandhu, R.S.; Pipinos, I.I. Isolated Iliac Artery Aneurysms. *Semin. Vasc. Surg.* **2005**, *18*, 209–215. [CrossRef] [PubMed]
6. Steenberge, S.P.; Caputo, F.J.; Rowse, J.W.; Lyden, S.P.; Quatromoni, J.G.; Kirksey, L.; Smolock, C.J. Natural History and Growth Rates of Isolated Common Iliac Artery Aneurysms. *J. Vasc. Surg.* **2022**, *76*, 461–465. [CrossRef] [PubMed]
7. Charisis, N.; Bouris, V.; Rakic, A.; Landau, D.; Labropoulos, N. A Systematic Review on Endovascular Repair of Isolated Common Iliac Artery Aneurysms and Suggestions Regarding Diameter Thresholds for Intervention. *J. Vasc. Surg.* **2021**, *74*, 1752–1762.e1. [CrossRef] [PubMed]

8. Honjo, O.; Yamada, Y.; Kuroko, Y.; Kushida, Y.; Une, D.; Hioki, K. Spontaneous Dissection and Rupture of Common Iliac Artery in a Patient with Fibromuscular Dysplasia: A Case Report and Review of the Literature on Iliac Artery Dissections Secondary to Fibromuscular Dysplasia. *J. Vasc. Surg.* **2004**, *40*, 1032–1036. [CrossRef]
9. Hayman, E.; Abayazeed, A.; Moghadamfalahi, M.; Cain, D. Vascular Type Ehlers-Danlos Syndrome with Fatal Spontaneous Rupture of a Right Common Iliac Artery Dissection: Case Report and Review of Literature. *J. Radiol. Case Rep.* **2014**, *8*, 63. [CrossRef]
10. Sakaue, Y.; Nomura, T.; Ono, K.; Wada, N.; Keira, N.; Tatsumi, T. Enlarged False Lumen Following Spontaneous External Iliac Artery Dissection-Induced Chronic Limb Threatening Ischemia. *Cardiovasc. Interv. Ther.* **2022**, *37*, 583–584. [CrossRef]
11. Chaer, R.A.; Barbato, J.E.; Lin, S.C.; Zenati, M.; Kent, K.C.; McKinsey, J.F. Isolated Iliac Artery Aneurysms: A Contemporary Comparison of Endovascular and Open Repair. *J. Vasc. Surg.* **2008**, *47*, 708–713.e1. [CrossRef] [PubMed]
12. Statistik Der Stationären Betriebe Des. Gesundheitswesens. Krankenhaustypologie. [Internet]. 2013. Volume 9 p. 2006. Available online: https://www.bfs.admin.ch/bfs/de/home/statistiken/gesundheit/erhebungen/ks.assetdetail.23546402.html (accessed on 11 April 2024).
13. von Elm, E.; Altman, D.G.; Egger, M.; Pocock, S.J.; Gøtzsche, P.C.; Vandenbroucke, J.P. The Strengthening the Reporting of Observational Studies in Epidemiology (STROBE) Statement: Guidelines for Reporting Observational Studies. *Int. J. Surg.* **2014**, *12*, 1495–1499. [CrossRef] [PubMed]
14. van Walraven, C.; Austin, P.C.; Jennings, A.; Quan, H.; Forster, A.J. A Modification of the Elixhauser Comorbidity Measures Into a Point System for Hospital Death Using Administrative Data. *Med. Care* **2009**, *47*, 626–633. [CrossRef] [PubMed]
15. Gasparini, A. Comorbidity: An R Package for Computing Comorbidity Scores. *J. Open Source Softw.* **2018**, *3*, 648. [CrossRef]
16. Meuli, L.; Menges, A.-L.; Steigmiller, K.; Kuehnl, A.; Reutersberg, B.; Held, U.; Zimmermann, A. Hospital Incidence and Mortality of Patients Treated for Abdominal Aortic Aneurysms in Switzerland—A Secondary Analysis of Swiss DRG Statistics Data. *Swiss Med. Wkly.* **2022**, *152*, w30191. [CrossRef] [PubMed]
17. Demografische Bilanz nach Alter. Bundesamt für Statistik [Internet]. Available online: https://www.pxweb.bfs.admin.ch/pxweb/de/px-x-0102020000_103/-/px-x-0102020000_103.px/ (accessed on 11 April 2024).
18. Altman, D.; Machin, D.; Bryant, T.; Gardner, M. *Statistics with Confidence: Confidence Intervals and Statistical Guidelines*, 2nd ed.; Wiley: Hoboken, NJ, USA, 2000.
19. R Core Team. R: A Language and Environment for Statistical Computing. 2013. Available online: http://www.R-Project.Org/ (accessed on 11 April 2024).
20. Meuli, L.; Menges, A.L.; Stoklasa, K.; Steigmiller, K.; Reutersberg, B.; Zimmermann, A. Inter-Hospital Transfer of Patients With Ruptured Abdominal Aortic Aneurysm in Switzerland. *Eur. J. Vasc. Endovasc. Surg.* **2023**, *65*, 484–492. [CrossRef]
21. Nachbur, B.H.; Inderbitzi, R.G.C.; Bär, W. Isolated Iliac Aneurysms. *Eur. J. Vasc. Surg.* **1991**, *5*, 375–381. [CrossRef] [PubMed]
22. Gouveia e Melo, R.; Fenelli, C.; Fernández Prendes, C.; Öz, T.; Stavroulakis, K.; Rantner, B.; Stana, J.; Tsilimparis, N. A Cross-Sectional Study on the Anatomic Feasibility of Iliac Side Branch Grafts in a Real-World Setting. *J. Vasc. Surg.* **2022**, *76*, 724–732. [CrossRef] [PubMed]
23. Oussoren, F.K.; Maldonado, T.S.; Reijnen, M.M.P.J.; Heyligers, J.M.M.; Akkersdijk, G.; Attisani, L.; Bellosta, R.; Heyligers, J.M.M.; Hoencamp, R.; Garrard, L.; et al. Solitary Iliac Branch Endoprosthesis Placement for Iliac Artery Aneurysms. *J. Vasc. Surg.* **2022**, *75*, 1268–1275.e1. [CrossRef]
24. Evangelista, A.; Isselbacher, E.M.; Bossone, E.; Gleason, T.G.; Di Eusanio, M.; Sechtem, U.; Ehrlich, M.P.; Trimarchi, S.; Braverman, A.C.; Myrmel, T.; et al. Insights From the International Registry of Acute Aortic Dissection. *Circulation* **2018**, *137*, 1846–1860. [CrossRef]
25. Kritpracha, B.; Pigott, J.P.; Price, C.I.; Russell, T.E.; Corbey, M.J.; Beebe, H.G. Distal Internal Iliac Artery Embolization: A Procedure to Avoid. *J. Vasc. Surg.* **2003**, *37*, 943–948. [CrossRef] [PubMed]
26. Yu, B.; Ko, R.-E.; Yoo, K.; Gil, E.; Choi, K.-J.; Park, C.-M. Non-Occlusive Mesenteric Ischemia in Critically Ill Patients. *PLoS ONE* **2022**, *17*, e0279196. [CrossRef] [PubMed]
27. Molyneux, K.; Beck-Esmay, J.; Koyfman, A.; Long, B. High Risk and Low Prevalence Diseases: Mesenteric Ischemia. *Am. J. Emerg. Med.* **2023**, *65*, 154–161. [CrossRef] [PubMed]
28. Zhorzel, S.; Busch, A.; Trenner, M.; Reutersberg, B.; Salvermoser, M.; Eckstein, H.-H.; Zimmermann, A. Open Versus Endovascular Repair of Isolated Iliac Artery Aneurysms. *Vasc. Endovasc. Surg.* **2019**, *53*, 12–20. [CrossRef]
29. Trenner, M.; Eckstein, H.-H.; Kallmayer, M.A.; Reutersberg, B.; Kühnl, A. Secondary Analysis of Statutorily Collected Routine Data. *Gefässchirurgie* **2019**, *24*, 220–227. [CrossRef]

Disclaimer/Publisher's Note: The statements, opinions and data contained in all publications are solely those of the individual author(s) and contributor(s) and not of MDPI and/or the editor(s). MDPI and/or the editor(s) disclaim responsibility for any injury to people or property resulting from any ideas, methods, instructions or products referred to in the content.

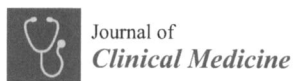 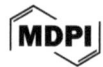

Article

Long-Term Health-Related Quality of Life following Acute Type A Aortic Dissection with a Focus on Male–Female Differences: A Cross Sectional Study

Frederike Meccanici [1], Carlijn G. E. Thijssen [1,2], Arjen L. Gökalp [3], Annemijn W. Bom [1], Guillaume S. C. Geuzebroek [4], Joost F. ter Woorst [5], Roland R. J. van Kimmenade [1,2], Marco C. Post [6,7], Johanna J. M. Takkenberg [3] and Jolien W. Roos-Hesselink [1,*]

1 Department of Cardiology, Erasmus MC, 3015 GD Rotterdam, The Netherlands
2 Department of Cardiology, Radboud University Medical Center, 6525 GA Nijmegen, The Netherlands
3 Department of Cardiothoracic Surgery, Erasmus MC, 3015 GD Rotterdam, The Netherlands
4 Department of Cardiothoracic Surgery, Radboud University Medical Center, 6525 GA Nijmegen, The Netherlands
5 Department of Cardiothoracic Surgery, Catharina Ziekenhuis Eindhoven, 5623 EJ Eindhoven, The Netherlands
6 Department of Cardiology, St. Antonius Ziekenhuis, 3435 CM Nieuwegein, The Netherlands
7 Department of Cardiology, University Medical Center Utrecht, 3584 CX Utrecht, The Netherlands
* Correspondence: j.roos@erasmusmc.nl; Tel.: +31-10-7032432

Citation: Meccanici, F.; Thijssen, C.G.E.; Gökalp, A.L.; Bom, A.W.; Geuzebroek, G.S.C.; ter Woorst, J.F.; van Kimmenade, R.R.J.; Post, M.C.; Takkenberg, J.J.M.; Roos-Hesselink, J.W. Long-Term Health-Related Quality of Life following Acute Type A Aortic Dissection with a Focus on Male–Female Differences: A Cross Sectional Study. *J. Clin. Med.* **2024**, *13*, 2265. https://doi.org/10.3390/jcm13082265

Academic Editors: Benedikt Reutersberg and Matthias Trenner

Received: 26 February 2024
Revised: 9 April 2024
Accepted: 11 April 2024
Published: 13 April 2024

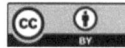

Copyright: © 2024 by the authors. Licensee MDPI, Basel, Switzerland. This article is an open access article distributed under the terms and conditions of the Creative Commons Attribution (CC BY) license (https://creativecommons.org/licenses/by/4.0/).

Abstract: Objectives: Acute type A aortic dissection (ATAAD) is a life-threatening cardiovascular emergency, of which the long-term impact on health-related quality of life (HRQoL) and male–female-specific insights remain inadequately clarified. **Methods**: Consecutive adult ATAAD patients who underwent surgery were retrospectively included between 2007 and 2017 in four referral centers in the Netherlands, and baseline data were collected. The 36-Item Short-Form (SF-36) Health Survey was sent to all survivors between 2019 and 2021 and compared to validated SF-36 scores of the Dutch general population stratified by age group and sex. **Results**: In total, 324/555 surviving patients returned the SF-36 questionnaire (response rate 58%), of which 40.0% were female; the median follow-up was 6.5 years (range: 1.7–13.9, IQR: 4.0–9.4) after surgery for ATAAD. In comparison to the general population, ATAAD patients scored significantly lower on 6/8 SF-36 subdomains and higher on bodily pain. Differences in HRQoL domains compared to the sex-matched data were largely comparable between sexes, apart from bodily pain. In the age-matched subgroups impaired HRQoL was most pronounced in younger patients aged 41–60 (5/8 impaired domains). Female ATAAD patients scored significantly worse on 5/8 SF-36 subdomains and the physical component summary (PCS) scores than male patients. Age at ATAAD, female sex, hypertension, COPD, and prior thoracic aortic aneurysm were associated with worse PCS scores. **Conclusions**: Long-term HRQoL was impaired in both male and female ATAAD patients when compared to the general population. Further studies on the nature of this impairment and on interventions to improve HRQoL after ATAAD are clearly warranted, with special attention to females and younger patients.

Keywords: acute type A aortic dissection; health-related quality of life; outcomes; cross-sectional; sex and gender

1. Introduction

Acute type A aortic dissection (ATAAD) is an urgent cardiovascular event, requiring immediate diagnosis and emergency surgery. Although early mortality has significantly decreased over time for ATAAD, the in-hospital mortality is still around 20% [1,2]. The recovery process after ATAAD is often challenging: postoperative complications such as bleeding, stroke, and renal failure [3] can prolong hospitalization and impact health-related quality of life (HRQoL). Also, patients require lifelong imaging follow-up, and reintervention on the aorta may be warranted [4]. All these factors might cause fear and influence the performance of normal daily activities significantly, which raises the question whether more personalized attention for patients' mental and physical wellbeing during clinical follow-up visits after ATAAD is required.

Recent literature has explored male–female differences in clinical presentation and management for ATAAD [5], yet a nuanced examination of how male and female patients perceive and experience HRQoL following ATAAD remains largely unexplored [6]. HRQoL has proven to be different for males and females in the general population as well as in patients with thoracic aortic disease [7,8], highlighting the need for a sex-specific evaluation of long-term HRQoL. Through examining male–female differences in various dimensions of HRQoL, including physical, emotional, and social well-being, this research can provide implications for tailored post-operative care strategies, risk stratification protocols, and patient-centered interventions to improve HRQoL.

Therefore, the primary objective was to investigate long-term HRQoL in adult ATAAD survivors in a large multicenter cross-sectional study in comparison with the Dutch general population. The secondary objectives were to examine male–female differences in HRQoL for the ATAAD population and to explore associations with patient and surgical characteristics and the physical and mental component summary scores.

2. Materials and Methods

2.1. Study Design and Study Population

Based on a multicenter retrospective cohort, a cross-sectional survey study was performed following the STROBE guidelines for cross-sectional studies [9]. All consecutive patients (≥18 years old) who presented with ATAAD between the 1 January 2007 and the 31 December 2017 in 4 tertiary referral centers in the Netherlands (the Erasmus University Medical Center in Rotterdam, the Catharina Medical Center in Eindhoven, Radboud University Medical Center in Nijmegen and St. Antonius Hospital in Nieuwegein) were eligible for inclusion. Exclusion criteria included: asymptomatic chronic type A aortic dissection, and iatrogenic or traumatic dissection. This multicenter study was designed, conducted, and controlled complying local and international good clinical practice guidelines and was approved by the local medical ethics committees with a waiver for informed consent for the retrospective data collection of all presenting ATAAD patients (MEC-2018-1535). Written informed consent was obtained from all surviving ATAAD patients for the collection of the HRQoL questionnaires.

2.2. Data Collection

Eligible patients were identified with the institutional aortic surgery databases and the hospitals' diagnosis registration systems. Additionally, the files of all patients with diagnostic treatment codes (DBCs) pertaining to any thoracic aortic disease were checked manually to ensure the comprehensiveness of the patient selection.

All study data were documented in an anonymized standardized case report form using OpenClinica (OpenClinica, LLC, version 3.6, Needham, MA, USA). The patient files were used to collect data on demographic, clinical presentation, and treatment characteristics. All patient characteristics at baseline with their definitions are shown in Appendix SI. Prior to sending the questionnaire, a mortality check was performed in the municipal data registry. In the period from July 2019 to February 2021, the 36-Item Short-Form Health Survey (SF-36) [10–12] including an informed consent form on paper was sent to all ATAAD survivors. To improve the response rate, all patients who had not returned the questionnaire were contacted by telephone. After exhausting all the aforementioned attempts to elicit a response, the patient was classified as a 'non-responder'.

2.3. HRQoL Questionnaire

The SF-36 questionnaire, comprising 36 items, is a widely employed tool for assessing HRQoL. It encompasses eight domains, namely: Physical Functioning (PF), Role limitations due to the Physical health problems (RP), Bodily Pain (BP), General Health perceptions (GH), Vitality (VT), Social Functioning (SF), Role limitations due to Emotional problems (RE), and general Mental Health (MH) (psychological distress) [7,12]. From these eight subdomains, two higher-ordered clusters are calculated: the Physical Component Summary (PCS) and the Mental Component Summary (MCS). The PCS and MCS are calculated by calculating the z-scores of each domain, followed by aggregation of scale scores and transformation of summary scores (T-scores). The first four domains (PF, RP, BP, GH) correlate most highly with the PCS, while the last four domains (VT, SF, RE, MH) are strongly correlated with the MCS [13]. The score range for all subdomains of SF-36 is 0–100, and for the PCS and MCS the mean score is 50 with a standard deviation of 10, with higher scores indicating better HRQoL.

Previous studies have utilized the SF-36 questionnaire as tool to examine HRQoL in patients with type A aortic dissection [6]. The SF-36 has been translated, validated, and normed in the Dutch population, as well as for the total population, and stratified by sex and age groups, which can be considered as normative data [7]. In order to compare the study data with the Dutch general population, the age categories used by Aaronson et al. [7] were applied to this study: age 16–40 years, 41–60 years, 61–70 years, and more than 70 years old.

2.4. Statistical Analysis

Data were analyzed using the statistical and computing program R (R Foundation for Statistical Computing, Vienna, Austria. Version 4.2.1). Continuous data were presented as mean and standard deviation (SD) when normally distributed and as median with interquartile range (IQR) when skewed. Normality was checked visually with histograms and tested with use of the Shapiro–Wilk test. Males and females were compared with an unpaired Student's *t*-test when normally distributed, and a Mann–Whitney U test was used when data were not normally distributed. Categorical data were presented as counts and frequencies, and males and females were compared with χ^2 test or Fisher's exact test, as appropriate.

Furthermore, two subgroup comparisons were made with the Dutch normative data: (1) sex-matched, and (2) age-matched (per age category as reported by Aaronson et al. [7]). In the comparison with the normative data, means and standard deviations were reported and a one-sample Student's *t*-test was used.

Associations with the PCS and the MCS were explored using univariable linear regression analyses with follow-up time, age at ATAAD, sex, comorbidities, and concomitant aortic valve and aortic arch surgery at ATAAD repair based on previous research and clinical relevance [6] in a complete case analysis. Multivariable analyses were performed adjusting for age and sex, and interactions with sex and the independent variables were checked. In an additional analysis, the association between postoperative cerebrovascular accidents and the PCS and MCS were explored in a univariable linear regression analysis.

To investigate non-responder and survival bias, the patient characteristics of responders were compared with non-responders of the total cohort using the aforementioned descriptive statistics for continuous and categorical data.

If the participant failed to fill in any data for one or more questions in a subdomain, the entire subdomain was regarded as missing. As a result, patients who had any incomplete subdomains would also have a missing end score of the PCS and MCS. If the participant did not provide the completion date for the questionnaire, the study center's median date was used as an estimate.

A two-sided *p*-value of <0.05 was considered statistically significant.

3. Results

In Figure 1, the flowchart of the patient selection is shown. The questionnaires were sent to 555 ATAAD survivors, of which 324 patients (40.0% females) completed the questionnaire and provided written informed consent, resulting in a response rate of 58.4%. In Table 1, the patient and surgical characteristics of all patients who completed the questionnaire (n = 324) are depicted stratified by sex. All ATAAD patients included in the present study had received surgical treatment at presentation. During admission or within 30 days after ATAAD surgery, cerebrovascular accidents were observed in 25 patients (7.9%, n = 8 females, n = 17 males) and transient ischemic attack in 2 patients (0.6%, n = 2 females). No significant male–female differences were observed in postoperative CVA/TIA incidence.

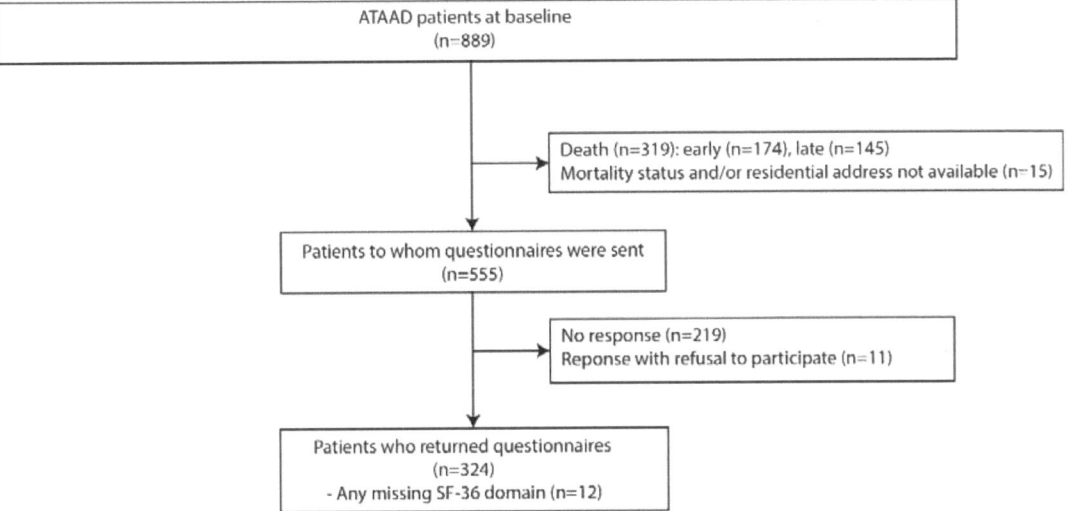

Figure 1. Flowchart of acute type A aortic dissection (ATAAD) patients.

In Figure 2, mean SF-36 subdomain scores are compared with the general Dutch population for the total study population (panel A), matched by sex (panel B) and matched by age (panel C). The crude data for these analyses are shown in Appendices SII and SIII. On 6/8 SF-36 subdomains, ATAAD patients scored significantly lower than the general population, whereas ATAAD patients scored higher for bodily pain (Figure 2, panel A). In the comparison with the sex-matched general population, both males and females scored significantly worse on physical functioning, role physical, general health, vitality, and social functioning, and the absolute differences with the general population seem greater for females on the physical functioning and role physical domain (Figure 2, panel B). Females scored significantly higher for bodily pain and males scored significantly lower for role emotional, when compared to the sex-matched data. In the age-matched subgroups, impaired HRQoL was especially observed in the youngest age category (41–60 years), with 5/8 domains significantly lower than the age-matched general population, compared to 2/8 impaired domains in the age group of 61–70 years and none in the age group of >70 years (Figure 2, panel C).

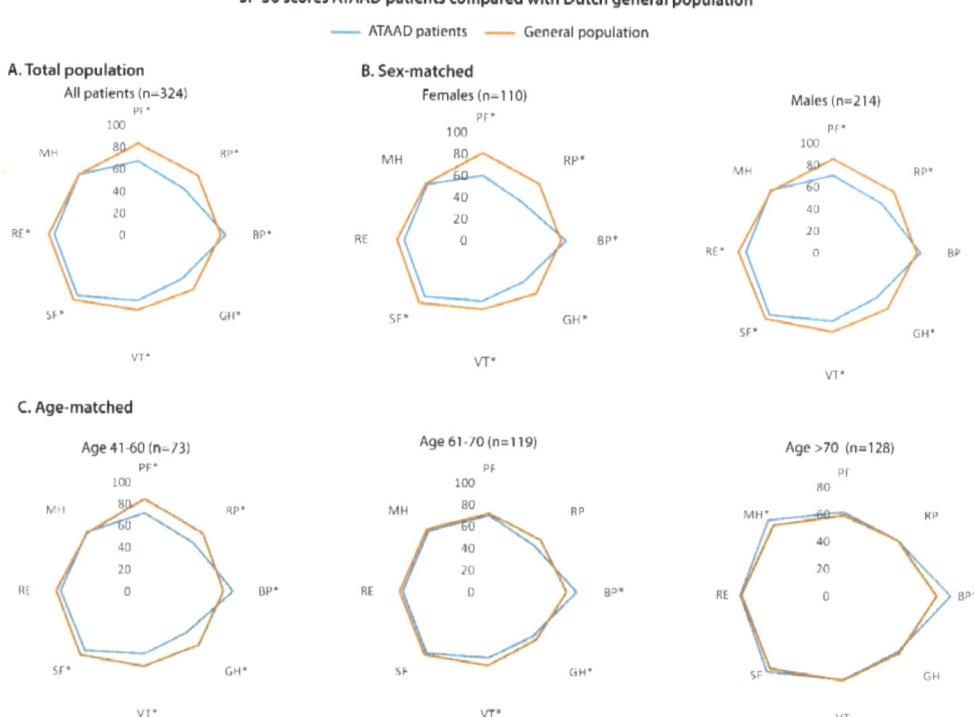

Figure 2. SF-36 scores of ATAAD patients compared with the Dutch general population. SF-36 subdomain scores are presented as the mean in order to compare the data with the general population data, which were reported as the mean. Three patients were in the age range of 16–40 years; therefore, these patients were not included in the age-matched analysis. * = p-value < 0.05 in one-sample Student's t-test compared with the general population. ATAAD = Acute type A aortic dissection, SF-36 = 36-Item Short-Form Health Survey, PF = physical functioning, RP = role physical, BP = bodily pain, GH = general health, VT = vitality, SF = social functioning, RE = role emotional, MH = mental health.

Table 1. Patient and surgical characteristics of ATAAD patients who completed the SF-36 questionnaire.

	All Patients (n = 324)	Females (n = 110)	Males (n = 214)	p-Value	Missing %
Age at questionnaire (median [IQR])—years	68.0 [61.0–74.0]	70.5 [64.3–77.0]	67.0 [60.0–73.0]	**0.001**	0.3
Follow-up time—years (median [IQR], (range)	6.5 [4.0–9.4], (1.7–14.2)	6.2 [3.9–9.3], (1.7–13.9)	6.6 [4.2–9.4], (1.7–14.2)	0.386	0.0
Patient demographics at ATAAD presentation					
Age at ATAAD (mean ± SD)—years	61.0 ± 10.1	63.7 ± 10.3	59.7 ± 9.7	**0.001**	0.3
BSA (mean ± SD)—m²	2.0 ± 0.2	1.8 ± 0.16	2.1 ± 0.2	**<0.001**	23.5
History of hypertension (%)	150 (48.9)	59 (55.7)	91 (45.3)	0.107	6.2
History of hyperlipidemia (%)	37 (11.7)	13 (12.1)	24 (11.5)	1.000	2.8
Diabetes mellitus (%)	3 (0.9)	2 (1.9)	1 (0.5)	0.268 ᶦ	2.2
COPD (%)	14 (4.4)	7 (6.4)	7 (3.3)	0.327	0.9
Current or past smoking ≥ 1 pack years	90 (62.9)	27 (56.2)	63 (66.3)	0.320	55.9
History of CVA or TIA (%)	14 (4.4)	6 (5.5)	8 (3.8)	0.686	0.9
History of MI (%)	7 (2.2)	3 (2.7)	4 (1.9)	0.695 ᶦ	1.2
Chronic kidney disease (%)	3 (0.9)	1 (0.9)	2 (0.9)	1.000 ᶦ	0.9

Table 1. Cont.

	All Patients (n = 324)	Females (n = 110)	Males (n = 214)	p-Value	Missing %
Prior TAA (%)	21 (6.6)	11 (10.1)	10 (4.7)	0.111	1.2
Prior aortic surgery (%)	5 (1.6)	0 (0.0)	5 (2.4)	0.170 [i]	1.5
Prior cardiac surgery (%)	13 (4.1)	3 (2.7)	10 (4.8)	0.554 [i]	1.2
Bicuspid aortic valve (%)	6 (2.1)	2 (2.0)	4 (2.2)	1.000 [i]	11.4
Known connective tissue disease (%) *	13 (10.7)	3 (7.9)	10 (12.0)		
No; no genetic testing performed	67 (55.4)	20 (52.6)	47 (56.6)	0.602 [i]	62.7
No; genetic testing performed but not found	41 (33.9)	15 (39.5)	26 (31.3)		
**Surgical procedures **					
Aortic valve surgery	210 (66.5)	75 (70.8)	135 (64.3)	0.306	2.5
Ascending aortic surgery	315 (97.2)	107 (97.3)	208 (97.2)	1.000	0.0
Aortic arch surgery	225 (70.8)	72 (67.9)	153 (72.2)	0.513	1.9
Descending aortic surgery	2 (0.6)	0 (0.0)	2 (0.9)	0.551 [i]	0.6
DHCA (%)	124 (39.7)	45 (42.1)	79 (38.5)	0.630	3.7

Normally distributed continuous variables are expressed as mean ± SD, skewed continuous variables are expressed as median and 25th–75th percentile, and categorical values are expressed as percentages. For follow-up time, the 25th–75th percentile as well as the range are reported. p-values < 0.05 are depicted in bold. * Known connective tissue disease at ATAAD presentation: Marfan syndrome (n = 2), Loeys–Dietz syndrome (n = 1), ACTA2 mutation (n = 3), other (n = 5). ** All patients received surgical treatment at ATAAD presentation. [i] = Fisher's exact test. IQR = interquartile range; BSA = body surface area; COPD = chronic obstructive pulmonary disease; CVA = cerebrovascular accident; DHCA = deep hypothermic circulatory arrest; MI = myocardial infarction; TAA = thoracic aortic aneurysm; TIA = transient ischemic attack.

Table 2 shows the SF-36 sub-domain scores and the PCS and MCS for the total study population and stratified by sex. Female patients scored significantly lower on 5/8 subdomains and on the PCS when compared to male patients.

Table 2. Health-related quality of life scores of the ATAAD study population for the 36-Item Short-Form Health Survey.

	All Patients (n = 324)	Females (n = 110)	Males (n = 214)	p-Value	Missing (%)
Physical Functioning	70.0 (53.8–85.0)	65.0 (42.5–80.0)	75.0 (60.0–90.0)	**<0.001**	1.2
Role Physical	75.0 (25.0–100.0)	50.0 (0.00–100.0)	75.0 (25.0–100.0)	**0.015**	2.2
Bodily Pain	90.0 (67.5–100.0)	82.5 (57.5–100.0)	90.0 (67.5–100.0)	0.142	0.3
General Health	60.0 (40.0–75.0)	52.5 (36.3–70.0)	60.0 (40.0–75.0)	0.103	0.0
Vitality	65.0 (45.0–80.0)	60.0 (40.0–75.0)	65.0 (45.0–80.0)	**0.035**	0.3
Social Functioning	87.5 (62.5–100.0)	75.0 (62.5–100.0)	87.5 (75.0–100.0)	**0.037**	0.9
Role Emotional	100.0 (66.7–100.0)	100.0 (33.3–100.0)	100.0 (66.7–100.0)	0.150	2.8
Mental Health	84.0 (68.0–92.0)	76.0 (64.0–88.0)	84.0 (72.0–92.0)	**0.006**	0.6
PCS	45.7 (36.7–53.5)	43.3 (35.0–50.3)	46.5 (39.1–53.8)	**0.008**	4.0
MCS	53.2 (44.2–58.2)	51.4 (41.6–58.0)	53.6 (45.1–58.3)	0.184	4.0

SF-36 subdomain scores and the Physical Component Summary and the Mental Component Summary are presented as median and 25th–75th percentile. p-values < 0.05 are depicted in bold. PCS = Physical Component Summary; MCS = Mental Component Summary.

Figure 3 shows the univariable analyses of patient and surgical characteristics with the PCS and the MCS for the total study population. As depicted in Appendix SIV, after correction for age and sex, the following variables remained significantly associated with lower PCS scores: history of hypertension ($p = 0.003$), COPD ($p = 0.012$), and prior thoracic aortic aneurysm ($p = 0.043$). For the MCS, no significant associations were found in univariable (Figure 3) and multivariable analysis (Appendix SIV). No significant interactions with sex and the independent variables were observed for both the PCS and MCS. Postoperative cerebrovascular accidents were not significantly associated with the PCS (beta estimate: −3.420 (95% CI −7.674–0.835), $p = 0.115$), nor with the MCS (beta estimate: 0.073 (95% CI −4.282–4.428), $p = 0.974$.

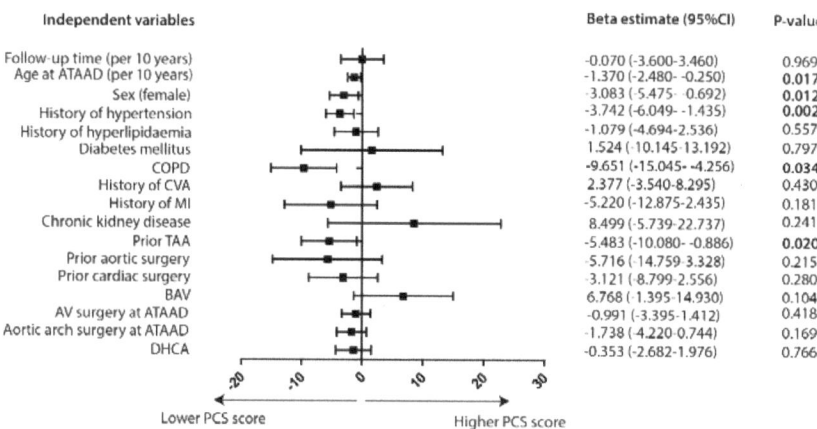
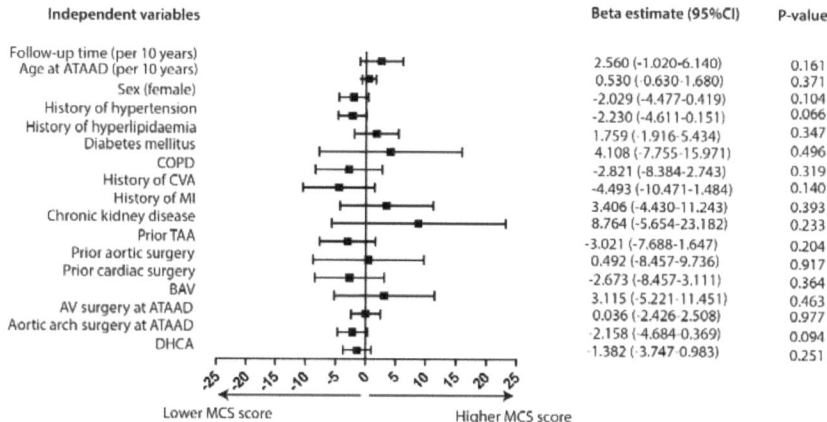

Figure 3. Associations with Physical Component Summary and Mental Component Summary scores. Beta coefficients and corresponding 95% CI are shown. Interpretation for beta coefficients: if the beta coefficient is positive, for every unit increase in the predictor variable, the outcome variable (PCS or MCS score) will increase by the beta coefficient value. p-values < 0.05 are depicted in bold. ATAAD = acute type A aortic dissection; PCS = physical component summary; MCS = mental component summary; COPD = chronic obstructive pulmonary disease; CVA = cerebrovascular accident; MI = myocardial infarction; TAA = thoracic aortic aneurysm; BAV = bicuspid aortic valve; AV = aortic valve; DHCA = deep hypothermic cardiac arrest.

In Table 3, responders (n = 324) are compared with non-responders (n = 231), showing a higher proportion of smoking in the non-responders (82.4 vs. 62.9, p = 0.001) and a lower proportion of concomitant aortic valve surgery (52.5 vs. 66.5, p = 0.002) when compared with responders.

Table 3. Sensitivity analysis: comparing ATAAD patient characteristics between responders and non-responders for the SF-36 questionnaire.

	Responders (n = 324)	Non-Responders (n = 231)	p-Value	Missing %
Patient demographics				
Female sex (%)	110 (34.0)	79 (34.2)	1.000	0.0
Age (median [IQR])—years	61.0 [54.0–68.0]	60.0 [51.0–67.8]	0.126	0.2
BSA (mean ± SD)—m^2	2.00 ± 0.21	1.98 ± 0.20	0.347	30.7
History of hypertension (%)	150 (48.9)	104 (47.1)	0.749	6.0
Hyperlipidemia (%)	37 (11.7)	20 (8.8)	0.330	4.3
Diabetes mellitus (%)	3 (0.9)	6 (2.6)	0.175 [i]	3.3
COPD (%)	14 (4.4)	11 (4.8)	0.979	3.0
Current or past smoking ≥ 1 pack years	90 (62.9)	89 (82.4)	**0.001**	58.2
History of CVA or TIA (%)	14 (4.4)	9 (4.0)	0.991	3.4
History of MI (%)	7 (2.2)	9 (4.0)	0.338	3.3
Chronic kidney disease (%)	3 (0.9)	4 (1.7)	0.458 [i]	3.3
Prior TAA (%)	21 (6.6)	15 (6.7)	1.000	4.0
Prior aortic surgery (%)	5 (1.6)	7 (3.1)	0.375	3.3
Prior cardiac surgery (%)	13 (4.1)	8 (3.5)	0.899	2.7
Bicuspid aortic valve (%)	6 (2.1)	6 (3.0)	0.754	13.5
Known connective tissue disease (%) *	67 (55.4)	40 (51.3)		
No; no genetic testing performed	41 (33.9)	29 (37.2)	0.852	65.8
No; genetic testing performed but not found	13 (10.7)	9 (11.5)		
Surgical procedures				
Aortic valve surgery	210 (66.5)	116 (52.5)	**0.002**	5.3
Ascending aortic surgery	315 (97.2)	226 (99.6)	0.053 [i]	2.6
Aortic arch surgery	225 (70.8)	148 (67.0)	0.400	4.7
Descending aortic surgery	2 (0.6)	2 (0.9)	1.000 [i]	2.5
DHCA	124 (39.7)	79 (37.1)	0.602	8.1

Normally distributed continuous variables are expressed as mean ± SD, skewed continuous variables are expressed as median and 25th–75th percentile, and categorical values are expressed as percentages. p-values < 0.05 are depicted in bold. * Connective tissue disease diagnosed before or after acute type B aortic dissection. [i] = Fisher's exact test. IQR = interquartile range; BMI = body mass index; BSA = body surface area; MI = myocardial infarction; TAA = thoracic aortic aneurysm; AAA = abdominal aortic aneurysm; DHCA = deep hypothermic circulatory arrest.

4. Discussion

In an era of advanced medical care and surgical techniques, patient-centered outcomes become more important. This is certainly true for patients with acute type A aortic dissection (ATAAD), for whom, historically, the most important outcome was survival. Through increased awareness of health-related quality of life (HRQoL) and potential sex differences, the current study will enhance a more personalized approach post-ATAAD. Female patients were older at surgery for ATAAD and at completion of the questionnaire and scored worse on 5/8 SF-36 subdomains when compared to male patients. Also, HRQoL was impaired in ATAAD patients when compared to the general population, especially in the younger age groups. In an explorative analysis, age at ATAAD, female sex, hypertension, COPD, and prior thoracic aortic aneurysm were associated with impaired physical component summary scores (PCS), whereas no significant associations with the mental component summary scores (MCS) were observed.

Overall, HRQoL in the study population was impaired when compared to the general population. Other literature comparing the HRQoL of ATAAD patients with age-adjusted normative data is conflicting: some studies show decreased HRQoL [14–17], while others show estimates comparable with the general population [18–20]. Patient age and follow-up duration, together with the sample size and statistical power in these studies, seem important factors to take into account. When measured longitudinally, Endlich and colleagues observed that HRQoL decreased during follow-up after ATAAD, especially concerning the mental component summary score in younger patients [15]. In a study investigating long-term HRQoL after cardiac surgery in general, a decay in HRQoL over time was more pronounced in older patients for 3/8 subdomains [21]. In the current study, measuring HRQoL at one moment during follow-up, the follow-up duration was not associated with either the physical or mental component summary score in linear regression.

Published evidence on HRQoL after ATAAD, unfortunately shows little attention to male–female differences [6]. The current study revealed that male ATAAD patients had higher scores than their female counterparts on 5/8 subdomains, reflecting a worse HRQoL in female ATAAD patients. However, this trend was also seen in the general Dutch population, where females had lower scores on even 7/8 subdomains [7]. The absolute difference with the general population seemed more pronounced in female patients on the physical domains, and female sex was associated with worse physical component summary scores. In a study on HRQoL in thoracic aortic disease patients, the physical domains also seemed more severely impaired in female patients compared to the sex-matched general population, than in male patients [8]. Of note, a study on physical activity after ATAAD found female sex to be an independent predictor for reduced physical activity [22]. Therefore, physical health warrants specific attention, and qualitative studies might explore the nature of this physical inactivity in female ATAAD patients.

Additionally, it is crucial to underscore the need to assess perceived physical impairments and mental health separately in survivors of ATAAD. With regard to physical status, in this cohort older age was associated with lower PCS scores, as described earlier [14,15,23]. Nevertheless, when compared with age-matched counterparts of the general population, comparable estimates on the physical domains for the age group >70 were observed, while worse scores were observed for the patients aged 41–60 years and 61–70 years. It could be possible that only the healthy elderly with little comorbidities have undergone surgery for ATAAD. These results underline the satisfactory HRQoL results for older patients after ATAAD surgery as reported [16,24].

A physically active lifestyle including mild to moderate exercise should be promoted in all adults but especially in ATAAD survivors [25], as it might improve their overall cardiovascular health by reducing blood pressure, maintaining a healthy body weight, and improving mental health [26]. Interestingly, a history of hypertension, prior thoracic aortic aneurysm, and COPD were associated with lower PCS scores, factors which have not been investigated in previous studies [6]. These conditions could reflect a poor cardiorespiratory condition with limited physical activity in these patients. It seems important to offer patient-tailored programs for different age categories, as the daily activities and expectation of physical health of a 60 year old differ greatly from those of an 80 year old. Also, patients could benefit from sex-specific programs, as females tend to be underrepresented in cardiac rehabilitation programs [27]. Future research should focus on the effect of clear exercise recommendations by healthcare providers and cardiac rehabilitation programs on the physical status of ATAAD surgery survivors.

Interestingly, ATAAD patients in general and female patients in particular had better scores for bodily pain when compared to the general population, indicating less pain and interference of pain with daily activities. In contrast, Jussli-Melchers et al. found that ATAAD patients scored worse on bodily pain [16]. Additionally, in a study on thoracic aortic disease, no significant differences were found in bodily pain scores when compared to the general population [8]. In long-term follow-up of adult congenital heart disease patients after surgical repair, generally better HRQoL scores were observed in comparison to normative data [28], reflecting a positive perception on life. Pain at ATAAD presentation is often described as 'worst-ever pain'. One could speculate that when having experienced such intense pain, all the painful experiences afterwards are put into perspective.

ATAAD is a life-threatening traumatic event, accompanied with excessive pain and followed by emergency surgery—a sequelae of events triggering anxiety and psychological distress [14,25,29]. In this study, role emotional, social functioning, and vitality were impaired when compared to the general population, reflecting a significant impact on patients' mental health. In the age-matched analysis, a pattern can be observed: with increasing age, mental-health-related domain scores increase relative to normative data. Endlich et al. observed a strong pattern of worse MCS in younger patients over time [15], indicating better coping with regard to mental wellbeing in older patients. Physicians should aim to provide guidance and understanding to younger patients, as the impact on their social environment and employment seems more significant than in older patients.

Interestingly, the subdomain of mental health, representing anxiety or depression, was not decreased compared to the general population. As the SF-36 is not designed to measure anxiety and psychological distress in depth, it might be underestimated in this study. It remains important for clinicians to screen patients after ATAAD for (unfounded) fears that might lead to inactivity and a decrease in HRQoL.

Surgical repair of ATAAD is usually a complex and lengthy procedure, which might impact HRQoL outcomes. A recent meta-analysis showed that females received less complex surgical repair than males and less frequently underwent aortic valve replacement at ATAAD presentation when compared to males [5]. There is an ongoing debate on the extent of the procedure in the acute phase of ATAAD, since reoperation on the distal aorta is common during follow-up. In one study on surgery of the proximal aorta, the use of DHCA was associated with worse HRQoL scores [20], which was not found in this study. Also, repair/replacement or arch repair were not significantly associated with PCS or MCS scores. Prospective HRQoL studies with measurements before and after intervention might provide more insight into a favorable approach with regard to HRQoL, although the effect of management on HRQoL is difficult to examine due to the inherent bias of observational studies.

5. Limitations

A few limitations need to be addressed. Since the study design is cross-sectional, no baseline or pre-dissection HRQoL were available, and HRQoL was assessed during follow-up at one time point, hampering a time-dependent analysis. In the current study, the response rate was 58%, comparable to other (online) questionnaires [30]. Some differences in baseline characteristics were observed between non-responders and responders, implicating non-responder bias. Furthermore, survival bias might be present: the relatively worse patients could have passed away preceding the follow-up moment. Also, the SF-36 might not capture all the disease-specific problems encountered by ATAAD survivors. Nonetheless, the SF-36 is a validated tool to measure HRQoL, which improves the comparison with other studies and the general population. As the baseline data collection was retrospective, we were unable to gather information on significant aspects related to HRQoL, such as cognitive abilities and psychiatric conditions.

6. Conclusions

In this large multicenter cross-sectional study, long-term HRQoL was clearly impaired in ATAAD patients when compared to the general population, and most pronounced in younger and female patients. Age- and sex-specific attention during follow-up after ATAAD might help improve HRQoL in these patients. Social aspects might be more important for younger patients than for older patients, while physical domains were especially affected in females and older patients. Due to the improvement in early mortality of ATAAD over the past years, ATAAD survivors will become lifelong patients, requiring a patient-tailored follow-up program and guidance. HRQoL could be improved by interventions such as clear lifestyle recommendations for patients and cardiac rehabilitation, with a more inclusive and holistic approach to patient care.

Supplementary Materials: The following supporting information can be downloaded at: https://www.mdpi.com/article/10.3390/jcm13082265/s1, Appendix SI: Variable definitions patient characteristics; Appendix SII: Scores of the study population compared with the general Dutch population stratified by sex; Appendix SIII: Scores of the study population compared with the general Dutch population stratified by age category; Appendix SIV: Multivariable linear regression analyses for the physical component summary (PCS) and mental component summary (MCS) scores adjusting for age and sex.

Author Contributions: Study design: F.M., C.G.E.T., A.L.G., J.J.M.T. and J.W.R.-H. Data collection: F.M., C.G.E.T., A.L.G. and A.W.B. Data analysis: F.M. Data interpretation: all authors. Manuscript draft: F.M. Critical revision, editing and approval of the final manuscript: all authors. All authors have read and agreed to the published version of the manuscript.

Funding: This study was supported by The Netherlands Organization for Health Research and Development ZonMW [Grant number 849200014].

Institutional Review Board Statement: The study was conducted in accordance with the Declaration of Helsinki, and approved by the Ethics Committee of the Erasmus University Medical Center (protocol code MEC-2018-1535 and date of approval 11 December 2018).

Informed Consent Statement: Informed consent was obtained from all subjects involved in the study.

Data Availability Statement: Data will be shared on request to the corresponding author with permission of the disSEXion study research group.

Acknowledgments: The authors would like to acknowledge the efforts of M.H.E.J. van Wijngaarden, M.F.A. Bierhuizen and G. Custers in the baseline data collection.

Conflicts of Interest: The authors declare no conflict of interest.

Abbreviations

ATAAD = acute type A aortic dissection; HRQoL = health-related quality of life.

References

1. Evangelista, A.; Isselbacher, E.M.; Bossone, E.; Gleason, T.G.; Eusanio, M.D.; Sechtem, U.; Ehrlich, M.P.; Trimarchi, S.; Braverman, A.C.; Myrmel, T.; et al. Insights from the International Registry of Acute Aortic Dissection: A 20-Year Experience of Collaborative Clinical Research. *Circulation* **2018**, *137*, 1846–1860. [CrossRef] [PubMed]
2. Smedberg, C.; Steuer, J.; Leander, K.; Hultgren, R. Sex differences and temporal trends in aortic dissection: A population-based study of incidence, treatment strategies, and outcome in Swedish patients during 15 years. *Eur. Heart J.* **2020**, *41*, 2430–2438. [CrossRef] [PubMed]
3. Hagan, P.G.; Nienaber, C.A.; Isselbacher, E.M.; Bruckman, D.; Karavite, D.J.; Russman, P.L.; Evangelista, A.; Fattori, R.; Suzuki, T.; Oh, J.K.; et al. The International Registry of Acute Aortic Dissection (IRAD): New insights into an old disease. *JAMA* **2000**, *283*, 897–903. [CrossRef] [PubMed]
4. Gariboldi, V.; Grisoli, D.; Kerbaul, F.; Giorgi, R.; Riberi, A.; Metras, D.; Mesana, T.G.; Collart, F. Long-term outcomes after repaired acute type A aortic dissections. *Interact. Cardiovasc. Thorac. Surg.* **2007**, *6*, 47–51. [CrossRef] [PubMed]
5. Carbone, A.; Ranieri, B.; Castaldo, R.; Franzese, M.; Rega, S.; Cittadini, A.; Czerny, M.; Bossone, E. Sex Differences in Type A Acute Aortic Dissection: A Systematic Review and Meta-Analysis. *Eur. J. Prev. Cardiol.* **2023**, *30*, 1074–1089. [CrossRef] [PubMed]
6. Eranki, A.; Wilson-Smith, A.; Williams, M.L.; Saxena, A.; Mejia, R. Quality of life following surgical repair of acute type A aortic dissection: A systematic review. *J. Cardiothorac. Surg.* **2022**, *17*, 118. [CrossRef] [PubMed]
7. Aaronson, N.K.; Muller, M.; Cohen, P.D.; Essink-Bot, M.L.; Fekkes, M.; Sanderman, R.; Sprangers, M.A.; te Velde, A.; Verrips, E. Translation, validation, and norming of the Dutch language version of the SF-36 Health Survey in community and chronic disease populations. *J. Clin. Epidemiol.* **1998**, *51*, 1055–1068. [CrossRef]
8. Thijssen, C.G.E.; Dekker, S.; Bons, L.R.; Gökalp, A.L.; Kauling, R.M.; van den Bosch, A.E.; Cuypers, J.; Utens, E.; van Kimmenade, R.R.L.; Takkenberg, J.J.M.; et al. Health-related quality of life and lived experiences in males and females with thoracic aortic disease and their partners. *Open Heart* **2020**, *7*, e001419. [CrossRef]
9. von Elm, E.; Altman, D.G.; Egger, M.; Pocock, S.J.; Gøtzsche, P.C.; Vandenbroucke, J.P.; Initiative, S. The Strengthening the Reporting of Observational Studies in Epidemiology (STROBE) Statement: Guidelines for reporting observational studies. *Int. J. Surg.* **2014**, *12*, 1495–1499. [CrossRef]
10. McHorney, C.A.; Ware, J.E., Jr.; Lu, J.F.; Sherbourne, C.D. The MOS 36-item Short-Form Health Survey (SF-36): III. Tests of data quality, scaling assumptions, and reliability across diverse patient groups. *Med. Care* **1994**, *32*, 40–66. [CrossRef]
11. McHorney, C.A.; Ware, J.E., Jr.; Raczek, A.E. The MOS 36-Item Short-Form Health Survey (SF-36): II. Psychometric and clinical tests of validity in measuring physical and mental health constructs. *Med. Care* **1993**, *31*, 247–263. [CrossRef] [PubMed]
12. Ware, J.E., Jr.; Sherbourne, C.D. The MOS 36-item short-form health survey (SF-36). I. Conceptual framework and item selection. *Med. Care* **1992**, *30*, 473–483. [CrossRef] [PubMed]
13. Ware, J.E., Jr. SF-36 health survey update. *Spine* **2000**, *25*, 3130–3139. [CrossRef] [PubMed]

14. Adam, U.; Habazettl, H.; Graefe, K.; Kuppe, H.; Wundram, M.; Kurz, S.D. Health-related quality of life of patients after surgery for acute Type A aortic dissection. *Interact. Cardiovasc. Thorac. Surg.* **2018**, *27*, 48–53. [CrossRef] [PubMed]
15. Endlich, M.; Hamiko, M.; Gestrich, C.; Probst, C.; Mellert, F.; Winkler, K.; Welz, A.; Schiller, W. Long-Term Outcome and Quality of Life in Aortic Type A Dissection Survivors. *Thorac. Cardiovasc. Surg.* **2016**, *64*, 91–99. [PubMed]
16. Jussli-Melchers, J.; Panholzer, B.; Friedrich, C.; Broch, O.; Renner, J.; Schöttler, J.; Rahimi, A.; Cremer, J.; Schoeneich, F.; Haneya, A. Long-term outcome and quality of life following emergency surgery for acute aortic dissection type A: A comparison between young and elderly adults. *Eur. J. Cardiothorac. Surg.* **2017**, *51*, 465–471. [CrossRef] [PubMed]
17. Immer, F.F.; Krähenbühl, E.; Immer-Bansi, A.S.; Berdat, P.A.; Kipfer, B.; Eckstein, F.S.; Saner, H.; Carrel, T.P. Quality of life after interventions on the thoracic aorta with deep hypothermic circulatory arrest. *Eur. J. Cardiothorac. Surg.* **2002**, *21*, 10–14. [CrossRef] [PubMed]
18. Santini, F.; Montalbano, G.; Messina, A.; D'Onofrio, A.; Casali, G.; Viscardi, F.; Luciani, G.B.; Mazzucco, A. Survival and quality of life after repair of acute type A aortic dissection in patients aged 75 years and older justify intervention. *Eur. J. Cardiothorac. Surg.* **2006**, *29*, 386–391. [CrossRef] [PubMed]
19. Sbarouni, E.; Georgiadou, P.; Manavi, M.; Analitis, A.; Beletsioti, C.; Niakas, D.; Iliodromitis, E.; Voudris, V. Long-term outcomes and quality of life following acute type A aortic dissection. *Hell. J. Cardiol.* **2021**, *62*, 463–465. [CrossRef]
20. Olsson, C.; Franco-Cereceda, A. Health-Related Quality of Life in Thoracic Aortic Disease: Part II. After Surgery on the Proximal (Root, Ascending, Arch) Aorta. *Aorta* **2013**, *1*, 162–170. [CrossRef]
21. Gjeilo, K.H.; Stenseth, R.; Wahba, A.; Lydersen, S.; Klepstad, P. Long-term health-related quality of life and survival after cardiac surgery: A prospective study. *J. Thorac. Cardiovasc. Surg.* **2018**, *156*, 2183–2190.e2182. [CrossRef]
22. Schachner, T.; Garrido, F.; Bonaros, N.; Krapf, C.; Dumfarth, J.; Grimm, M. Factors limiting physical activity after acute type A aortic dissection. *Wien. Klin. Wochenschr.* **2019**, *131*, 174–179. [CrossRef] [PubMed]
23. Tang, G.H.; Malekan, R.; Yu, C.J.; Kai, M.; Lansman, S.L.; Spielvogel, D. Surgery for acute type A aortic dissection in octogenarians is justified. *J. Thorac. Cardiovasc. Surg.* **2013**, *145* (Suppl. S3), S186–S190. [CrossRef] [PubMed]
24. Bojko, M.M.; Suhail, M.; Bavaria, J.E.; Bueker, A.; Hu, R.W.; Harmon, J.; Habertheuer, A.; Milewski, R.K.; Szeto, W.Y.; Vallabhajosyula, P. Midterm outcomes of emergency surgery for acute type A aortic dissection in octogenarians. *J. Thorac. Cardiovasc. Surg.* **2022**, *163*, 2–12.e7. [CrossRef] [PubMed]
25. Chaddha, A.; Kline-Rogers, E.; Braverman, A.C.; Erickson, S.R.; Jackson, E.A.; Franklin, B.A.; Woznicki, E.M.; Jabara, J.T.; Montgomery, D.G.; Eagle, K.A. Survivors of Aortic Dissection: Activity, Mental Health, and Sexual Function. *Clin. Cardiol.* **2015**, *38*, 652–659. [CrossRef] [PubMed]
26. Perk, J.; De Backer, G.; Gohlke, H.; Graham, I.; Reiner, Z.; Verschuren, M.; Albus, C.; Benlian, P.; Boysen, G.; Cifkova, R.; et al. European Guidelines on cardiovascular disease prevention in clinical practice (version 2012): The Fifth Joint Task Force of the European Society of Cardiology and Other Societies on Cardiovascular Disease Prevention in Clinical Practice (constituted by representatives of nine societies and by invited experts). *Eur. J. Prev. Cardiol.* **2012**, *19*, 585–667.
27. Smith, J.R.; Thomas, R.J.; Bonikowske, A.R.; Hammer, S.M.; Olson, T.P. Sex Differences in Cardiac Rehabilitation Outcomes. *Circ. Res.* **2022**, *130*, 552–565. [CrossRef] [PubMed]
28. Pelosi, C.; Kauling, R.M.; Cuypers, J.; van den Bosch, A.E.; Helbing, W.A.; Utens, E.; Legerstee, J.S.; Roos-Hesselink, J.W. Daily life and psychosocial functioning of adults with congenital heart disease: A 40–53 years after surgery follow-up study. *Clin. Res. Cardiol.* **2023**, *112*, 880–890. [CrossRef] [PubMed]
29. Pasadyn, S.R.; Roselli, E.E.; Artis, A.S.; Pasadyn, C.L.; Phelan, D.; Hurley, K.; Desai, M.Y.; Blackstone, E.H. From Tear to Fear: Posttraumatic Stress Disorder in Patients with Acute Type A Aortic Dissection. *J. Am. Heart Assoc.* **2020**, *9*, e015060. [CrossRef]
30. Ebert, J.F.; Huibers, L.; Christensen, B.; Christensen, M.B. Paper- or Web-Based Questionnaire Invitations as a Method for Data Collection: Cross-Sectional Comparative Study of Differences in Response Rate, Completeness of Data, and Financial Cost. *J. Med. Internet Res.* **2018**, *20*, e24. [CrossRef]

Disclaimer/Publisher's Note: The statements, opinions and data contained in all publications are solely those of the individual author(s) and contributor(s) and not of MDPI and/or the editor(s). MDPI and/or the editor(s) disclaim responsibility for any injury to people or property resulting from any ideas, methods, instructions or products referred to in the content.

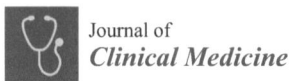

Review

Acute Aortic Syndromes from Diagnosis to Treatment—A Comprehensive Review

Cosmin M. Banceu [1,2,3], Diana M. Banceu [3,*], David S. Kauvar [4], Adrian Popentiu [5], Vladimir Voth [6], Markus Liebrich [6], Marius Halic Neamtu [7,8], Marvin Oprean [9], Daiana Cristutiu [3], Marius Harpa [1,2,3], Klara Brinzaniuc [1,10] and Horatiu Suciu [1,2,3]

[1] I.O.S.U.D., George Emil Palade University of Medicine, Pharmacy, Science, and Technology of Targu Mures, 540139 Targu Mures, Romania; cosmin.banceu@umfst.ro (C.M.B.)
[2] Department of Surgery M3, George Emil Palade University of Medicine, Pharmacy, Science, and Technology of Targu Mures, 540139 Targu Mures, Romania
[3] Emergency Institute for Cardiovascular Diseases and Transplantation Targu Mures, 540136 Targu Mures, Romania
[4] Department of Surgery, Division of Vascular Surgery, Stanford University School of Medicine, Palo Alto, CA 94305, USA
[5] Faculty of Medicine, University Lucian Blaga Sibiu, 550169 Sibiu, Romania
[6] Sana Cardiac Surgery, 70174 Stuttgart, Germany
[7] Swiss Federal Institute of Forest, Snow and Landscape Research WSL, 8903 Birmensdorf, Switzerland
[8] Institute of Environmental Engineering, ETH Zurich, 8039 Zurich, Switzerland
[9] Mathematics and Statistics Department, Amherst College, Amherst, MA 01002, USA
[10] Department of Anatomy, George Emil Palade University of Medicine, Pharmacy, Science, and Technology of Targu Mures, 540142 Targu Mures, Romania
* Correspondence: c_diana_maria@yahoo.com; Tel.: +40-74-663-851

Abstract: This work aims to provide a comprehensive description of the characteristics of a group of acute aortic diseases that are all potentially life-threatening and are collectively referred to as acute aortic syndromes (AASs). There have been recent developments in the care and diagnostic plan for AAS. A substantial clinical index of suspicion is required to identify AASs before irreversible fatal consequences arise because of their indefinite symptoms and physical indicators. A methodical approach to the diagnosis of AAS is addressed. Timely and suitable therapy should be started immediately after diagnosis. Improving clinical outcomes requires centralising patients with AAS in high-volume centres with high-volume surgeons. Consequently, the management of these patients benefits from the increased use of aortic centres, multidisciplinary teams and an "aorta code". Each acute aortic entity requires a different patient treatment strategy; these are outlined below. Finally, numerous preventive strategies for AAS are discussed. The keys to good results are early diagnosis, understanding the natural history of these disorders and, where necessary, prompt surgical intervention. It is important to keep in mind that chest pain does not necessarily correspond with coronary heart disease and to be alert to the possible existence of aortic diseases because once antiplatelet drugs are administered, a blocked coagulation system can complicate aortic surgery and affect prognosis. The management of AAS in "aortic centres" improves long-term outcomes and decreases mortality rates.

Keywords: acute aortic syndrome; acute aortic dissection; intramural hematoma; penetrating atherosclerotic ulcer; traumatic aortic injury; aortic centres; Stanford A; Stanford B; Stanford non-A non-B; aortic surgery

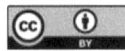

1. Introduction

Disorders of the thoracic and abdominal aorta known as acute aortic syndromes (AASs) are potentially life-threatening, typically symptomatic and necessitate prompt surgical assessment. The term AAS refers to a diverse group of disorders that share a common set of signs and symptoms, the most prominent of which is aortic discomfort. It was first used in 1998 [1] and thoroughly defined in 2001 [2]. Aortic dissection (AD), intramural hematoma (IMH), penetrating atherosclerotic ulcer (PAU) and traumatic AD (TAD) are the four acute aortic diseases considered as AAS, see Figure 1.

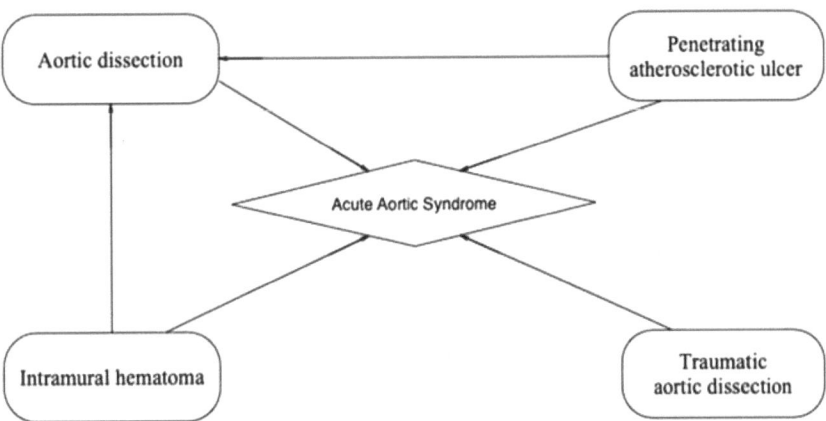

Figure 1. Acute Aortic Syndrome Spectrum.

Knowledge of the pathologic spectrum of AAS helps to clarify the origin and course of aortic lesions [3,4]. AAS can be categorised into two groups based on whether the ascending aorta is involved (Stanford type A) or not (Stanford type B). A unique disease known as non-A non-B AAS occurs when a lesion is limited to the aortic arch only or when a lesion that originated distal to the left subclavian artery retrogradely spreads to the arch instead of accessing the ascending aorta [5]. Any AD with an entrance tear that starts distal to the innominate artery ostium is classified as a type B AAS [6].

Acute AD is a highly prevalent and potentially deadly condition, necessitating prompt diagnosis and treatment. If not treated, mortality can be up to 90% after three months, and acute mortality can be 1–2% per hour after the onset of symptoms [7,8]. A tear in the aortic intima causes AD, which is characterised by a blood column entering the medial layer of the aorta and resulting in a "hydraulic endarterectomy" [9]. This creates a septum made of medial and intimal aortic tissue that separates the aorta's real and false lumens. In many people, the aorta's detached outer layer, which consists of adventitia and aortic medial tissue, is robust enough to prevent the aorta from rupturing into the pericardial cavity and causing fatal cardiac tamponade, or into the pleural cavities and causing deadly exsanguination. In these cases, aortic branch occlusion is determined by the size of the dissecting hematoma [10]. This hematoma can induce blockage of vital aortic branches, such as those supplying the brain, kidneys, abdominal viscera and limbs. The dissection flap arises from a tear in the proximal aorta and spreads distally for a varied length. Paraplegia can occur when the lumbar and intercostal arteries are occluded. When the dissecting hematoma grows near the aortic root, it may obstruct the coronary artery ostia, which could cause myocardial infarction or damage the aortic valve, which may then cause aortic regurgitation.

A highly prevalent trigger for acute AD is hypertension [7]. Approximately 20% of individuals have severe forms of cystic medial degeneration. Aortic coarctation, bicuspid valve, dilatation of the ascending aorta and aortic root, collagen vascular disorders, extreme isometric exertion, pregnancy and aortic inflammatory diseases are additional risk factors. Acute AD is most frequently characterised by abrupt, intense chest discomfort [7]. Acute AD may occur in the absence of pain, and additional variations of back and chest discomfort have been observed. The anterior chest is typically where type A dissection pain is felt, though it can also radiate to the back, neck or belly. The pain associated with type B dissection typically manifests as both posterior chest and abdominal pain. Additional symptoms include a coma induced by obstruction or serious blockage of the brachiocephalic arteries and syncope, which is caused by hypotension linked to cardiac tamponade or aortic rupture. Hypoperfusion of the renal and mesenteric arteries causes abdominal pain. In the context of acute AD, mesenteric ischemia can result in a death rate of up to 87% and renal failure in the range of 50–70% [7]. Obstruction of the infrarenal aorta and iliofemoral arteries causes acute limb pain and pulselessness.

2. Clinical Presentation and Diagnosis

2.1. Challenges of Diagnosis

To establish a correct diagnosis of AAS, an in-depth examination must be performed, which involves investigations allowing for the exclusion of several other conditions that are part of the differential diagnosis. The diagnosis of AAS is difficult due to three key factors: a modest prevalence, a lack of precise biomarkers and a highly varied clinical course [11,12]. Thus, the key to diagnosing AAS is to retain an elevated level of medical suspicion. Several initiatives—including AAS training sessions, educational materials, computerised diagnostic instruments and algorithms created especially for patients with chest pain—may increase the level of awareness [13–15]. A three-step process has been designed to make emergency room diagnosis easier.

2.1.1. Phase 1

The first phase of this process entails determining the likelihood of AAS using three categories: risk factors, physical examination results and characteristics of pain. Risk factors for AAS are widely recognised. The most common, severe chronic hypertension, is closely linked to the emergence of AAS. Indeed, individuals with hypertension have a risk of AAS more than twice as high as those without it, and 54% of the population has a risk of AAS due to hypertension [16]. Other risk factors that should be considered include bicuspid aortic valve, aortic valve disease, previous family history of aortic disease, Marfan syndrome and Loeys–Dietz syndrome. In addition to risk factors, a highly prevalent clinical complaint among patients with AAS is chest discomfort [13,17–19]. According to descriptions, the "aortic pain" is sudden, sharp, strong and tearing, and often radiates towards the destination of the lesion's advancement in accordance with the implicated aortic branches. Patients with type A AAS most often have pain in the chest, whereas patients with type B AAS typically experience aortic pain in the back. Experiencing AAS without discomfort is less common. Finally, a thorough physical examination may show common indications of AAS, such as an aortic regurgitation murmur or pulse deficit/asymmetric pulses. Acute aortic syndrome should be discussed in patients hospitalised for severe hypotension, syncope or shock, especially in those who additionally presented chest pain. This preliminary likelihood evaluation is advised for class I [13,15]. If more than one risk factor is found, this would prompt concerns about possible AAS and direct further action.

2.1.2. Phase 2

The second phase entails the standard diagnostic procedures that are required for any patient experiencing chest pain, including an electrocardiogram (ECG), a chest X-ray and laboratory testing for biomarkers [14,20]. This is a crucial step in the diagnostic procedure that allows differentiation between the two most common serious illnesses that cause chest pain: pulmonary embolism and acute coronary syndrome (ACS). ACS can be diagnosed with great sensitivity when troponin levels and ECG are combined [20]. Chest pain originating from the heart, such as in myocardial infarction, can be distinguished with an ECG. AAS and myocardial infarction can both manifest simultaneously, although cases like this require more research and cautious handling. Because antiplatelet medications required for ACS may complicate therapy and significantly decrease the prognosis of patients with AAS, differential diagnosis between AAS and ACS is crucial. However, a high troponin level does not mean that AAS is not present. Elevated troponin levels in patients with AAS can be attributable to myocardial ischemia worsened by acute aortic regurgitation or hypotension, or they can result in death if the dissection flap involves a coronary artery. The use of D-dimer values for AD diagnosis has been extensively demonstrated in numerous investigations [21–23]. D-dimer values boost the effectiveness of the diagnostic approach when they are combined with an evaluation of the likelihood of developing AAS [22,24]. As a result, the sensitivity and specificity are 98.8% and 57.3%, respectively, whenever a patient exhibits one or more risk factors for AAS and the D-dimer is negative. The negative likelihood ratio for developing AAS therefore amounts to nearly 100% [22].

2.1.3. Phase 3

The second stage is crucial because, in patients presenting with "aortic pain", elevated D-dimer values, normal troponins and a normal ECG, all suggest the possibility of AAS/pulmonary embolism, which necessitates imaging tests, i.e., the third stage, which will yield a conclusive diagnosis [15,25]. The core of the diagnostic process is imaging, which involves the application of magnetic resonance imaging (MRI), computed tomography (CT), ultrasound (US) or chest radiography. Basic chest radiography may detect AAS with up to 64% sensitivity and 86% specificity. The characteristics observed on a chest X-ray include tracheal shift, aortic kinking, widening of the mediastinum, widening of the aortic notch and a twofold increase in the frequency of the aortic shadow [26]. In the emergency room, CT is the favoured imaging diagnostic for confirming the development of AAS. This method is ideal because of several benefits: quick collection times, widespread accessibility in emergency rooms in most hospitals and comprehensive anatomic evaluation of the overall aorta and aortic branch vessels [25,27]. A CT scan can recognise AAS with a normative sensitivity of up to 95%. Observed values have ranged from 87–100% [28,29]. All patients with intermediate/high diagnosis of AAS should have a full aortic CT scan, regardless of the contrast [30].

2.2. Assessment Methods

Both transthoracic echocardiography (TTE) and transesophageal echocardiography (TEE) can aid in the diagnosis of AAS, but their efficacy differs greatly. TTE is useful for diagnosing both proximal dissection and its consequences in an acute scenario. However, there are numerous other locations throughout the entire aorta where views may be restricted. Focus TTE may also help to evaluate other pertinent conditions, such cardiac function, aortic valve regurgitation and pericardial effusion [13,31]. However, TEE enables the US tool to approach the aorta extremely closely, resulting in 99% sensitivity and 89% specificity in one study [32]. In an emergency situation, TEE becomes much less accessible and more operator-dependent. Additionally, an examination that necessitates esophageal intubation is significantly more intrusive. A bedside TTE and CT scan combination is a great diagnostic strategy, since it enables the assessment of likely problems related to AAS and a view of the entire length of the aorta.

Because there are few MRIs available for use during an emergency and because AASs are serious, MRIs are rarely employed as the main method of acute investigation. Whenever initial investigations are not definitive, this modality—which is a highly sensitive and specific means of identifying all forms of AAS—can be employed. TEE has been implemented during surgery to provide necessary information, and to promptly assess outcomes during open surgery and endovascular therapy [33].

In patients with AAS, the use of chest X-rays and ECGs is restricted to eliminating other conditions that manifest as chest discomfort. Chest X-rays for type A lesions can show enlarged mediastinum, although this result is absent in 20–28% of dissections [34,35]. AD cannot be diagnosed only by X-ray. Heart troponin T levels are often higher in patients with AAS and are linked to a later diagnosis [36]. TEE and CT or MRI are part of the first diagnostic assessment [37]. According to published research, TEE has greater specificity and sensitivity (86–100% and 90–100%, respectively) for acute dissection than CT (95–100%

and 94–98%, respectively) [28,38–42]. TTE, in contrast, performs less well, with a median sensitivity of 86.9–100.0% and a specificity of 81.2–91.0% (81.1%) [43,44].

Acute dissection must be diagnosed as soon as possible. When imaging is not an option (due to a lack of scanners or a patient's declining clinical condition, for example) serologic biomarkers that indicate nascent aortic wall injury are a desirable diagnostic tool. D-dimer is now the best researched among those biomarkers [21] and has a minimal threshold level of 0.5 µg/mL, a sensitivity of 51.7–100.0% (median, 93.5%) and a specificity of 32.8–89.2% (median, 54.0%) [21,45–48]. Moreover, higher in-hospital mortality has been linked to higher D-dimer levels [49]. The following biomarkers were also studied: matrix metalloproteinase [50], soluble lectin-like oxidised low-density lipoprotein receptor [51], smooth muscle myosin heavy chain [52] and soluble elastin fragments [53]. Nevertheless, the dearth of randomised controlled trials precludes any inferences about their capacity to boost results.

Between 35 and 37% of the ECGs in the International Registry of Aortic Dissection (IRAD) and another cohort were normal. Some studies have shown that 50–70% of patients had enlarged mediastina on their chest X-rays [34,54]; of those, 26% had pleural effusion [54]. The sensitivity and specificity of TEE were 96.5–99.6% and 92.3–98.5%, respectively [55–57]. After receiving medical attention for a mean of 450 days, 44 patients with a simple type B IMH were monitored; the disease advanced in 87% of the individuals exhibiting an early intimal abnormality, whereas this occurred in only 9% of individuals lacking such an abnormality ($p < 0.001$). One study found that 80% and 40% of patients with IMH with focal dissection showed five and eight years, respectively, without death linked to dissection (Table 1) [58].

Table 1. Diagnostic tools for acute aortic syndromes: sensitivity and specificity.

Diagnostic Tool	Sensitivity	Specificity
Computed tomography	100	100
Magnetic resonance imaging	95.0–100	94.0–98.0
Transesophageal echocardiography	86.0–100	90.0–100
Transthoracic echocardiography	73.7–100	71.2–91.0
Intravascular ultrasound	100	100
D-dimer	51.7–100	32.8–89.2
Elastin degradation products	99.8	99.8
Matrix metalloproteinase 8/9	100	9.5
Smooth muscle myosin heavy chain	90	97
Soluble lectin-like oxidised low-density lipoprotein receptor 1	89.5	94.3

CT and MRI are the gold standards for the diagnosis of IMH. Furthermore, CT identification of intimal defects (erosion of the vessel wall in discrete locations) in patients with IMH is associated with progression to dissection [59].

3. Treatment of Patients with AAS

The two types of AAS are those that impact the ascending and descending aortas. Surgical intervention is the final therapy for situations affecting the ascending aorta. Immediate surgical intervention is required only for rapidly progressing static AAS impacting the descending aorta and causing organ or limb malperfusion, unbearable pain or danger of rupture. Static AASs affecting the descending aorta are typically managed conservatively [60].

To halt the advancement of the dissection or prevent aortic rupture, early therapy for patients with AAS in emergencies concentrates on lowering systolic blood pressure below 120 mmHg and lowering the rate of change of blood pressure (dP/dt). An injectable beta-blocker, like labetalol, is the cornerstone of medical therapy for keeping the heart rate around 60, which is called "impulse control". Non-dihydropyridine calcium channel blockers could be an option for patients who cannot tolerate beta-blockers. Vasodilators may be administered in addition to these.

In the examined trials, the observed 30-day or in-hospital mortality for type A acute AD ranged from 13–17% for open surgical treatment and from 0–16% for thoracic endovascular aneurysm repair (TEVAR). For people with type A AAS, urgent open surgical correction is the recommended course of action. The primary goals are to prevent aortic rupture, fix aortic regurgitation and reroute blood flow to the correct lumen [14]. A supracoronary tube graft, with or without valve replacement or repair, may be adequate to accomplish this purpose provided the aortic root is unaffected. The standard procedure for treating aortic root inclusion is a Bentall–De Bono operation, which can be combined with a mechanical or biological valve replacement [61,62].

Nevertheless, high-volume centres and skilled surgeons must consider various other approaches. In certain patients, valve-sparing aortic root surgeries, including the David or Yacoub approaches, can be explored [62,63]. Aortic root substitution using a composite valve tube or aortic valve resuspension is necessary for people with aortic annulus growth or entry tears at the aortic root and for the majority of people with connective tissue illnesses.

An open method has historically been used to treat ascending AD. The goal of treatment is to close or excise the most proximal intimal tear and all successive tears in order to eradicate the false lumen. As an alternative, artificial grafts may be used to strengthen the aortic wall. Aortic valve inadequacy and coronary artery injury can result from proximal extension into the aortic valve. These can be fixed either by replacing the complete valve or by resuspending the valve.

In patients with type A AAS, "hemiarch" replacement of the aortic arch with no involvement of the supra-aortic trunks remains the conventional surgical technique. The safety and efficacy of total arch replacement are becoming more and more clear [64–66]. Therefore, in centres with appropriate expertise, a total arch replacement procedure must be considered in the event of any of the following conditions: a dilated aortic arch, an entry tear at the aortic arch, arch or proximal descending re-entrance tears or a dilated proximal descending aorta [14,66,67]. This strategy enables distal aortic remodelling and shields against additional operations. Employing a hybrid prosthesis, the "frozen elephant trunk" method proved to be a workable solution in AAS scenarios, resulting in positive outcomes. By joining more endoprostheses to the distal portion of the hybrid prosthesis, it also becomes feasible to implement an endovascular restoration of the distal descending and abdominal aorta. The challenge of managing dissection affecting the aortic valve and root is the main drawback of the endovascular method.

In the IRAD, surgical intervention was used to treat 72% of patients with type A acute AD. When a patient was too old, had too many coexisting conditions, refused treatment or passed away before a scheduled surgery, medical intervention was employed. In-hospital mortality following open surgery was 26%, whereas that following medical management was 58% [38]. IRAD data were used to identify four different periods—hyperacute (0–24 h), acute (2–7 days), subacute (8–30 days) and chronic ($\geq$30 days)—for the onset of symptoms and emergency department attendance. Nevertheless, the observational study design limits these findings [68]. Twenty to thirty percent of 2317 individuals with acute type A dissection in a large German registry had neurological impairment at presentation; 12.3% of these patients recovered after surgery and 9.5% of these individuals had additional neurological problems after surgery. A fresh episode of postoperative neurological impairment was associated with longer operating time, dissection of the supra-aortic arteries and malperfusion syndrome [69]. Between 2006 and 2015, nine off-label and five on-label procedures were conducted in the sole US Food and Drug Administration-approved, physician-sponsored investigational device exemption study of endovascular therapy for type A AD [70]. Acute and chronic type A ADs affected six patients and five patients, respectively. All surgeries were practically effective, with a 7.1% 30-day mortality rate.

For type B AAS, problems such as hemodynamic instability, malperfusion, rapid aortic dilation and aortic rupture should be addressed by TEVAR. Additional dangerous conditions that must be considered include refractory discomfort or hypertension, a large proximal entrance tear, an aortic diameter greater than 44 mm and a false lumen diameter greater than 22 mm [6,13]. Since TEVAR has demonstrated positive outcomes and few periprocedural problems, it can be postponed whenever feasible [71,72]. All other patients with type B AAS should be treated.

For type B acute AD, 30-day or in-hospital mortality ranged from 0–27%, 13–17% and 0–18% for medicinal treatment, open surgical surgery and TEVAR, respectively. In the IRAD study, in-hospital mortality for type B acute AD managed with medicinal therapy was 9.5%, but it reached 29% for the surgical cohort [73]. Malperfusion syndrome or indications of a periaortic hematoma in the surgical cohort suggested the need for surgery. Therefore, it is possible that the two groups' different levels of illness severity affected the outcomes.

In a propensity-matched study, Fattori et al. [74] compared 276 patients receiving TEVAR to 853 patients receiving medical treatment for type B dissection. Although TEVAR patients had more problems upon admission, hospital mortality did not differ between the two groups, and TEVAR patients had a decreased five-year cumulative risk of death (15.5% vs. 29.0%; $p = 0.02$) [74]. An experimental device exemption study using TEVAR for complex type B dissections reported a 30-day mortality rate of 8% (Table 2) [75].

Table 2. Reported results of treatment for acute aortic syndromes (AASs).

	Medical	Open Surgical Procedure	TEVAR [1]
Mortality range of AAS (%)	0–29	0–50	0–21

[1] Thoracic endovascular aneurysm repair.

In patients with uncomplicated acute type B AD, the Level IB Acute Dissection: Stent Graft or Best Medical Treatment (ADSORB) trial compared medical therapy with TEVAR in a randomised controlled study. "Favourable aortic remodelling" at one year was the main goal. There were no aortic ruptures in either group and the amount of aortic dilatation was comparable in the two groups. In contrast to patients receiving TEVAR, participants receiving medical therapy had a lower rate of false lumen thrombosis (97% vs. 43%; $p < 0.001$). Additionally, compared to the medically treated group, the TEVAR group showed better aortic remodelling at the one-year follow-up [76]. Despite addressing chronic type B dissections, the Investigative Study of Stent Grafts in Aortic Dissection with Extended Length of Follow-up (INSTEAD-XL) trial offers some of the finest Level IB evidence for long-term results following TEVAR in uncomplicated type B dissection [71]. INSTEAD-XL found that, at the five-year assessment, TEVAR was linked to improved results compared to solely medical treatment for both disease progression (4.1% vs. 28.1%; $p = 0.004$) and endpoint (6.9% vs. 19.3%; $p = 0.04$). However, aorta-specific mortality for TEVAR was higher in the first 12 months (7.5 vs. 3.0). TEVAR failed to lower the all-cause mortality rate (11.1% vs. 19.3%; $p = 0.13$) [71].

Aortic intramural hematoma (AIH) requires particular attention in a few areas. Though less common than ascending AD, AIHs are managed similarly because of the possibilities of progression to dissection, aneurysm formation or aortic rupture. Whenever feasible, endovascular stenting is used for AIH impacting the ascending aorta, while surgery or watch-and-wait therapy is used for instances impacting the descending aorta [77]. In asymptomatic individuals with type A AIH, early medicinal therapy combined with a careful waiting approach may be a safe course of action. In such a scenario, it is necessary to provide serial clinical and radiological assessment and to conduct surgery in the event of hemodynamic deterioration or the emergence of high-risk imaging signals [14,78,79]. Additionally, for people with type B AIH, the standard unidentified variables in TEVAR include the lack of a healthy aortic proximal landing zone and an evident entrance tear that needs to be closed. Patients with type B AIH are often treated medically, and the development of ulcer-like projections warrants close imaging monitoring because they are linked to an increased risk of complications, particularly if they are detected on the first CT scan [80–82].

Medicinal therapy was found to be appropriate for patients with "moderate" IMHs in a study involving 86 cases of AAS. Patients with moderate hematomas include patients without hemodynamic instability, persistent pain, impending rupture and ruptured aneurysm. Definitive surgical treatment was recommended for patients with "severe" IMHs who exhibited these symptoms. Of 26 patients who were treated medically, six (23%) experienced spontaneous regression and seven (27%) ultimately underwent surgery [83]. Among 27 patients who had conservative care for a type B IMH and were monitored for an average of 33 months, 47% experienced regression, 14% stayed stable and 39% advanced to AD or enlargement [34]. In a different trial, medical therapy plus TEVAR was compared to early medical therapy for IMHs complicated by intimal erosion. Ninety percent of medically treated patients showed regression at a mean follow-up of 17.6 months, and 45% of patients had full clearance of their IMH. Every patient receiving TEVAR experienced resolution [84].

Song et al. examined 127 individuals with type A and type B IMHs. Patients with type A IMHs had greater mortality rates than type B patients (7% vs. 1%) and more frequent pericardial and pleural effusions [85]. Nevertheless, rates of regression and progression to dissection were comparable. For type A IMH in the IRAD, the in-hospital mortality rates were 24% for surgical therapy and 40% for medical therapy. The in-hospital mortality rates for type B hematoma were 20% for surgical therapy and 4% for medicinal treatment [54]. TEVAR and medical therapy were compared for 56 individuals with type B IMHs. Patients who had sustained chest or back pain despite receiving the most aggressive medical care, had a maximum aortic diameter greater than 45 mm or had hematoma thickness greater than 10 mm were eligible for TEVAR. There was neither mortality nor progression in the TEVAR group, leading to 100% clinical success.

Medical therapy is a safe way to treat isolated asymptomatic PAU, which is frequently incidentally discovered on imaging obtained for other purposes. Aortic rupture, pseudoaneurysm formation and aneurysm formation are more likely to occur in cases of symptomatic PAU. Surgical therapy is often necessary because of the comorbidities and advanced age of patients who are commonly diagnosed with PAU. Endovascular surgery with stent grafts provides the largest reduction in mortality, over non-interventional management [86]. However, because these studies are observational, the quality of evidence is limited.

4. Discussion

4.1. The Role of Multidisciplinary Teams in Treating AAS

Treatment for acute aortic pathology should be centralised in "aortic centres" due to substantial evidence for a volume–outcome link [87–89]. The goals are very clear: lower early mortality, prevent repeat surgeries and improve long-term results.

The "aorta code", an organised emergency care approach that is always accessible and can be initiated from emergency rooms of low-volume hospitals, should be developed to overcome the obstacles that impede early detection and efficient management of AAS. The aorta code serves three main purposes: (1) In order to diagnose AAS earlier, emergency care providers should be more knowledgeable about it. (2) Patients should be transferred to an aortic centre as soon as possible to shorten the time between diagnosis and treatment. (3) By employing highly skilled aortic surgeons, the best course of action can be provided, thereby improving clinical outcomes.

The objective of this code is to provide patients with AAS with standardised, optimised care using a systematic procedure, from the emergency department to the operating room [90,91]. An "aorta team" is employed for diagnosis, treatment and aftercare [15]. Practitioners from multiple areas of expertise, such as clinical cardiologists, cardiac imaging specialists, cardiac surgeons, vascular surgeons, radiologists, vascular interventional radiologists, anesthesiologists and others, are required to possess a high level of knowledge about the care of patients with AAS. The multidisciplinary group needs to work together well. To determine the optimal course of treatment for each patient—open surgery, hybrid vascular and endovascular operations, a full endovascular approach or conservative management—early consultation with the aortic team is crucial [13,15]. Following initial hospitalisation, every patient should undergo systematic monitoring and surveillance at a clinic experienced in aortic care.

Apart from preventive measures, the best way to enhance clinical results is by centralising treatment of AAS (high-volume surgeons in high-volume centres) [17,92–95]. It should be made clear, nonetheless, that the experience of an individual surgeon is very important for achieving the best results [93,95,96]. Having low-volume surgeons treat patients with AAS at a high-volume centre is not ideal.

4.2. Prevention of AAS

Preventive surgery, medical therapy, controlling hypertension and gathering a thorough family history are all essential preventive procedures that can detect individuals who are at risk for AAS.

It has become widely known that certain aortic problems can be inherited [97,98]. Regardless of the presence of symptoms related to aortic disease, a family history of AD is an important risk factor for AAS. The general likelihood of developing AAS is influenced by both genetic and environmental factors; therefore, it is prudent to perform regular imaging and genetic screening of individuals with a family history of both AAS and aortic aneurysm. Tight supervision of risk factors and close observation of patients with AAS could reduce the incidence of this medical condition.

One established indication of risk of AAS is aortic aneurysm [13]. As a result, suggestions for preventive aortic restoration, with a focus on aneurysm diameter, in such patients are provided by the guidelines of professional associations [13,15,99]. Nevertheless, their effectiveness in lowering the prevalence of AAS in the general population is unknown. The diagnosis of aortic aneurysm has become more common over time, and surgical repair rates have also increased [100,101]. However, interventions for AAS continue to rise concurrently [102,103].

Since most patients with type A acute ADs have ascending aortic diameters less than 55 mm, the guidelines' suggestions appear to be overly cautious. Based on the available data, the likelihood of having an aortic diameter larger than 55 mm is approximately 20% and, if the diameter is lower, it is less than one in a million [104]. With a diameter less than 3.5 cm, the normal aorta often presents a deceiving appearance. The prevalence of individuals falling within this smaller size range contributes to the aortic size paradox [105]. Setting a limit of 50 mm or below would undoubtedly prevent some AAS, but doing so would bring higher risks of morbidity and death from ascending aortic surgery. Furthermore, after adjusting for body surface area, the Genetically Triggered Thoracic Aortic Aneurysms and Cardiovascular Conditions (GenTAC) registry revealed that women experienced dissection at narrower aortic diameters than men despite having comparable aortic sizes [106]. Women's body sizes are often smaller than men's; therefore, it is possible that women are receiving less treatment since present guidelines depend on aortic diameters. Regardless, relying only on the size criterion to decide on when to address an aortic aneurysm is inadequate.

A history of hypertension has been shown to be a reliable indicator of type A acute AD [104]. Controlling blood pressure thus becomes vitally important. Given that half of all people with hypertension globally are ignorant of their blood pressure, it appears that patient and clinician education regarding blood pressure is required [107]. Given that AASs are uncommon but many individuals have hypertension, it is critical to identify the underlying mechanism causing AAS. Progress in genetics and translational research may be useful in forecasting future risks of AAS.

The goal of using stabilising aortic wall medications, such as statins, beta-blockers or angiotensin receptor blockers, early in the course of a medical condition is to prevent the aneurysm from progressing [108]. Clinical investigations have demonstrated that statins have a preventive function in AD development and therapy. It has been established that the action of statins on AD seems unlikely to be dependent on the primary action of reducing cholesterol levels. In contrast, minichromosome maintenance proteins, a class of proteins that statins target, are increased in the tissues of the torn aorta wall and are crucial for controlling the cell cycle and mitosis in patients with AD. They have been used to stop the course of aortic illnesses, and there is growing evidence that they can reduce aortic enlargement and rupture [109]. It is still not readily apparent whether these or other medications reduce the risk of AAS in individuals without connective tissue disorders and with or without hypertension; this requires more investigation. The use of fluoroquinolones has been linked to an elevated risk of acute AD and aortic aneurysm, according to population-based research [110]. Furthermore, when these individuals are administered this type of antibiotic, they risk experiencing negative effects [107]. Thus, fluoroquinolones should be avoided in patients at risk for AAS if another treatment option is available [111].

5. Conclusions

Over the past 20 years, there have been significant changes in the diagnosis and management of AAS. AAS must be considered and identified as soon as possible in patients who present with acute chest or back pain and high blood pressure, due to high rates of mortality and morbidity. For AAS, CTA is the preferred diagnostic method. Improved surgical outcomes have led to a considerable decrease in mortality in patients with type A AAS. Because endovascular treatment has become more widely available, the use of medical treatment alone has declined for patients with type B AAS, but in-hospital mortality has not decreased considerably. Furthermore, there are still numerous unanswered questions about the diagnosis and management of AAS. To improve our understanding of the architectural and functional characteristics of the aortic wall, innovations and basic research should be prioritised. To find the disease early, precise biomarkers of AAS are required. It is advisable to expand access to centres for aortic surgery and institutional protocols specific to AAS. To determine the course of treatment for patients with less prevalent types of AAS, more research is required. The effectiveness of preventive therapies in the context of aortic problems needs to be tested by prospective multi-centre clinical trials and, more practically, mandatory registries.

Author Contributions: Conceptualisation, C.M.B. and H.S.; methodology, C.M.B., D.M.B. and A.P.; validation, H.S., D.S.K. and K.B.; formal analysis, C.M.B., V.V. and M.L.; investigation, C.M.B., D.M.B., D.C. and M.O.; data curation, C.M.B., H.S., M.H. and D.M.B.; writing—original draft preparation, C.M.B.; writing—review and editing, D.S.K., A.P., V.V., M.L. and H.S.; visualisation, K.B. and M.H.N.; supervision, D.S.K. and H.S.; project administration, C.M.B. All authors have read and agreed to the published version of the manuscript.

Funding: This research received no external funding.

Institutional Review Board Statement: Not applicable.

Informed Consent Statement: Not applicable.

Data Availability Statement: The data supporting this study's findings are available from the corresponding author upon request.

Conflicts of Interest: The authors declare no conflicts of interest.

References

1. Vilacosta, I.; San Román, J.A.; Aragoncillo, P.; Aragoncillo, P.; Ferreirós, J.; Mendez, R.; Graupner, C.; Batlle, E.; Serrano, J.; Pinto, A.; et al. Penetrating atherosclerotic aortic ulcer: Documentation by transesophageal echocardiography. *J. Am. Coll. Cardiol.* **1998**, *32*, 83–89. [CrossRef] [PubMed]
2. Vilacosta, I.; San Román, J.A. Acute aortic syndrome. *Heart* **2001**, *85*, 365–368. [CrossRef] [PubMed]

3. Vilacosta, I.; Aragoncillo, P.; Cañadas, V.; San Román, J.A.; Ferreirós, J.; Rodríguez, E. Acute aortic syndrome: A new look at an old conundrum. *Heart* **2009**, *95*, 1130–1139. [CrossRef] [PubMed]
4. Macura, K.J.; Corl, F.M.; Fishman, E.K.; Bluemke, D.A. Pathogenesis in acute aortic syndromes: Aortic dissection, intramural hematoma, and penetrating atherosclerotic aortic ulcer. *AJR Am. J. Roentgenol.* **2003**, *181*, 309–316. [CrossRef]
5. Carino, D.; Singh, M.; Molardi, A.; Agostinelli, A.; Goldoni, M.; Pacini, D.; Nicolini, F. Non-A non-B aortic dissection: A systematic review and meta-analysis. *Eur. J. Cardiothorac. Surg.* **2019**, *55*, 653–659. [CrossRef] [PubMed]
6. Lombardi, J.V.; Hughes, G.C.; Appoo, J.J.; Bavaria, J.E.; Beck, A.W.; Cambria, R.P.; Charlton-Ouw, K.; Eslami, M.H.; Kim, K.M.; Leshnower, B.G.; et al. Society for Vascular Surgery (SVS) and Society of Thoracic Surgeons (STS) reporting standards for type B aortic dissections. *J. Vasc. Surg.* **2020**, *71*, 723–747. [CrossRef]
7. Tsai, T.T.; Nienaber, C.A.; Eagle, K.A. Acute aortic syndromes. *Circulation* **2005**, *112*, 3802–3813. [CrossRef]
8. Kouchoukos, N.T.; Dougenis, D. Surgery of the thoracic aorta. *N. Engl. J. Med.* **1997**, *336*, 1876–1888. [CrossRef]
9. Murphy, M.C.; Castner, C.F.; Kouchoukos, N.T. Acute aortic syndromes: Diagnosis and treatment. *Mo. Med.* **2017**, *114*, 458–463.
10. Sweeney, M.S.; Lewis, C.T.; Murphy, M.C.; Williams, J.P.; Frazier, O.H. Cardiac surgical emergencies. *Crit. Care Clin.* **1989**, *5*, 659–678. [CrossRef]
11. Salmasi, M.Y.; Al-Saadi, N.; Hartley, P.; Jarral, O.A.; Raja, S.; Hussein, M.; Redhead, J.; Rosendahl, U.; Nienaber, C.A.; Pepper, J.R.; et al. The risk of misdiagnosis in acute thoracic aortic dissection: A review of current guidelines. *Heart* **2020**, *106*, 885–891. [CrossRef] [PubMed]
12. Zaschke, L.; Habazettl, H.; Thurau, J.; Matschilles, C.; Göhlich, A.; Montagner, M.; Falk, V.; Kurz, S.D. Acute type A aortic dissection: Aortic Dissection Detection Risk Score in emergency care—Surgical delay because of initial misdiagnosis. *Eur. Heart J. Acute Cardiovasc. Care* **2020**, *9*, S40–S47. [CrossRef] [PubMed]
13. Erbel, R.; Aboyans, V.; Boileau, C.; Bossone, E.; Bartolomeo, R.D.; Eggebrecht, H.; Evangelista, A.; Falk, V.; Frank, H.; Gaemperli, O.; et al. 2014 ESC Guidelines on the diagnosis and treatment of aortic diseases: Document covering acute and chronic aortic diseases of the thoracic and abdominal aorta of the adult. The Task Force for the Diagnosis and Treatment of Aortic Diseases of the European Society of Cardiology (ESC). *Eur. Heart J.* **2014**, *35*, 2873–2926, reprinted in *Eur. Heart J.* **2015**, *36*, 2779. [CrossRef]
14. Vilacosta, I.; San Román, J.A.; di Bartolomeo, R.; Eagle, K.; Estrera, A.L.; Ferrera, C.; Kaji, S.; Nienaber, C.A.; Riambau, V.; Schäfers, H.J.; et al. Acute aortic syndrome revisited: JACC State-of-the-Art Review. *J. Am. Coll. Cardiol.* **2021**, *78*, 2106–2125. [CrossRef] [PubMed]
15. Hiratzka, L.F.; Bakris, G.L.; Beckman, J.A.; Bersin, R.M.; Carr, V.F.; Casey, D.E., Jr.; Eagle, K.A.; Hermann, L.K.; Isselbacher, E.M.; Kazerooni, E.A.; et al. 2010 ACCF/AHA/AATS/ACR/ASA/SCA/SCAI/SIR/STS/SVM guidelines for the diagnosis and management of patients with thoracic aortic disease: A report of the American College of Cardiology Foundation/American Heart Association Task Force on Practice Guidelines, American Association for Thoracic Surgery, American College of Radiology, American Stroke Association, Society of Cardiovascular Anesthesiologists, Society for Cardiovascular Angiography and Interventions, Society of Interventional Radiology, Society of Thoracic Surgeons, and Society for Vascular Medicine. *J. Am. Coll. Cardiol.* **2010**, *55*, e27–e129, reprinted in *J. Am. Coll. Cardiol.* **2013**, *62*, 1039–1040. [CrossRef]
16. Landenhed, M.; Engström, G.; Gottsäter, A.; Caulfield, M.P.; Hedblad, B.; Newton-Cheh, C.; Melander, O.; Smith, J.G. Risk profiles for aortic dissection and ruptured or surgically treated aneurysms: A prospective cohort study. *J. Am. Heart Assoc.* **2015**, *4*, e001513. [CrossRef]
17. Pape, L.A.; Awais, M.; Woznicki, E.M.; Suzuki, T.; Trimarchi, S.; Evangelista, A.; Myrmel, T.; Larsen, M.; Harris, K.M.; Greason, K. Presentation, diagnosis, and outcomes of acute aortic dissection: 17-year trends from the International Registry of Acute Aortic Dissection. *J. Am. Coll. Cardiol.* **2015**, *66*, 350–358. [CrossRef]
18. Evangelista Masip, A.; López-Sainz, Á.; Barros Membrilla, A.J.; RESA centers. Spanish Registry of Acute Aortic Syndrome (RESA). Changes in therapeutic management and lower mortality in acute aortic syndrome. *Rev. Esp. Cardiol. Engl. Ed.* **2022**, *75*, 816–824. [CrossRef]
19. Qanadli, S.D.; Malekzadeh, S.; Villard, N.; Jouannic, A.M.; Bodenmann, D.; Tozzi, P.; Rotzinger, D.C. A new clinically driven classification for acute aortic dissection. *Front. Surg.* **2020**, *7*, 37. [CrossRef]
20. Stepinska, J.; Lettino, M.; Ahrens, I.; Bueno, H.; Garcia-Castrillo, L.; Khoury, A.; Lancellotti, P.; Mueller, C.; Muenzel, T.; Oleksiak, A.; et al. Diagnosis and risk stratification of chest pain patients in the emergency department: Focus on acute coronary syndromes. A position paper of the Acute Cardiovascular Care Association. *Eur. Heart J. Acute Cardiovasc. Care* **2020**, *9*, 76–89. [CrossRef]
21. Suzuki, T.; Distante, A.; Zizza, A.; Trimarchi, S.; Villani, M.; Salerno Uriarte, J.A.; De Luca Tupputi Schinosa, L.; Renzulli, A.; Sabino, F. Diagnosis of acute aortic dissection by D-dimer: The International Registry of Acute Aortic Dissection Substudy on Biomarkers (IRAD-Bio) experience. *Circulation* **2009**, *119*, 2702–2707. [CrossRef]
22. Nazerian, P.; Mueller, C.; Soeiro, A.M.; Leidel, B.A.; Salvadeo, S.A.T.; Giachino, F.; Vanni, S.; Grimm, K.; Oliveira, M.T., Jr.; Pivetta, E.; et al. Diagnostic accuracy of the aortic dissection detection risk score plus D-dimer for acute aortic syndromes: The ADvISED prospective multicenter study. *Circulation* **2018**, *137*, 250–258. [CrossRef] [PubMed]
23. Watanabe, H.; Horita, N.; Shibata, Y.; Minegishi, S.; Ota, E.; Kaneko, T. Diagnostic test accuracy of D-dimer for acute aortic syndrome: Systematic review and meta-analysis of 22 studies with 5000 subjects. *Sci. Rep.* **2016**, *6*, 26893. [CrossRef] [PubMed]

24. Gorla, R.; Erbel, R.; Kahlert, P.; Tsagakis, K.; Jakob, H.; Mahabadi, A.A.; Schlosser, T.; Eggebrecht, H.; Bossone, E.; Jánosi, R.A. Accuracy of a diagnostic strategy combining aortic dissection detection risk score and D-dimer levels in patients with suspected acute aortic syndrome. *Eur. Heart J. Acute Cardiovasc. Care* **2017**, *6*, 371–378. [CrossRef]
25. Vardhanabhuti, V.; Nicol, E.; Morgan-Hughes, G.; Roobottom, C.A.; Roditi, G.; Hamilton, M.C.; Bull, R.K.; Pugliese, F.; Williams, M.C.; Stirrup, J.; et al. Recommendations for accurate CT diagnosis of suspected acute aortic syndrome (AAS)—On behalf of the British Society of Cardiovascular Imaging (BSCI)/British Society of Cardiovascular CT (BSCCT). *Br. J. Radiol.* **2016**, *89*, 20150705. [CrossRef]
26. Von Kodolitsch, Y.; Nienaber, C.A.; Dieckmann, C.; Schwartz, A.G.; Hofmann, T.; Brekenfeld, C.; Nicolas, V.; Berger, J.; Meinertz, T. Chest radiography for the diagnosis of acute aortic syndrome. *Am. J. Med.* **2004**, *116*, 73–77. [CrossRef] [PubMed]
27. Murillo, H.; Molvin, L.; Chin, A.S.; Fleischmann, D. Aortic dissection and other acute aortic syndromes: Diagnostic imaging findings from acute to chronic longitudinal progression. *Radiographics* **2021**, *41*, 425–446. [CrossRef]
28. Sommer, T.; Fehske, W.; Holzknecht, N.; Smekal, A.V.; Keller, E.; Lutterbey, G.; Kreft, B.; Kuhl, C.; Gieseke, J.; Abu-Ramadan, D.; et al. Aortic dissection: A comparative study of diagnosis with spiral CT, multiplanar transesophageal echocardiography, and MR imaging. *Radiology* **1996**, *199*, 347–352. [CrossRef]
29. Nienaber, C.A.; von Kodolitsch, Y. Diagnostic imaging of aortic diseases. *Radiologe* **1997**, *37*, 402–409. [CrossRef]
30. Chao, C.P.; Walker, T.G.; Kalva, S.P. Natural history and CT appearances of aortic intramural hematoma. *Radiographics* **2009**, *29*, 791–804. [CrossRef]
31. Pare, J.R.; Liu, R.; Moore, C.L.; Sherban, T.; Kelleher, M.S.; Thomas, S., Jr.; Taylor, R.A. Emergency physician focused cardiac ultrasound improves diagnosis of ascending aortic dissection. *Am. J. Emerg. Med.* **2016**, *34*, 486–492. [CrossRef] [PubMed]
32. Erbel, R.; Engberding, R.; Daniel, W.; Roelandt, J.; Visser, C.; Rennollet, H. Echocardiography in diagnosis of aortic dissection. *Lancet* **1989**, *1*, 457–461. [CrossRef] [PubMed]
33. Castro-Verdes, M.; Yuan, X.; Mitsis, A.; Li, W.; Nienaber, C.A. Transesophageal ultrasound guidance for endovascular interventions on the aorta. *Aorta* **2022**, *10*, 3–12. [CrossRef] [PubMed]
34. Falconi, M.; Oberti, P.; Krauss, J.; Domenech, A.; Cesáreo, V.; Bracco, D.; Pizarro, R. Different clinical features of aortic intramural hematoma versus dissection involving the descending thoracic aorta. *Echocardiography* **2005**, *22*, 629–635. [CrossRef]
35. Harris, K.M.; Strauss, C.E.; Eagle, K.A.; Hirsch, A.T.; Isselbacher, E.M.; Tsai, T.T.; Shiran, H.; Fattori, R.; Evangelista, A.; Cooper, J.V.; et al. Correlates of delayed recognition and treatment of acute type A aortic dissection: The International Registry of Acute Aortic Dissection (IRAD). *Circulation* **2011**, *124*, 1911–1918. [CrossRef] [PubMed]
36. Vagnarelli, F.; Corsini, A.; Bugani, G.; Lorenzini, M.; Longhi, S.; Bacchi Reggiani, M.L.; Biagini, E.; Graziosi, M.; Cinti, L.; Norscini, G.; et al. Troponin T elevation in acute aortic syndromes: Frequency and impact on diagnostic delay and misdiagnosis. *Eur. Heart J. Acute Cardiovasc. Care* **2016**, *5*, 61–71. [CrossRef] [PubMed]
37. Moore, A.G.; Eagle, K.A.; Bruckman, D.; Moon, B.S.; Malouf, J.F.; Fattori, R.; Evangelista, A.; Isselbacher, E.M.; Suzuki, T.; Nienaber, C.A.; et al. Choice of computed tomography, transesophageal echocardiography, magnetic resonance imaging, and aortography in acute aortic dissection: International Registry of Acute Aortic Dissection (IRAD). *Am. J. Cardiol.* **2002**, *89*, 1235–1238. [CrossRef]
38. Hagan, P.G.; Nienaber, C.A.; Isselbacher, E.M.; Bruckman, D.; Karavite, D.J.; Russman, P.L.; Evangelista, A.; Fattori, R.; Suzuki, T.; Oh, J.K.; et al. The International Registry of Acute Aortic Dissection (IRAD): New insights into an old disease. *JAMA* **2000**, *283*, 897–903. [CrossRef]
39. Panting, J.R.; Norell, M.S.; Baker, C.; Nicholson, A.A. Feasibility, accuracy and safety of magnetic resonance imaging in acute aortic dissection. *Clin. Radiol.* **1995**, *50*, 455–458. [CrossRef]
40. Di Cesare, E.; Giordano, A.V.; Cerone, G.; De Remigis, F.; Deusanio, G.; Masciocchi, C. Comparative evaluation of TEE, conventional MRI and contrast-enhanced 3D breath-hold MRA in the post-operative follow-up of dissecting aneurysms. *Int. J. Card. Imaging* **2000**, *16*, 135–147. [CrossRef]
41. Laissy, J.P.; Blanc, F.; Soyer, P.; Assayag, P.; Sibert, A.; Tebboune, D.; Arrivé, L.; Brochet, E.; Hvass, U.; Langlois, J. Thoracic aortic dissection: Diagnosis with transesophageal echocardiography versus MR imaging. *Radiology* **1995**, *194*, 331–336. [CrossRef]
42. Evangelista, A.; Garcia-del-Castillo, H.; Gonzalez-Alujas, T.; Dominguez-Oronoz, R.; Salas, A.; Permanyer-Miralda, G.; Soler-Soler, J. Diagnosis of ascending aortic dissection by transesophageal echocardiography: Utility of M-mode in recognizing artifacts. *J. Am. Coll. Cardiol.* **1996**, *27*, 102–107. [CrossRef]
43. Evangelista, A.; Avegliano, G.; Aguilar, R.; Cuellar, H.; Igual, A.; González-Alujas, T.; Rodríguez-Palomares, J.; Mahia, P.; García-Dorado, D. Impact of contrast-enhanced echocardiography on the diagnostic algorithm of acute aortic dissection. *Eur. Heart J.* **2010**, *31*, 472–479. [CrossRef] [PubMed]
44. Nazerian, P.; Vanni, S.; Castelli, M.; Morello, F.; Tozzetti, C.; Zagli, G.; Giannazzo, G.; Vergara, R.; Grifoni, S. Diagnostic performance of emergency transthoracic focus cardiac ultrasound in suspected acute type A aortic dissection. *Intern. Emerg. Med.* **2014**, *9*, 665–670. [CrossRef] [PubMed]
45. Akutsu, K.; Sato, N.; Yamamoto, T.; Morita, N.; Takagi, H.; Fujita, N.; Tanaka, K.; Takano, T.L. A rapid bedside D-dimer assay (cardiac D-dimer) for screening of clinically suspected acute aortic dissection. *Circ. J.* **2005**, *69*, 397–403. [CrossRef] [PubMed]
46. Sbarouni, E.; Georgiadou, P.; Marathias, A.; Geroulanos, S.; Kremastinos, D.T. D-dimer and BNP levels in acute aortic dissection. *Int. J. Cardiol.* **2007**, *122*, 170–172. [CrossRef] [PubMed]

47. Shao, N.; Xia, S.; Wang, J.; Shao, N.; Xia, S.; Wang, J.; Zhou, X.; Huang, Z.; Zhu, W.; Chen, Y. The role of D-dimers in the diagnosis of acute aortic dissection. *Mol. Biol. Rep.* **2014**, *41*, 6397–6403. [CrossRef] [PubMed]
48. Wen, D.; Du, X.; Dong, J.Z.; Zhou, X.L.; Ma, C.S. Value of D-dimer and C reactive protein in predicting inhospital death in acute aortic dissection. *Heart* **2013**, *99*, 1192–1197. [CrossRef] [PubMed]
49. Huang, B.; Yang, Y.; Lu, H.; Zhao, Z.; Zhang, S.; Hui, R.; Fan, X. Impact of D-dimer levels on admission on inhospital and long-term outcome in patients with type A acute aortic dissection. *Am. J. Cardiol.* **2015**, *115*, 1595–1600. [CrossRef]
50. Giachino, F.; Loiacono, M.; Lucchiari, M.; Manzo, M.; Battista, S.; Saglio, E.; Lupia, E.; Moiraghi, C.; Hirsch, E.; Mengozzi, G. Rule out of acute aortic dissection with plasma matrix metalloproteinase 8 in the emergency department. *Crit. Care* **2013**, *17*, R33. [CrossRef]
51. Kobayashi, N.; Hata, N.; Kume, N.; Yokoyama, S.; Takano, M.; Shinada, T.; Tomita, K.; Shirakabe, A.; Inami, T.; Seino, Y.; et al. Detection of acute aortic dissection by extremely high soluble lectin-like oxidized LDL receptor-1 (sLOX-1) and low troponin T levels in blood. *Int. J. Cardiol.* **2013**, *165*, 557–559. [CrossRef] [PubMed]
52. Suzuki, T.; Katoh, H.; Watanabe, M.; Kurabayashi, M.; Hiramori, K.; Hori, S.; Nobuyoshi, M.; Tanaka, H.; Kodama, K.; Sato, H.; et al. Novel biochemical diagnostic method for aortic dissection: Results of a prospective study using an immunoassay of smooth muscle myosin heavy chain. *Circulation* **1996**, *93*, 1244–1249. [CrossRef] [PubMed]
53. Shinohara, T.; Suzuki, K.; Okada, M.; Shiigai, M.; Shimizu, M.; Maehara, T.; Ohsuzu, F. Soluble elastin fragments in serum are elevated in acute aortic dissection. *Arterioscler. Thromb. Vasc. Biol.* **2003**, *23*, 1839–1844. [CrossRef] [PubMed]
54. Harris, K.M.; Braverman, A.C.; Eagle, K.A.; Woznicki, E.M.; Pyeritz, R.E.; Myrmel, T.; Peterson, M.D.; Voehringer, M.; Fattori, R.; Januzzi, J.L.; et al. Acute aortic intramural hematoma: An analysis from the International Registry of Acute Aortic Dissection. *Circulation* **2012**, *126*, S91–S96. [CrossRef] [PubMed]
55. Keren, A.; Kim, C.B.; Hu, B.S.; Eyngorina, I.; Billingham, M.E.; Mitchell, R.S.; Miller, D.C.; Popp, R.L.; Schnittger, I. Accuracy of biplane and multiplane transesophageal echocardiography in diagnosis of typical acute aortic dissection and intramural hematoma. *J. Am. Coll. Cardiol.* **1996**, *28*, 627–636. [CrossRef] [PubMed]
56. Kang, D.H.; Song, J.K.; Song, M.G.; Lee, I.S.; Song, H.; Lee, J.W.; Park, S.W.; Kim, Y.H.; Lim, T.H.; Park, S.J. Clinical and echocardiographic outcomes of aortic intramural hemorrhage compared with acute aortic dissection. *Am. J. Cardiol.* **1998**, *81*, 202–206. [CrossRef] [PubMed]
57. Pepi, M.; Campodonico, J.; Galli, C.; Tamborini, G.; Barbier, P.; Doria, E.; Maltagliati, A.; Alimento, M.; Spirito, R. Rapid diagnosis and management of thoracic aortic dissection and intramural haematoma: A prospective study of advantages of multiplane vs. biplane transoesophageal echocardiography. *Eur. J. Echocardiogr.* **2000**, *1*, 72–79. [CrossRef]
58. Winnerkvist, A.; Lockowandt, U.; Rasmussen, E.; Rådegran, K. A prospective study of medically treated acute type B aortic dissection. *Eur. J. Vasc. Endovasc. Surg.* **2006**, *32*, 349–355. [CrossRef]
59. Schlatter, T.; Auriol, J.; Marcheix, B.; Lebbadi, M.; Marachet, M.A.; Dang-Tran, K.D.; Tran, M.; Honton, B.; Gardette, V.; Rousseau, H. Type B intramural hematoma of the aorta: Evolution and prognostic value of intimal erosion. *J. Vasc. Interv. Radiol.* **2011**, *22*, 533–541. [CrossRef]
60. Nienaber, C.A.; Powell, J.T. Management of acute aortic syndromes. *Eur. Heart J.* **2012**, *33*, 26–35. [CrossRef]
61. Khachatryan, Z.; Leontyev, S.; Magomedov, K.; Haunschild, J.; Holzhey, D.M.; Misfeld, M.; Etz, C.D.; Borger, M.A. Management of aortic root in type A dissection: Bentall approach. *J. Card. Surg.* **2021**, *36*, 1779–1785. [CrossRef]
62. Kallenbach, K.; Büsch, C.; Rylski, B.; Dohle, D.S.; Krüger, T.; Holubec, T.; Brickwedel, J.; Pöling, J.; Noack, T.; Hagl, C.; et al. Treatment of the aortic root in acute aortic dissection type A: Insights from the German Registry for Acute Aortic Dissection Type A. *Eur. J. Cardiothorac. Surg.* **2022**, *20*, ezac261. [CrossRef] [PubMed]
63. Soto, M.E.; Ochoa-Hein, E.; Anaya-Ayala, J.E.; Ayala-Picazo, M.; Koretzky, S.G. Systematic review and meta-analysis of aortic valve-sparing surgery versus replacement surgery in ascending aortic aneurysms and dissection in patients with Marfan syndrome and other genetic connective tissue disorders. *J. Thorac. Dis.* **2021**, *13*, 4830–4844. [CrossRef]
64. Norton, E.L.; Wu, X.; Farhat, L.; Kim, K.M.; Patel, H.J.; Deeb, G.M.; Yang, B. Dissection of arch branches alone: An indication for aggressive arch management in type A dissection. *Ann. Thorac. Surg.* **2020**, *109*, 487–494. [CrossRef] [PubMed]
65. Di Bartolomeo, R.; Pacini, D.; Savini, C.; Pilato, E.; Martin-Suarez, S.; Di Marco, L.; Di Eusanio, M. Complex thoracic aortic disease: Single-stage procedure with the frozen elephant trunk technique. *J. Thorac. Cardiovasc. Surg.* **2010**, *140*, S81–S91. [CrossRef] [PubMed]
66. Beckmann, E.; Martens, A.; Kaufeld, T.; Natanov, R.; Krueger, H.; Rudolph, L.; Haverich, A.; Shrestha, M. Frozen elephant trunk in acute aortic type A dissection: Risk analysis of concomitant root replacement. *Eur. J. Cardiothorac. Surg.* **2022**, *62*, ezac051. [CrossRef] [PubMed]
67. Czerny, M.; Schmidli, J.; Adler, S.; van den Berg, J.C.; Bertoglio, L.; Carrel, T.; Chiesa, R.; Clough, R.E.; Eberle, B.; Etz, C.; et al. Current options and recommendations for the treatment of thoracic aortic pathologies involving the aortic arch: An expert consensus document of the European Association for Cardio-Thoracic surgery (EACTS) and the European Society for Vascular Surgery (ESVS). *Eur. J. Cardiothorac. Surg.* **2019**, *55*, 133–162. [CrossRef] [PubMed]
68. Booher, A.M.; Isselbacher, E.M.; Nienaber, C.A.; Trimarchi, S.; Evangelista, A.; Montgomery, D.G.; Froehlich, J.B.; Ehrlich, M.P.; Oh, J.K.; Januzzi, J.L.; et al. The IRAD classification system for characterizing survival after aortic dissection. *Am. J. Med.* **2013**, *126*, 730.e19–730.e24. [CrossRef]

69. Conzelmann, L.O.; Hoffmann, I.; Blettner, M.; Kallenbach, K.; Karck, M.; Dapunt, O.; Borger, M.A.; Weigang, E.; GERAADA Investigators. Analysis of risk factors for neurological dysfunction in patients with acute aortic dissection type A: Data from the German Registry for Acute Aortic Dissection Type A (GERAADA). *Eur. J. Cardiothorac. Surg.* **2012**, *42*, 557–565. [CrossRef]
70. Muehle, A.; Chou, D.; Shah, A.; Khoynezhad, A. Experiences with ascending aortic endografts using FDA IDE approved devices. What has been done, what lesions can be treated and what challenges remain. *J. Cardiovasc. Surg.* **2015**, *56*, 11–18.
71. Nienaber, C.A.; Kische, S.; Rousseau, H.; Eggebrecht, H.; Rehders, T.C.; Kundt, G.; Glass, A.; Scheinert, D.; Czerny, M.; Kleinfeldt, T.; et al. Endovascular repair of type B aortic dissection: Long-term results of the randomized investigation of stent grafts in aortic dissection trial. *Circ. Cardiovasc. Interv.* **2013**, *6*, 407–416. [CrossRef]
72. Munshi, B.; Doyle, B.J.; Ritter, J.C.; Jansen, S.; Parker, L.P.; Riambau, V.; Bicknell, C.; Norman, P.E.; Wanhainen, A. Surgical decision making in uncomplicated type B aortic dissection: A survey of Australian/New Zealand and European surgeons. *Eur. J. Vasc. Endovasc. Surg.* **2020**, *60*, 194–200. [CrossRef] [PubMed]
73. Evangelista, A.; Mukherjee, D.; Mehta, R.H.; O'Gara, P.T.; Fattori, R.; Cooper, J.V.; Smith, D.E.; Oh, J.K.; Hutchison, S.; Sechtem, U.; et al. Acute intramural hematoma of the aorta: A mystery in evolution. *Circulation* **2005**, *111*, 1063–1070. [CrossRef] [PubMed]
74. Fattori, R.; Montgomery, D.; Lovato, L.; Kische, S.; Di Eusanio, M.; Ince, H.; Eagle, K.A.; Isselbacher, E.M.; Nienaber, C.A. Survival after endovascular therapy in patients with type B aortic dissection: A report from the International Registry of Acute Aortic Dissection (IRAD). *JACC Cardiovasc. Interv.* **2013**, *6*, 876–882. [CrossRef] [PubMed]
75. Bavaria, J.E.; Brinkman, W.T.; Hughes, G.C.; Khoynezhad, A.; Szeto, W.Y.; Azizzadeh, A.; Lee, W.A.; White, R.A. Outcomes of thoracic endovascular aortic repair in acute type B aortic dissection: Results from the Valiant United States investigational device exemption study. *Ann. Thorac. Surg.* **2015**, *100*, 802–809. [CrossRef] [PubMed]
76. Brunkwall, J.; Kasprzak, P.; Verhoeven, E.; Heijmen, R.; Taylor, P.; ADSORB Trialists; Alric, P.; Canaud, L.; Janotta, M.; Raithel, D.; et al. Endovascular repair of acute uncomplicated aortic type B dissection promotes aortic remodelling: 1 year results of the ADSORB trial. *Eur. J. Vasc. Endovasc. Surg.* **2014**, *48*, 285–291, reprinted in *Eur. J. Vasc. Endovasc. Surg.* **2015**, *50*, 130. [CrossRef] [PubMed]
77. Houben, I.B.; van Bakel, T.M.J.; Patel, H.J. Type B intramural hematoma: Thoracic endovascular aortic repair (TEVAR) or conservative approach? *Ann. Cardiothorac. Surg.* **2019**, *8*, 483–487. [CrossRef] [PubMed]
78. Kitai, T.; Kaji, S.; Yamamuro, A.; Tani, T.; Tamita, K.; Kinoshita, M.; Ehara, N.; Kobori, A.; Nasu, M.; Okada, Y.; et al. Clinical outcomes of medical therapy and timely operation in initially diagnosed type A aortic intramural hematoma: A 20-year experience. *Circulation* **2009**, *120*, S292–S298. [CrossRef]
79. Song, J.K.; Yim, J.H.; Ahn, J.M.; Kim, D.H.; Kang, J.W.; Lee, T.Y.; Song, J.M.; Choo, S.J.; Kang, D.H.; Chung, C.H.; et al. Outcomes of patients with acute type A aortic intramural hematoma. *Circulation* **2009**, *120*, 2046–2052. [CrossRef]
80. Kitai, T.; Kaji, S.; Yamamuro, A.; Tani, T.; Kinoshita, M.; Ehara, N.; Kobori, A.; Kim, K.; Kita, T.; Furukawa, Y. Detection of intimal defect by 64-row multidetector computed tomography in patients with acute aortic intramural hematoma. *Circulation* **2011**, *124*, S174–S178. [CrossRef]
81. Ferrera, C.; Vilacosta, I.; Cabeza, B.; Cobiella, J.; Martínez, I.; Saiz-Pardo Sanz, M.; Bustos, A.; Serrano, F.J.; Maroto, L. Diagnosing aortic intramural hematoma: Current perspectives. *Vasc. Health Risk Manag.* **2020**, *16*, 203–213. [CrossRef] [PubMed]
82. Ferrera, C.; Vilacosta, I.; Gómez-Polo, J.C.; Villanueva-Medina, S.; Cabeza, B.; Ortega, L.; Cañadas, V.; Carnero-Alcázar, M.; Martínez-López, I.; Maroto-Castellanos, L.; et al. Evolution and prognosis of intramural aortic hematoma. Insights from a midterm cohort study. *Int. J. Cardiol.* **2017**, *249*, 410–413. [CrossRef] [PubMed]
83. Motoyoshi, N.; Moizumi, Y.; Komatsu, T.; Tabayashi, K. Intramural hematoma and dissection involving ascending aorta: The clinical features and prognosis. *Eur. J. Cardiothorac. Surg.* **2003**, *24*, 237–242. [CrossRef] [PubMed]
84. Zhang, G.; Feng, Q.; Zheng, D.; Ma, L.; Li, R.; Jiang, J.; Ni, Y. Early aggressive medical treatment associated with selective prophylactic aortic stent-grafting for aortic intramural hematoma. *Thorac. Cardiovasc. Surg.* **2011**, *59*, 342–348. [CrossRef] [PubMed]
85. Song, J.K.; Kim, H.S.; Song, J.M.; Kang, D.H.; Ha, J.W.; Rim, S.J.; Chung, N.; Kim, K.S.; Park, S.W.; Kim, Y.J. Outcomes of medically treated patients with aortic intramural hematoma. *Am. J. Med.* **2002**, *113*, 181–187. [CrossRef] [PubMed]
86. Li, D.L.; Zhang, H.K.; Cai, Y.Y.; Jin, W.; Chen, X.D.; Tian, L.; Li, M. Acute type B aortic intramural hematoma: Treatment strategy and the role of endovascular repair. *J. Endovasc. Ther.* **2010**, *17*, 617–621. [CrossRef]
87. Czerny, M.; Schmidli, J.; Bertoglio, L.; Carrel, T.; Chiesa, R.; Clough, R.E.; Grabenwöger, M.; Kari, F.A.; Mestres, C.A.; Rylski, B.; et al. Clinical cases referring to diagnosis and management of patients with thoracic aortic pathologies involving the aortic arch: A companion document of the 2018 European Association for Cardio-Thoracic Surgery (EACTS) and the European Society for Vascular Surgery (ESVS) expert consensus document addressing current options and recommendations for the treatment of thoracic aortic pathologies involving the aortic arch. *Eur. J. Cardio-Thorac. Surg. Off. J. Eur. Assoc. Cardio-Thorac. Surg.* **2019**, *55*, 163–171. [CrossRef]
88. Andersen, N.D.; Ganapathi, A.M.; Hanna, J.M.; Williams, J.B.; Gaca, J.G.; Hughes, G.C. Outcomes of acute type A dissection repair before and after implementation of a multidisciplinary thoracic aortic surgery program. *J. Am. Coll. Cardiol.* **2014**, *63*, 1796–1803. [CrossRef]
89. Ferrera, C.; Vilacosta, I.; Busca, P.; Martínez, A.M.; Serrano, F.J.; Maroto, L.C. Código Aorta: Proyecto piloto de una red asistencial para la atención al paciente con síndrome aórtico agudo. *Rev. Esp. Cardiol.* **2021**, *75*, 95–98. [CrossRef]

90. Harris, K.M.; Strauss, C.E.; Duval, S.; Unger, B.T.; Kroshus, T.J.; Inampudi, S.; Cohen, J.D.; Kapsner, C.; Boland, L.L.; Eales, F.; et al. Multidisciplinary standardized care for acute aortic dissection: Design and initial outcomes of a regional care model. *Circ. Cardiovasc. Qual. Outcomes* **2010**, *3*, 424–430. [CrossRef]
91. Vaja, R.; Talukder, S.; Norkunas, M.; Hoffman, R.; Nienaber, C.; Pepper, J.; Rosendahl, U.; Asimakopoulos, G.; Quarto, C. Impact of a streamlined rotational system for the management of acute aortic syndrome: Sharing is caring. *Eur. J. Cardiothorac. Surg.* **2019**, *55*, 984–989. [CrossRef] [PubMed]
92. Chikwe, J.; Cavallaro, P.; Itagaki, S.; Seigerman, M.; Diluozzo, G.; Adams, D.H. National outcomes in acute aortic dissection: Influence of surgeon and institutional volume on operative mortality. *Ann. Thorac. Surg.* **2013**, *95*, 1563–1569. [CrossRef] [PubMed]
93. Andersen, N.D.; Benrashid, E.; Ross, A.K.; Pickett, L.C.; Smith, P.K.; Daneshmand, M.A.; Schroder, J.N.; Gaca, J.G.; Hughes, G.C. The utility of the aortic dissection team: Outcomes and insights after a decade of experience. *Ann. Cardiothorac. Surg.* **2016**, *5*, 194–201. [CrossRef] [PubMed]
94. Bashir, M.; Harky, A.; Fok, M.; Shaw, M.; Hickey, G.L.; Grant, S.W.; Uppal, R.; Oo, A. Acute type A aortic dissection in the United Kingdom: Surgeon volume-outcome relation. *J. Thorac. Cardiovasc. Surg.* **2017**, *154*, 398–406. [CrossRef] [PubMed]
95. Umana-Pizano, J.B.; Nissen, A.P.; Sandhu, H.K.; Miller, C.C.; Loghin, A.; Safi, H.J.; Eisenberg, S.B.; Estrera, A.L.; Nguyen, T.C. Acute type A dissection repair by high-volume vs low-volume surgeons at a high-volume aortic center. *Ann. Thorac. Surg.* **2019**, *108*, 1330–1336. [CrossRef]
96. Khan, H.; Hussain, A.; Chaubey, S.; Sameh, M.; Salter, I.; Deshpande, R.; Baghai, M.; Wendler, O. Acute aortic dissection type A: Impact of aortic specialists on short and long term outcomes. *J. Card. Surg.* **2021**, *36*, 952–958. [CrossRef] [PubMed]
97. Chen, S.W.; Kuo, C.F.; Huang, Y.T.; Lin, W.T.; Chien-Chia Wu, V.; Chou, A.H.; Lin, P.J.; Chang, S.H.; Chu, P.H. Association of family history with incidence and outcomes of aortic dissection. *J. Am. Coll. Cardiol.* **2020**, *76*, 1181–1192. [CrossRef]
98. Raunsø, J.; Song, R.J.; Vasan, R.S.; Bourdillon, M.T.; Nørager, B.; Torp-Pedersen, C.; Gislason, G.H.; Xanthakis, V.; Andersson, C. Familial clustering of aortic size, aneurysms, and dissections in the community. *Circulation* **2020**, *142*, 920–928. [CrossRef]
99. Riambau, V.; Böckler, D.; Brunkwall, J.; Cao, P.; Chiesa, R.; Coppi, G.; Czerny, M.; Fraedrich, G.; Haulon, S.; Jacobs, M.J.; et al. Editor's Choice—Management of descending thoracic aorta diseases: Clinical practice guidelines of the European Society for Vascular Surgery (ESVS). *Eur. J. Vasc. Endovasc. Surg.* **2017**, *53*, 4–52. [CrossRef]
100. Olsson, C.; Thelin, S.; Ståhle, E.; Ekbom, A.; Granath, F. Thoracic aortic aneurysm and dissection: Increasing prevalence and improved outcomes reported in a nationwide population-based study of more than 14,000 cases from 1987 to 2002. *Circulation* **2006**, *114*, 2611–2618. [CrossRef]
101. Wang, G.J.; Jackson, B.M.; Foley, P.J.; Damrauer, S.M.; Goodney, P.P.; Kelz, R.R.; Wirtalla, C.; Fairman, R.M. National trends in admissions, repair, and mortality for thoracic aortic aneurysm and type B dissection in the National Inpatient Sample. *J. Vasc. Surg.* **2018**, *67*, 1649–1658. [CrossRef] [PubMed]
102. Mullan, C.W.; Mori, M.; Bin Mahmood, S.U.; Yousef, S.; Mangi, A.A.; Elefteriades, J.A.; Geirsson, A. Incidence and characteristics of hospitalization for proximal aortic surgery for acute syndromes and for aneurysms in the USA from 2005 to 2014. *Eur. J. Cardiothorac. Surg.* **2020**, *58*, 583–589. [CrossRef] [PubMed]
103. Paruchuri, V.; Salhab, K.F.; Kuzmik, G.; Gubernikoff, G.; Gubernikoff, G.; Fang, H.; Rizzo, J.A.; Ziganshin, B.A.; Elefteriades, J.A. Aortic Size Distribution in the General Population: Explaining the Size Paradox in Aortic Dissection. *Cardiology* **2015**, *131*, 265–272, Erratum in *Cardiology* **2015**, *132*, 44. [CrossRef] [PubMed]
104. Elbadawi, A.; Elgendy, I.Y.; Jimenez, E.; Omer, M.A.; Shahin, H.I.; Ogunbayo, G.O.; Paniagua, D.; Jneid, H. Trends and outcomes of elective thoracic aortic repair and acute thoracic aortic syndromes in the United States. *Am. J. Med.* **2021**, *134*, 902–909.e5. [CrossRef] [PubMed]
105. Pape, L.A.; Tsai, T.T.; Isselbacher, E.M.; Oh, J.K.; O'gara, P.T.; Evangelista, A.; Fattori, R.; Meinhardt, G.; Trimarchi, S.; Bossone, E. Aortic diameter ≥ 5.5 cm is not a good predictor of type A aortic dissection: Observations from the International Registry of Acute Aortic Dissection (IRAD). *Circulation* **2007**, *116*, 1120–1127. [CrossRef] [PubMed]
106. Holmes, K.W.; Maslen, C.L.; Kindem, M.; Kroner, B.L.; Song, H.K.; Ravekes, W.; Dietz, H.C.; Weinsaft, J.W.; Roman, M.J.; Devereux, R.B.; et al. GenTAC registry report: Gender differences among individuals with genetically triggered thoracic aortic aneurysm and dissection. *Am. J. Med. Genet. A* **2013**, *161*, 779–786. [CrossRef] [PubMed]
107. Salata, K.; Syed, M.; Hussain, M.A.; de Mestral, C.; Greco, E.; Mamdani, M.; Tu, J.V.; Forbes, T.L.; Bhatt, D.L.; Verma, S.; et al. Statins Reduce Abdominal Aortic Aneurysm Growth, Rupture, and Perioperative Mortality: A Systematic Review and Meta-Analysis. *J. Am. Heart Assoc.* **2018**, *7*, e008657. [CrossRef]
108. Whelton, P.K.; Carey, R.M.; Aronow, W.S.; Casey, D.E., Jr.; Collins, K.J.; Dennison Himmelfarb, C.; DePalma, S.M.; Gidding, S.; Jamerson, K.A.; Jones, D.W. 2017 ACC/AHA/AAPA/ABC/ACPM/AGS/APhA/ASH/ASPC/NMA/PCNA guideline for the prevention, detection, evaluation, and management of high blood pressure in adults: A report of the American College of Cardiology/American Heart Association Task Force on Clinical Practice Guidelines. *Hypertension* **2018**, *71*, 1269–1324; reprinted in *J. Am. Coll. Cardiol.* **2018**, *71*, 2275–2279. [CrossRef]
109. Chen, S.W.; Chan, Y.H.; Chien-Chia Wu, V.; Cheng, Y.T.; Chen, D.Y.; Lin, C.P.; Hung, K.C.; Chang, S.H.; Chu, P.H.; Chou, A.H. Effects of fluoroquinolones on outcomes of patients with aortic dissection or aneurysm. *J. Am. Coll. Cardiol.* **2021**, *77*, 1875–1887. [CrossRef]

110. Chen, C.; Patterson, B.; Simpson, R.; Li, Y.; Chen, Z.; Lv, Q.; Guo, D.; Li, X.; Fu, W.; Guo, B. Do fluoroquinolones increase aortic aneurysm or dissection incidence and mortality? A systematic review and meta-analysis. *Front. Cardiovasc. Med.* **2022**, *9*, 949538. [CrossRef]
111. Ribeiro, N.V.; Melo, R.G.; Guerra, N.C.; Nobre, Â.; Fernandes, R.M.; Pedro, L.M.; Costa, J.; Pinto, F.J.; Caldeira, D. Fluoroquinolones Are Associated with Increased Risk of Aortic Aneurysm or Dissection: Systematic Review and Meta-analysis. *Semin. Thorac. Cardiovasc. Surg.* **2021**, *33*, 907–918. [CrossRef]

Disclaimer/Publisher's Note: The statements, opinions and data contained in all publications are solely those of the individual author(s) and contributor(s) and not of MDPI and/or the editor(s). MDPI and/or the editor(s) disclaim responsibility for any injury to people or property resulting from any ideas, methods, instructions or products referred to in the content.

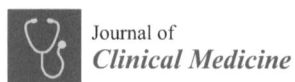 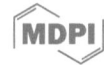

Article

Factors Associated with Early Mortality in Acute Type A Aortic Dissection—A Single-Centre Experience

Panagiotis Doukas [1,*], Nicola Dalibor [1], András Keszei [2], Jelle Frankort [1], Julia Krabbe [3], Rachad Zayat [4], Michael J. Jacobs [1], Alexander Gombert [1], Payam Akhyari [4] and Arash Mehdiani [4]

1. European Vascular Center Aachen-Maastricht, Department of Vascular Surgery, RWTH University Hospital Aachen, Pauwelsstraße 30, 52074 Aachen, Germany; nicola.dalibor@rwth-aachen.de (N.D.); jefrankort@ukaachen.de (J.F.); mjacobs@ukaachen.de (M.J.J.); agombert@ukaachen.de (A.G.)
2. Center for Translational & Clinical Research Aachen (CTC-A), RWTH Aachen University, Pauwelsstraße 30, 52074 Aachen, Germany; akeszei@ukaachen.de
3. Institute of Occupational, Social and Environmental Medicine, Medical Faculty, RWTH Aachen University, Pauwelsstraße 30, 52074 Aachen, Germany
4. Clinic for Cardiac Surgery, University Hospital RWTH Aachen, Pauwelsstraße 30, 52074 Aachen, Germany; rzayat@ukaachen.de (R.Z.); pakhyari@ukaachen.de (P.A.); amehdiani@ukaachen.de (A.M.)
* Correspondence: pdoukas@ukaachen.de; Tel.: +49-241-8080832

Citation: Doukas, P.; Dalibor, N.; Keszei, A.; Frankort, J.; Krabbe, J.; Zayat, R.; Jacobs, M.J.; Gombert, A.; Akhyari, P.; Mehdiani, A. Factors Associated with Early Mortality in Acute Type A Aortic Dissection—A Single-Centre Experience. *J. Clin. Med.* 2024, *13*, 1023. https://doi.org/10.3390/jcm13041023

Academic Editor: Reinhard Kopp

Received: 24 January 2024
Revised: 31 January 2024
Accepted: 8 February 2024
Published: 10 February 2024

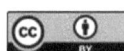

Copyright: © 2024 by the authors. Licensee MDPI, Basel, Switzerland. This article is an open access article distributed under the terms and conditions of the Creative Commons Attribution (CC BY) license (https://creativecommons.org/licenses/by/4.0/).

Abstract: Background: Acute aortic dissection type A (AADA) is a surgical emergency with relevant mortality and morbidity despite improvements in current management protocols. Identifying patients at risk of a fatal outcome and controlling the factors associated with mortality remain of paramount importance. Methods: In this retrospective observational study, we reviewed the medical records of 117 patients with AADA, who were referred to our centre and operated on between 2005 and 2021. Preoperative, intraoperative, and postoperative variables were analysed and tested for their correlation with in-hospital mortality. Results: The overall survival rate was 83%. Preoperatively, factors associated with mortality were age ($p = 0.02$), chronic hypertension ($p = 0.02$), any grade of aortic valve stenosis in the patient's medical history ($p = 0.03$), atrial fibrillation ($p = 0.04$), and oral anticoagulation ($p = 0.04$). Non-survivors had significantly longer operative times ($p = 0.002$). During the postoperative phase, mortality was strongly associated with acute kidney injury (AKI) ($p < 0.001$), acute heart failure ($p < 0.001$), stroke ($p = 0.02$), focal neurological deficits ($p = 0.02$), and sepsis ($p = 0.001$). In the multivariate regression analysis, the onset of postoperative focal neurological deficits was the best predictor of a fatal outcome after adjusting for ARDS (odds ratio: 5.8, 95%-CI: 1.2–41.7, $p = 0.04$). Conclusions: In this retrospective analysis, atrial fibrillation, oral anticoagulation, hypertension, and age were significantly correlated with mortality. Postoperatively, acute kidney injury, acute heart failure, sepsis, and focal neurological deficits were correlated with in-hospital mortality, and focal neurological deficit has been identified as a significant predictor of fatal outcomes. Early detection and interdisciplinary management of at-risk patients remain crucial throughout the postoperative phase.

Keywords: aortic dissection; type A; management; outcomes; complications

1. Introduction

Aortic dissection involving the ascending aorta and/or the aortic arch, defined as type A aortic dissection according to the Stanford classification, remains an acute, critical pathology requiring emergent surgical treatment. Although diagnostic and treatment protocols have been continuously improved and optimized through the years, the associated mortality rates are still significant (17.7% to 22% in-hospital mortality and a 65% survival rate over the following 10 years) [1,2]. Many aspects of the surgical management of acute aortic dissections type A (AADA), such as the extent of distal aortic reconstruction and management of the aortic root, among others, remain the subject of debate among clinicians [3], since reducing the complexity of surgery may improve early outcomes on the one hand, but may lead to increased risk of reoperation on the other [4].

Furthermore, complications in the postoperative phase after this challenging procedure may lead to adverse events, potentially affecting the patients' prognosis and survival [5]. Prompt identification of patients at risk for complications and early intervention may improve outcomes and reduce in-hospital mortality.

In this retrospective observational study, we report our experience with AADA cases at our centre over the last 16 years. This study aimed to identify the factors that may influence the postoperative prognosis.

2. Materials and Methods

2.1. Patients

In this study, we retrospectively reviewed the medical records of 117 patients with acute AADA, who were referred to our centre and underwent surgery between 2005 and 2021. The exclusion criteria were subacute type A aortic dissection, defined as older than 2 weeks; chronic aortic dissection, defined as older than 90 days [6]; patients declared dead on arrival in the emergency department; and patients that did not undergo surgery. The study was reviewed and approved by the ethics committee of the University Hospital RWTH Aachen (EK 20-003) and was designed according to the STROBE criteria and the Declaration of Helsinki.

2.2. Surgery

After the initial clinical evaluation in the emergency department and radiologic confirmation of diagnosis through an ECG-gated CT scan, the patients were brought to the operating room. The operating team consisted of two experienced surgeons and a senior resident. The surgical protocol was initiated with median sternotomy and establishment of cardiopulmonary bypass (CBP) under full heparinization. The right subclavian, right axillary, or left femoral artery was used as an access site for arterial cannulation. In some cases, direct cannulation of the aorta was possible. A two-stage venous cannula was placed in most cases in the right atrium, with femoral venous cannulation as a second option, according to the standard procedure as described in the literature [7]. Cerebral perfusion was established unilaterally or bilaterally in an antegrade manner. During the early phase of the investigated period, patients with pathologies limited to the ascending aorta did not undergo selective cerebral perfusion. After initiation of the CBP, depending on the extent of the planned distal reconstruction, the procedure was performed under hypothermic circulatory arrest and the patient was cooled down to 18 °C. Antegrade cardioplegia with Bretschneider cardioplegia solution (Custodiol®, Dr. F. Köhler Chemie GmbH., Bensheim, Germany) was used to protect the myocardium. Aortic root management was dependent on valve functionality and on whether the aortic root was affected by the dissection. If possible, the aortic root was managed conservatively or with valve-sparing reconstruction using the David technique. The extent of distal repair was decided depending on the state of the aortic arch and descending aorta. Total arch repair was performed in cases of complex tears in the aortic arch, aneurysmatic expansion, or rupture of the arch. The supra-aortic vessels were reimplanted individually or using the island technique. In cases of extensive pathologies involving the descending aorta, the frozen elephant trunk technique was performed. After completion of the distal part of the reconstruction, the air was removed from the graft, antegrade perfusion was resumed, and systemic rewarming was initiated. The period from the removal of the aortic clamp until systemic rewarming is complete is subsequently referred to as the "reperfusion time". Cerebral perfusion was monitored throughout the procedure using near-infrared spectroscopy (NIRS) [8,9].

2.3. Definitions

If the sequential organ failure assessment score (SOFA) was increased by two or more points from the previous day and clinical suspicion of infection was in place, the diagnosis of sepsis was confirmed [10]. Compromised function of the liver (spontaneous international normalized ratio of >1.5) and acute jaundice satisfied the criteria for the diagnosis of acute liver failure [11]. Acute kidney injury (AKI) was diagnosed according to the Kidney Disease Improving Global Outcomes (KDIGO) criteria [12]. Acute heart failure was diagnosed in patients with the clinical presentation of cardiogenic shock, pulmonary oedema, or congestive heart failure [13]. Shock was defined as having a systolic blood pressure below 90 mmHg or necessitating mechanical or pressor support to uphold values above this threshold [14]. Spinal ischaemia was assessed with the modified Tarlov scale [15]. Postoperative ischaemic strokes were detected using either CT or MRI scans [16], and focal neurological deficits were assessed through clinical examination by a neurologist. The gastrointestinal complications reported in this study summarize cases of gastrointestinal bleeding and/or mesenteric ischaemia [17]. The diagnosis of acute respiratory distress syndrome (ARDS) and its classification were made based on the Berlin criteria [18]. Failure of two or more vital organ systems fulfilled the criteria for the diagnosis of multiple organ dysfunction syndrome (MODS) [19]. Dissection-related obstruction of the aortic branches and the following hypoperfusion of the end-organ were defined as malperfusion [20]. Gastrointestinal complications ranged from gastrointestinal bleeds to transmural intestinal necrosis [21].

2.4. Statistics

Continuous variables were described using the mean and standard deviation. Categorical variables were tabulated using frequencies and percentages. The occurrence of death was modelled using logistic regression models. Predefined sets of independent variables were used in the models. Missing observations of categorical variables were modelled as separate categories. Missing continuous variables were imputed using multiple imputations with chained equations using predictive mean matching. Fifty imputed datasets were generated, and Rubin's rule was used to pool the parameter estimates. Data analysis was performed using the R language and environment for statistical computing (Version 4.1.0 R Foundation for Statistical Computing, Vienna, Austria. URL (accessed on 11 November 2023) https://www.R-project.org/). Best subset model selection was performed using the glmulti package (Version 1.0.8) [22], and the mice package (Version 3.14.0) [23] was used for imputations.

3. Results

3.1. Demographics and Clinical Presentation

Between March 2005 and October 2021, on average, 7.3 patients per year were operated on (Figure 1). Most patients were admitted at noon (Figure 1). The median duration from hospital admission to surgery was 91 min [IQR 69-145]. The majority of patients (50.3%) were directly transported to the emergency room of our centre after an ambulance was alerted about their symptoms, while 52 patients (44.4%) were transferred from other hospitals following diagnosis confirmation. Urgent referrals from primary care institutions and general practitioners accounted for five patients (4.2%). Transportation to the emergency room was predominantly via ambulance for most patients (91.4%), with medical air rescue utilized in ten cases (8.6%). In two instances, treatment was delayed due to the patient's initial admission to another ward with a different primary diagnosis.

Of the 117 analysed patients, 31 were women (26%). There was a significant difference in age between survivors and non-survivors (58.4 ± 11.4 vs. 65.3 ± 11; $p = 0.02$). Patients on anticoagulants ($p = 0.04$), those with chronic atrial fibrillation ($p = 0.04$), and those with chronic hypertension ($p = 0.02$) had a significantly increased risk of fatal outcomes. We also observed a positive association between mortality and aortic valve stenosis ($p = 0.03$). The clinical presentation of spinal ischaemia varied across the cohort and ranged from mild paraparesis in seven patients (modified Tarlov scale score of four) to complete paraplegia in four patients (modified Tarlov scale score of zero). Additionally, five patients presented a moderate form of paraplegia (modified Tarlov score of two). The details of the patient demographics and clinical presentations at admission are summarized in Table 1. Using the classification system proposed by the Society for Vascular Surgery (SVS) and the Society of Thoracic Surgeons (STS) [24,25], entry tears were found in the vast majority of cases in Zone 0. In one case, the tear was in Zone 1, and in two cases, the entries were found in Zone 2 or further below in the descending aorta and progressed retrogradely to involve the ascending aorta. In most cases, dissection progressed to the aortoiliac bifurcation. We did not find any association between the localization of the entry tear or extent of dissection and mortality. Cerebral and renovisceral malperfusion—as revealed by CT scans [26]—were also not significantly correlated with in-hospital mortality (Supplementary Table S1).

Table 1. Patient demographics and clinical presentation.

	Survivors n = 97 (%)	Non-Survivors n = 20 (%)	Analysed Cases (n)	Association with Mortality (p-Value)
Demographics				
Age (years)	58.4 ± 11.4	65.3 ± 11	117	0.02 *
Women	28 (29)	3 (15)	117	0.31
BMI (kg/m^2)	26.9 ± 5.3	27.6 ± 3.3	117	0.52
Smoking	32 (53)	8 (73)	117	0.38
Hypertension	57 (53)	18 (73)	117	0.02 *
Chronic obstructive pulmonary disease	3 (3)	2 (10)	117	0.14
Chronic limb ischaemia	1 (1)	1 (5)	117	0.78
Chronic kidney disease	6 (6)	2 (10)	117	0.92
Creatinine, preoperative (mg/dL)	1.2 ± 1.2	1 ± 0.4	117	0.25
Connective tissue disease	6 (6)	0 (0)	117	0.54
Atrial fibrillation	6 (6)	4 (20)	117	0.04 *
Heart or vascular implants	5 (5)	0 (0)	117	0.65
Heart failure	0 (0)	0 (0)	117	NA
Aortic valve insufficiency in history	4 (4)	2 (10)	117	0.63
Aortic valve stenosis in history	0 (0)	2 (10)	117	0.03 *
Prior CABG	0 (0)	0 (0)	117	NA
Prior valve reconstruction	1 (1)	0 (0)	117	1
Medication at Admission				
Beta blockers	9 (23)	1 (17)	45	1
ACE inhibitors	9 (22)	1 (17)	46	1
ARBs	3 (7)	1 (14)	48	1
Acetylsalicylic acid	4 (10)	0 (0)	47	0.88
Oral anticoagulants	6 (6)	4 (20)	117	0.04 *
Clinical Presentation				
Thoracic pain	76 (88)	15 (94)	102	0.84
Cardiac arrest	4 (4)	0 (0)	116	0.83
Pericardial effusion	38 (48)	9 (53)	97	0.23
Aortic regurgitation	46 (55)	7 (44)	99	0.56
Unconscious at admission	17 (20)	3 (19)	100	1
Spinal ischaemia	14 (16)	3 (17)	105	1
Acute limb ischaemia	17 (20)	7 (41)	104	0.1
Acute kidney injury	0 (0)	0 (0)	106	NA
Shock	26 (36)	8 (67)	84	0.09

BMI: body mass index; CABG: coronary artery bypass grafting; ACE inhibitor: angiotensin-converting enzyme inhibitors; ARBs: angiotensin II receptor blockers. Statistical significance for p-values < 0.05 is marked with *. NA: not applicable

3.2. Operative Details

In the total of the present cohort, aortic reconstruction was limited to the ascending aorta in 35 patients (30%). Hemiarch replacement was performed in 28 cases (24%), extensive distal reconstruction with total arch replacement was performed in 5 cases (4%), and the frozen elephant trunk technique was performed in 49 cases (42%). If simultaneous valve repair was necessary, biological valve conduits were the most common, with

29 cases (25%), followed by mechanical Bentall repairs (28 cases, 24%). Nine patients (8%) underwent valve-sparing aortic root repair. There was no significant correlation between different operative modalities and patient mortality (Table 2). We observed significantly longer operation times in the non-survivor group (minutes: 364.6 ± 97.1 vs. 449.1 ± 141.7, $p = 0.002$). Nineteen patients required operative revision for bleeding, a complication observed in 25% of the cases with fatal outcomes. The origin of the bleeding remained elusive in seven cases, while in nine cases, it presented as diffuse. Additionally, in two cases, the bleeding emanated directly from the right ventricle, and in one case, it originated from the proximal anastomosis.

Table 2. Operative details.

	Survivors n = 97 (%)	Non-Survivors n = 20 (%)	Analysed Cases (n)	Association with Mortality (p-Value)
Duration of operation	364.6 ± 97.1	449.1 ± 141.7	117	0.002 *
CBP temperature (°C)	19 ± 2.4	19.6 ± 2.7	112	0.37
Aortic cross clamp time (minutes)	123.8 ± 46	135.1 ± 72.1	85	0.58
Circulatory arrest time (minutes)	44.2 ± 22.1	53.4 ± 23.5	97	0.18
Reperfusion time (minutes)	83.3 ± 40.6	98.4 ± 40.5	72	0.25
Total bypass time (minutes)	215.8 ± 73.6	256.2 ± 125.9	88	0.26
Arterial canulation site			100	0.92
Subclavial/Axillary	56 (67)	10 (63)		
Femoral	20 (24)	4 (25)		
Aorta	8 (9)	2 (12)		
Venous canulation site			99	0.05
Right atrium	77 (93)	12 (75)		
Femoral	5 (6)	4 (25)		
Bicaval	1 (1)	0 (0)		
Cerebral perfusion			98	0.11
None	19 (23)	1 (6)		
Unilateral	45 (55)	8 (50)		
Bilateral	18 (22)	7 (44)		
Operative Modalities				
Ascending aorta repair	29 (30)	6 (30)	117	1
Ascending aorta and hemiarch repair	25 (26)	3 (15)	117	0.46
Ascending aorta and complete arch repair	4 (4)	1 (5)	117	1
Frozen elephant trunk	39 (40)	10 (50)	117	0.65
Conservative root management	46 (47)	13 (65)	117	0.24
Valve-sparing aortic root repair	9 (9)	0 (0)	117	0.34
Bio-Bentall	17 (18)	4 (20)	117	0.96
Mechan. Bentall	25 (26)	3 (15)	117	0.46
Intraoperative CABG	8 (8)	3 (15)	117	0.4
Postoperative Complications				
Rethoracotomy: bleeding	14 (14)	5 (25)	117	0.4
Wound infection	6 (6)	0 (0)	117	0.58
N. recurens paralysis	10 (10)	0 (0)	117	0.48

CBP: cardiopulmonary bypass; CABG: coronary artery bypass grafting. Statistical significance for p-values < 0.05 is marked with *.

3.3. Postoperative Phase

Twenty patients died in hospital. Cardiogenic shock and postoperative stroke were the most common causes of death in our cohort, accounting for 60% of the fatal outcomes, followed by septic shock in five cases (Table 3). The time points of the registered deaths, along with their respective causalities, are shown in Figure 2.

AKI and acute heart failure ($p < 0.001$ for both), sepsis ($p = 0.04$), and focal neurological deficits ($p = 0.02$) were strongly associated with in-hospital mortality. ARDS of all stages was more common in the non-survivor group (24% vs. 6%; $p = 0.06$). Acute limb ischaemia was found to be strongly associated with poor prognosis (18% vs. 3%; $p = 0.06$). Details of the postoperative complications and their association with mortality are presented in Table 3.

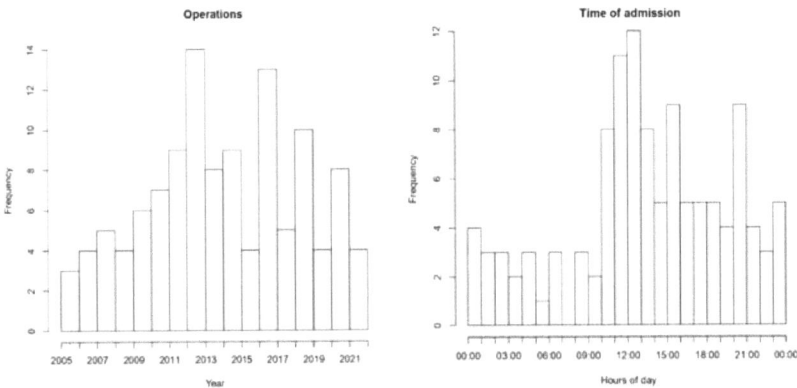

Figure 1. Frequency of operations per year and time of patient admission.

Table 3. Postoperative complications.

	Survivors n = 97 (%)	Non-Survivors n = 20 (%)	Analysed Cases (n)	Association with Mortality (p-Value)
In-hospital mortality		20 (17)	117	
Cause of death			20	
Bleeding		1 (5)		
Postoperative stroke		6 (30)		
Cardiogenic shock		6 (30)		
Septic shock		5 (25)		
Multi-organ failure		1 (5)		
Hospital stay (days)	21.5 ± 13.3	9.5 ± 8	117	0.002 *
ICU stay (days)	12.9 ± 10.6	8.3 ± 8.8	117	0.04 *
Invasive ventilation (hours)	151.1 ± 225.6	156.5 ± 159.5	117	0.9
AKI post-op	31 (32)	16 (80)	117	<0.001 *
RRT	19 (20)	15 (80)	117	<0.001 *
Arrhythmia post-op	48 (49)	10 (50)	117	1
Permanent pacemaker	3 (3)	2 (10)	117	0.43
Atrioventricular block	2 (2)	1 (5)	117	0.44
Aortic valve insufficiency post-op	46 (55)	7 (44)	99	0.56
Acute heart failure	11 (11)	9 (45)	117	<0.001 *
Postoperative stroke	18 (19)	8 (47)	114	0.02 *
Focal neurological deficits	31 (32)	7 (78)	106	0.02 *
Delirium	51 (53)	3 (50)	103	1
Acute limb ischaemia	3 (3)	3 (18)	114	0.06
Pneumonia	54 (56)	16 (64)	112	1
ARDS	7 (7)	4 (27)	112	0.06
Pulmonary artery embolism	2 (2)	0 (0)	114	1
Tracheostomy	24 (25)	3 (27)	99	0.97
GI complications	11 (11)	4 (24)	114	0.32
Liver failure	1 (1)	2 (10)	117	0.13
Sepsis	23 (24)	8 (53)	112	0.04 *

ICU: intensive care unit; AKI: acute kidney injury; RRT: renal replacement therapy; ARDS: acute respiratory distress syndrome; GI: gastrointestinal. Statistical significance for p-values < 0.05 is marked with *.

Clinical factors associated with poor outcomes and end-organ damage were included in a univariate regression model (Supplementary Table S2). After evaluating every possible subset combination, the best fitting model of mortality included the onset of focal neurological deficits and ARDS (Supplementary Table S3). Patients with focal neurological deficits had an odds ratio of 5.8 (95% confidence interval: 1.2–41.7; $p = 0.04$) for mortality adjusted for ARDS.

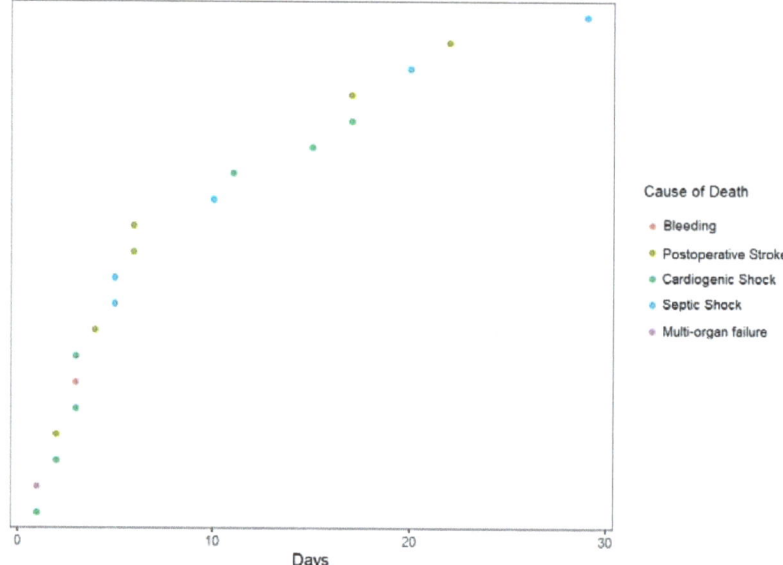

Figure 2. Causes and time points of fatal outcomes.

4. Discussion

Despite modern advancements in its detection and treatment, AADA remains a challenging aortic pathology, with relevant mortality rates. A recent study investigating the epidemiologic characteristics of AADA in the Danish population revealed an incidence rate of 2.2/100.000 and a 30-day mortality rate of 22% [27], confirming the rather uncommon but fatal nature of the disease. The risk factors usually associated with AADA are hypertension, atherosclerosis, aneurysmatic degeneration of the aorta, and connective tissue disease [2,28]. In this retrospective, observational study, we examined the pre- and perioperative parameters of patients admitted with AADA in our centre, as well as their postoperative course and complications, in order to elucidate the correlations of the parameters associated with poor outcomes and identify the patients at risk.

Regarding the preoperative characteristics of our patient cohort, hypertension was the most common comorbidity (64% of all patients), and it was significantly correlated with mortality ($p = 0.02$). This observation is in line with the findings of Wang et al., who described hypertension as an independent risk factor for long-term modality [29]. Another factor associated with early mortality is atrial fibrillation [30]. Patients with atrial fibrillation and acute aortic syndrome reportedly have a higher in-hospital mortality than do those without atrial fibrillation [30]. These patients are often on oral anticoagulation, which has also been described as a risk factor for bleeding and haemodynamic instability after AADA surgery [31]. In line with these findings, our results indicated both atrial fibrillation ($p = 0.04$) and oral anticoagulation ($p = 0.04$) to be strongly associated with mortality. Postoperative bleeding was observed in 25% of the non-survivors in our cohort and was a relevant complication in 19 patients requiring surgical revision.

The duration of extracorporeal circulation correlates with patients' survival [5,32]. Survivors in our study showed a trend for shorter reperfusion times (minutes: 83.3 ± 40.6 vs. 98.4 ± 40.5; $p = 0.25$) and total CBP times (minutes: 215.8 ± 73.6 vs. 256.2 ± 125.9; $p = 0.26$) with a significantly shorter total operation time (minutes: 364.6 ± 97.1 vs. 449.1 ± 141.7; $p = 0.002$). Longer applications of extracorporeal circulation reflect the severity of the dissection on the one hand and the patients' cardiovascular capacity to negotiate reperfusion on the other. Moreover, CBP disrupts the integrity of red blood cells, causing haemolysis; in this way, it may affect microcirculation and organ perfusion [33]. To improve patient outcomes, understanding and optimizing the underlying mechanisms of extracorporeal circulation remain of paramount importance. Simplifying the operation technique might influence the patient's outcome; in particular, the indication for patients treated with FET should be well justified. In the new era of acute aortic surgery, the application of FET in case of AADA without an entry in the aortic arch is a matter of ongoing discussion.

Organ dysfunction during the postoperative phase may severely affect patient recovery and is associated with adverse outcomes. In our cohort, cardiogenic shock was the most common cause of death, accounting for 30% of all fatal outcomes. In all, 45% of non-survivors were diagnosed with acute heart failure, which was strongly associated with mortality ($p < 0.001$). AKI and a need for renal replacement therapy were also strongly associated with mortality in our cohort ($p < 0.001$), confirming the observations of Huo et al. [5]. AKI after aortic surgery is potentially limiting in terms of patients' prognosis [34–37]. In line with this, patients with preoperatively impaired renal function [38] or those with renal malperfusion [39] carry a higher risk of postoperative renal failure. Furthermore, based on the results of the current cohort, chronic kidney disease was not a relevant factor for mortality, and both survivors and non-survivors had comparable serum creatinine levels at admission (survivors: 1.2 ± 1.2 mg/dL; non-survivors: 1 ± 0.4 mg/dL). These findings underline the importance of early detection of postoperative AKI [40] and undeferred initiation of nephroprotective measures to contain damage to the kidney tissue and allow for a quick organ recovery.

Persistent focal neurological deficits and postoperative stroke were also significantly associated with mortality ($p = 0.02$ for both). Multivariate regression analysis revealed an odds ratio of 5.8 for a fatal outcome in cases of focal neurological deficits. Although the interpretation of this analysis is limited due to the small sample size of the presented cohort, it is in line with clinical observations in the literature. Neurological deficits, with or without evidence of stroke, complicate the patient's recovery and are associated with high mortality and hospitalization [16], particularly in the elderly [41]. Although intraoperative protocols have been adjusted to monitor and contain cerebral malperfusion, through tedious blood pressure management and intraoperative NIRS monitoring, postoperative neurological complications remain a significant cause of morbidity and mortality [42]. Procedures involving the aortic arch display increased stroke rates [43], and the different arterial cannulation sites have not been found to bring certain benefits in stroke prevention [44]. Identifying and treating affected patients early in the postoperative phase with an interdisciplinary team may improve the overall outcome during the hospital stay and after the patient's discharge.

This study is subject to several limitations inherent in retrospective, non-randomized research. The data extraction process was confined to the information available in medical records, which inherently imposes constraints on the depth and comprehensiveness of the dataset. Given that AADA is an emergent pathology, the documentation of patients' medical history upon admission, and, to a lesser extent, the recording of intraoperative parameters, is frequently found to be insufficient and incomplete. To mitigate potential biases arising from missing data, our statistical analysis considered the absence of observations for categorical variables. Additionally, we employed imputation techniques to address missing values in continuous variables, thereby enhancing the robustness and reliability of our findings. The interpretation of the analysis results should take into account the additional limitation posed by the small sample size within the analysed cohort. Moreover, some of the discoveries presented in this report echo those found in prior publications. Nevertheless, the current study distinguishes itself by providing a comprehensive overview of perioperative predictors of mortality and emphasizes the significance of early postoperative assessment and the screening of end-organ damage, offering a nuanced and detailed exploration of these crucial aspects. Furthermore, the absence of long-term follow-up data for a considerable number of patients post-discharge limits our ability to provide an extended analysis of outcomes. Future trials with robust follow-up mechanisms are warranted to address this limitation and contribute to a more thorough understanding of the extended implications of the surgical modalities for the treatment of AADA.

5. Conclusions

Despite improvements in the surgical management of AADA, it still holds relevant mortality and morbidity rates. In this retrospective analysis, we found that atrial fibrillation, oral anticoagulation, and hypertension were significantly correlated with mortality. Postoperatively, acute kidney injury, acute heart failure, and persistent focal neurological deficits were identified as significant predictors of fatal outcomes. Early detection and interdisciplinary management of the patients at risk remain crucial throughout the postoperative phase.

Supplementary Materials: The following supporting information can be downloaded at: https://www.mdpi.com/article/10.3390/jcm13041023/s1, Table S1: CT angiography findings on admission. Table S2: Univariate logistic regression model. Table S3: Summary of logistic regression coefficients after best subset selection.

Author Contributions: Conceptualization, P.D., A.G., R.Z. and J.F.; methodology, P.D., N.D., A.G., A.K. and A.M.; software, A.K.; validation, A.K., J.K., P.A., A.M., A.G. and M.J.J.; formal analysis, P.D. and A.K.; investigation, P.D. and N.D.; data curation, N.D.; writing—original draft preparation, P.D.; writing—review and editing, A.G., A.M., P.A. and M.J.J.; visualization, A.K.; supervision, A.G., A.M., M.J.J. and P.A.; project administration, P.D. and A.G. All authors have read and agreed to the published version of the manuscript.

Funding: This research received no external funding.

Institutional Review Board Statement: The study was conducted in accordance with the Declaration of Helsinki and approved by the Ethics Committee of the University Hospital RWTH Aachen (EK 20-003), Approved Date: 29/4/2020.

Informed Consent Statement: Informed consent was obtained from all subjects involved in the study.

Data Availability Statement: The data that support the findings of this study are available from the corresponding author, P.D., upon reasonable request.

Conflicts of Interest: The authors declare no conflicts of interest.

References

1. Biancari, F.; Juvonen, T.; Fiore, A.; Perrotti, A.; Hervé, A.; Touma, J.; Pettinari, M.; Peterss, S.; Buech, J.; Dell'aquila, A.M.; et al. Current Outcome after Surgery for Type A Aortic Dissection. *Ann. Surg.* **2023**, *278*, e885–e892. [CrossRef]
2. Evangelista, A.; Isselbacher, E.M.; Bossone, E.; Gleason, T.G.; Eusanio, M.D.; Sechtem, U.; Ehrlich, M.P.; Trimarchi, S.; Braverman, A.C.; Myrmel, T.; et al. Insights From the International Registry of Acute Aortic Dissection: A 20-Year Experience of Collaborative Clinical Research. *Circulation* **2018**, *137*, 1846–1860. [CrossRef] [PubMed]
3. Sayed, A.; Munir, M.; Bahbah, E.I. Aortic Dissection: A Review of the Pathophysiology, Management and Prospective Advances. *Curr. Cardiol. Rev.* **2021**, *17*, e230421186875. [CrossRef]
4. Fattori, R.; Bacchi-Reggiani, L.; Bertaccini, P.; Napoli, G.; Fusco, F.; Longo, M.; Pierangeli, A.; Gavelli, G. Evolution of aortic dissection after surgical repair. *Am. J. Cardiol.* **2000**, *86*, 868–872. [CrossRef] [PubMed]
5. Huo, Y.; Zhang, H.; Li, B.; Zhang, K.; Li, B.; Guo, S.-H.; Hu, Z.-J.; Zhu, G.-J. Risk Factors for Postoperative Mortality in Patients with Acute Stanford Type A Aortic Dissection. *Int. J. Gen. Med.* **2021**, *14*, 7007–7015. [CrossRef] [PubMed]
6. Erbel, R.; Aboyans, V.; Boileau, C.; Bossone, E.; Di Bartolomeo, R.; Eggebrecht, H.; Evangelista, A.; Falk, V.; Frank, H.; Gaemperli, O.; et al. 2014 ESC Guidelines on the diagnosis and treatment of aortic diseases: Document covering acute and chronic aortic diseases of the thoracic and abdominal aorta of the adult. The Task Force for the Diagnosis and Treatment of Aortic Diseases of the European Society of Cardiology (ESC). *Eur. Heart J.* **2014**, *35*, 2873–2926, Erratum in *Eur. Heart J.* **2015**, *36*, 2779.
7. Cabasa, A.; Pochettino, A. Surgical management and outcomes of type A dissection—The Mayo Clinic experience. *Ann. Cardiothorac. Surg.* **2016**, *5*, 296–309. [CrossRef] [PubMed]
8. Zheng, F.; Sheinberg, R.; Yee, M.S.; Ono, M.; Zheng, Y.; Hogue, C.W. Cerebral near-infrared spectroscopy monitoring and neurologic outcomes in adult cardiac surgery patients: A systematic review. *Anesth. Analg.* **2013**, *116*, 663–676. [CrossRef] [PubMed]
9. Bennett, S.R.; Abukhodair, A.W.; Alqarni, M.S.; Fernandez, J.A.; Fernandez, A.J.; Bennett, M.R. Outcomes in Cardiac Surgery Based on Preoperative, Mean Intraoperative and Stratified Cerebral Oximetry Values. *Cureus* **2021**, *13*, e17123. [CrossRef]

10. Singer, M.; Deutschman, C.S.; Seymour, C.W.; Shankar-Hari, M.; Annane, D.; Bauer, M.; Bellomo, R.; Bernard, G.R.; Chiche, J.-D.; Coopersmith, C.M.; et al. The Third International Consensus Definitions for Sepsis and Septic Shock (Sepsis-3). *Jama* **2016**, *315*, 801–810. [CrossRef]
11. EASL Clinical Practice Guidelines: Management of hepatocellular carcinoma. *J. Hepatol.* **2018**, *69*, 182–236. [CrossRef] [PubMed]
12. Thomas, M.E.; Blaine, C.; Dawnay, A.; Devonald, M.A.; Ftouh, S.; Laing, C.; Latchem, S.; Lewington, A.; Milford, D.V.; Ostermann, M. The definition of acute kidney injury and its use in practice. *Kidney Int.* **2015**, *87*, 62–73. [CrossRef] [PubMed]
13. Mebazaa, A.; A Pitsis, A.; Rudiger, A.; Toller, W.; Longrois, D.; Ricksten, S.-E.; Bobek, I.; De Hert, S.; Wieselthaler, G.; Schirmer, U.; et al. Clinical review: Practical recommendations on the management of perioperative heart failure in cardiac surgery. *Crit. Care* **2010**, *14*, 201. [CrossRef] [PubMed]
14. Thiele, H.; de Waha-Thiele, S.; Freund, A.; Zeymer, U.; Desch, S.; Fitzgerald, S. Management of cardiogenic shock. *EuroIntervention* **2021**, *17*, 451–465. [CrossRef] [PubMed]
15. Bisdas, T.; Panuccio, G.; Sugimoto, M.; Torsello, G.; Austermann, M. Risk factors for spinal cord ischemia after endovascular repair of thoracoabdominal aortic aneurysms. *J. Vasc. Surg.* **2015**, *61*, 1408–1416. [CrossRef]
16. Raffa, G.M.; Agnello, F.; Occhipinti, G.; Miraglia, R.; Re, V.L.; Marrone, G.; Tuzzolino, F.; Arcadipane, A.; Pilato, M.; Luca, A. Neurological complications after cardiac surgery: A retrospective case-control study of risk factors and outcome. *J. Cardiothorac. Surg.* **2019**, *14*, 23. [CrossRef]
17. Viana, F.F.; Chen, Y.; Almeida, A.A.; Baxter, H.D.; Cochrane, A.D.; Smith, J.A. Gastrointestinal complications after cardiac surgery: 10-year experience of a single Australian centre. *ANZ J. Surg.* **2013**, *83*, 651–656. [CrossRef]
18. Meyer, N.J.; Gattinoni, L.; Calfee, C.S. Acute respiratory distress syndrome. *Lancet* **2021**, *398*, 622–637. [CrossRef]
19. Rossaint, J.; Zarbock, A. Pathogenesis of Multiple Organ Failure in Sepsis. *Crit. Rev. Immunol.* **2015**, *35*, 277–291. [CrossRef]
20. Yang, B.; Patel, H.J.; Williams, D.M.; Dasika, N.L.; Deeb, G.M. Management of type A dissection with malperfusion. *Ann. Cardiothorac. Surg.* **2016**, *5*, 265–274. [CrossRef]
21. Chor, C.Y.T.; Mahmood, S.; Khan, I.H.; Shirke, M.; Harky, A. Gastrointestinal complications following cardiac surgery. *Asian Cardiovasc. Thorac. Ann.* **2020**, *28*, 621–632. [CrossRef] [PubMed]
22. Bürkner, P.-C. brms: An R Package for Bayesian Multilevel Models Using Stan. *J. Stat. Softw.* **2017**, *80*, 1–28. [CrossRef]
23. van Buuren, S.; Groothuis-Oudshoorn, K. mice: Multivariate Imputation by Chained Equations in R. *J. Stat. Softw.* **2011**, *45*, 1–67. [CrossRef]
24. Lombardi, J.V.; Hughes, G.C.; Appoo, J.J.; Bavaria, J.E.; Beck, A.W.; Cambria, R.P.; Charlton-Ouw, K.; Eslami, M.H.; Kim, K.M.; Leshnower, B.G.; et al. Society for Vascular Surgery (SVS) and Society of Thoracic Surgeons (STS) reporting standards for type B aortic dissections. *J. Vasc. Surg.* **2020**, *71*, 723–747. [CrossRef] [PubMed]
25. Writing Committee Members; Isselbacher, E.M.; Preventza, O.; Hamilton Black, J., III; Augoustides, J.G.; Beck, A.W.; Bolen, M.A.; Braverman, A.C.; Bray, B.E.; Brown-Zimmerman, M.M.; et al. 2022 ACC/AHA Guideline for the Diagnosis and Management of Aortic Disease: A Report of the American Heart Association/American College of Cardiology Joint Committee on Clinical Practice Guidelines. *Circulation* **2022**, *146*, e334–e482. [CrossRef] [PubMed]
26. Kamman, A.V.; Yang, B.; Kim, K.M.; Williams, D.M.; Michael Deeb, G.; Patel, H.J. Visceral Malperfusion in Aortic Dissection: The Michigan Experience. *Semin. Thorac. Cardiovasc. Surg.* **2017**, *29*, 173–178. [CrossRef]
27. Obel, L.M.; Lindholt, J.S.; Lasota, A.N.; Jensen, H.K.; Benhassen, L.L.; Mørkved, A.L.; Srinanthalogen, R.; Christiansen, M.; Bundgaard, H.; Liisberg, M. Clinical Characteristics, Incidences, and Mortality Rates for Type A and B Aortic Dissections: A Nationwide Danish Population-Based Cohort Study From 1996 to 2016. *Circulation* **2022**, *146*, 1903–1917. [CrossRef]
28. Wundram, M.; Falk, V.; Eulert-Grehn, J.-J.; Herbst, H.; Thurau, J.; Leidel, B.A.; Göncz, E.; Bauer, W.; Habazettl, H.; Kurz, S.D. Incidence of acute type A aortic dissection in emergency departments. *Sci. Rep.* **2020**, *10*, 7434. [CrossRef]
29. Wang, Z.; Ge, M.; Chen, T.; Chen, C.; Zong, Q.; Lu, L.; Wang, D. Impact of hypertension on short- and long-term survival of patients who underwent emergency surgery for type A acute aortic dissection. *J. Thorac. Dis.* **2020**, *12*, 6618–6628. [CrossRef]
30. Campia, U.; Rizzo, S.M.; Snyder, J.E.; Pfefferman, M.A.; Morrison, R.B.; Piazza, G.; Goldhaber, S.Z. Impact of Atrial Fibrillation on In-Hospital Mortality and Stroke in Acute Aortic Syndromes. *Am. J. Med.* **2021**, *134*, 1419–1423. [CrossRef]
31. Sromicki, J.; Van Hemelrijck, M.; O Schmiady, M.; Krüger, B.; Morjan, M.; Bettex, D.; Vogt, P.R.; Carrel, T.P.; Mestres, C.-A. Prior intake of new oral anticoagulants adversely affects outcome following surgery for acute type A aortic dissection. *Interact. CardioVascular Thorac. Surg.* **2022**, *35*, ivac037. [CrossRef]
32. Yuan, H.; Sun, Z.; Zhang, Y.; Wu, W.; Liu, M.; Yang, Y.; Wang, J.; Lv, Q.; Zhang, L.; Li, Y.; et al. Clinical Analysis of Risk Factors for Mortality in Type A Acute Aortic Dissection: A Single Study From China. *Front. Cardiovasc. Med.* **2021**, *8*, 728568. [CrossRef]
33. Govender, K.; Jani, V.P.; Cabrales, P. The Disconnect Between Extracorporeal Circulation and the Microcirculation: A Review. *Asaio J.* **2022**, *68*, 881–889. [CrossRef]
34. Vives, M.; Hernandez, A.; Parramon, F.; Estanyol, N.; Pardina, B.; Muñoz, A.; Alvarez, P.; Hernandez, C. Acute kidney injury after cardiac surgery: Prevalence, impact and management challenges. *Int. J. Nephrol. Renov. Dis.* **2019**, *12*, 153–166. [CrossRef]
35. Meng, W.; Li, R.; Lihua, E.; Zha, N. Postoperative acute kidney injury and early and long-term mortality in acute aortic dissection patients: A meta-analysis. *Medicine* **2021**, *100*, 23426. [CrossRef]
36. Ko, T.; Higashitani, M.; Sato, O.; Uemura, Y.; Norimatsu, T.; Mahara, K.; Takamisawa, I.; Seki, A.; Shimizu, J.; Tobaru, T.; et al. Impact of Acute Kidney Injury on Early to Long-Term Outcomes in Patients Who Underwent Surgery for Type A Acute Aortic Dissection. *Am. J. Cardiol.* **2015**, *116*, 463–468. [CrossRef]

37. Tsai, H.-S.; Tsai, F.-C.; Chen, Y.-C.; Wu, L.-S.; Chen, S.-W.; Chu, J.-J.; Lin, P.-J.; Chu, P.-H. Impact of acute kidney injury on one-year survival after surgery for aortic dissection. *Ann. Thorac. Surg.* **2012**, *94*, 1407–1412. [CrossRef]
38. Chien, T.-M.; Wen, H.; Huang, J.-W.; Hsieh, C.-C.; Chen, H.-M.; Chiu, C.-C.; Chen, Y.-F. Significance of preoperative acute kidney injury in patients with acute type A aortic dissection. *J. Formos. Med. Assoc.* **2019**, *118*, 815–820. [CrossRef] [PubMed]
39. Qian, S.-C.; Ma, W.-G.; Pan, X.-D.; Liu, H.; Zhang, K.; Zheng, J.; Liu, Y.-M.; Zhu, J.-M.; Sun, L.-Z. Renal malperfusion affects operative mortality rather than late death following acute type A aortic dissection repair. *Asian J. Surg.* **2020**, *43*, 213–219. [CrossRef] [PubMed]
40. Averdunk, L.; Rückbeil, M.V.; Zarbock, A.; Martin, L.; Marx, G.; Jalaie, H.; Jacobs, M.J.; Stoppe, C.; Gombert, A. SLPI—A Biomarker of Acute Kidney Injury after Open and Endovascular Thoracoabdominal Aortic Aneurysm (TAAA) Repair. *Sci. Rep.* **2020**, *10*, 3453. [CrossRef] [PubMed]
41. Ngaage, D.L.; Cowen, M.E.; Griffin, S.; Guvendik, L.; Cale, A.R. Early neurological complications after coronary artery bypass grafting and valve surgery in octogenarians. *Eur. J. Cardio-Thorac. Surg.* **2008**, *33*, 653–659. [CrossRef] [PubMed]
42. McDonagh, D.L.; Berger, M.; Mathew, J.P.; Graffagnino, C.; A Milano, C.; Newman, M.F. Neurological complications of cardiac surgery. *Lancet Neurol.* **2014**, *13*, 490–502. [CrossRef] [PubMed]
43. Kremer, J.; Preisner, F.; Dib, B.; Tochtermann, U.; Ruhparwar, A.; Karck, M.; Farag, M.l. Aortic arch replacement with frozen elephant trunk technique—A single-center study. *J. Cardiothorac. Surg.* **2019**, *14*, 147. [CrossRef] [PubMed]
44. osinski, B.F.; Idrees, J.J.; Roselli, E.E.; Germano, E.; Pasadyn, S.R.; Lowry, A.M.; Blackstone, E.H.; Johnston, D.R.; Soltesz, E.G.; Navia, J.L.; et al. Cannulation strategies in acute type A dissection repair: A systematic axillary artery approach. *J. Thorac. Cardiovasc. Surg.* **2019**, *158*, 647–659.e5. [CrossRef]

Disclaimer/Publisher's Note: The statements, opinions and data contained in all publications are solely those of the individual author(s) and contributor(s) and not of MDPI and/or the editor(s). MDPI and/or the editor(s) disclaim responsibility for any injury to people or property resulting from any ideas, methods, instructions or products referred to in the content.

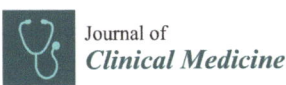

Article

Relative Thrombus Burden Ratio Reveals Overproportioned Intraluminal Thrombus Growth—Potential Implications for Abdominal Aortic Aneurysm

Joscha Mulorz [†], Agnesa Mazrekaj [†], Justus Sehl, Amir Arnautovic, Waseem Garabet, Kim-Jürgen Krott, Hubert Schelzig, Margitta Elvers and Markus Udo Wagenhäuser *

Clinic for Vascular and Endovascular Surgery, Medical Faculty and University Hospital Düsseldorf, 40225 Düsseldorf, Germany
* Correspondence: markus.wagenhaeuser@med.uni-duesseldorf.de
† These authors contributed equally to this work.

Citation: Mulorz, J.; Mazrekaj, A.; Sehl, J.; Arnautovic, A.; Garabet, W.; Krott, K.-J.; Schelzig, H.; Elvers, M.; Wagenhäuser, M.U. Relative Thrombus Burden Ratio Reveals Overproportioned Intraluminal Thrombus Growth—Potential Implications for Abdominal Aortic Aneurysm. *J. Clin. Med.* **2024**, *13*, 962. https://doi.org/10.3390/jcm13040962

Academic Editors: Ralf Kolvenbach, Benedikt Reutersberg and Matthias Trenner

Received: 11 January 2024
Revised: 29 January 2024
Accepted: 6 February 2024
Published: 8 February 2024

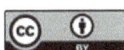

Copyright: © 2024 by the authors. Licensee MDPI, Basel, Switzerland. This article is an open access article distributed under the terms and conditions of the Creative Commons Attribution (CC BY) license (https:// creativecommons.org/licenses/by/ 4.0/).

Abstract: Background: An intraluminal, non-occlusive thrombus (ILT) is a common feature in an abdominal aortic aneurysm (AAA). This study investigated the relative progression of ILT vs. AAA volume using a novel parameter, the so-called thrombus burden ratio (TBR), in non-treated AAAs. Parameters potentially associated with TBR progression were analyzed and TBR progression in large vs. small and fast- vs. slow-growing AAAs was assessed. **Methods:** This retrospective, single-center study analyzed sequential contrast-enhanced computed tomography angiography (CTA) scans between 2009 and 2018 from patients with an AAA before surgical treatment. Patients' medical data and CTA scans were analyzed at two given time points. The TBR was calculated as a ratio of ILT and AAA volume, and relative TBR progression was calculated by normalization for time between sequential CTA scans. Spearman's correlation was applied to identify morphologic parameters correlating with TBR progression, and multivariate linear regression analysis was used to evaluate the association of clinical and morphological parameters with TBR progression. **Results:** A total of 35 patients were included. The mean time between CT scans was 16 ± 15.9 months. AAA volume progression was 12 ± 3% and ILT volume progression was 36 ± 13%, resulting in a TBR progression of 11 ± 4%, suggesting overproportioned ILT growth. TBR progression was 0.8 ± 0.8% per month. Spearman's correlation verified ILT growth as the most relevant parameter contributing to TBR progression (R = 0.51). Relative TBR progression did not differ significantly in large vs. small and fast- vs. slow-growing AAAs. In the multivariate regression analysis, none of the studied factors were associated with TBR progression. **Conclusion:** TBR increases during AAA development, indicating an overproportioned ILT vs. AAA volume growth. The TBR may serve as a useful parameter, as it incorporates the ILT volume growth relative to the AAA volume, therefore combining two important parameters that are usually reported separately. Yet, the clinical relevance in helping to identify potential corresponding risk factors and the evaluation of patients at risk needs to be further validated in a larger study cohort.

Keywords: aortic aneurysm; intraluminal thrombus; aneurysm research; aneurysm growth

1. Introduction

Abdominal aortic aneurysm (AAA) constitutes a significant burden to public health with a prevalence up to 12.5% in males and 5.2% in females [1]. AAA treatment remains challenging as rupture is associated with high morbidity and mortality [2]. Importantly, there is a correlation between AAA and cardiovascular disease (CVD), e.g., stroke or myocardial infarction, with a significantly higher incidence of CVD in patients with an AAA compared to other populations [3].

An AAA is considered a chronic inflammatory and atherothrombotic disease of the aortic wall, accompanied by the formation of a non-occlusive intraluminal thrombus (ILT) in most cases [4–6]. Despite a high ILT prevalence, there is ongoing scientific dispute regarding its role during AAA initiation and progression. Earlier studies described the ILT as reducing peak wall stress, which may protect from aortic rupture [7,8]. In contrast, more recent findings linked the presence of an ILT to increased elastolysis, a lower density of smooth muscle cells in the media layer, and increased immuno-inflammation in the adventitia [6,9].

Currently, the clinical diagnosis and initiation of open or endovascular surgical therapy is based on the AAA diameter and/or its progression, usually without consideration of the ILT and its potential risks. There have been various attempts to untangle the relationship between AAA diameter progression and the ILT. A recent study nominated the ILT as an independent predictor of AAA growth [10]. Another meta-analysis found ILT volume to be associated with AAA rupture [11]. Importantly these studies reported the maximum aortic and ILT diameter or volume separately, and only few studies have reported ILT size relative to aneurysm size [12].

Taking a step forward, we suggest a novel parameter, the so-called *thrombus burden ratio* (TBR), which is defined as a ratio between AAA and ILT volume, which may be more relevant than the ILT volume itself. Such a ratio and its changes over time have only been poorly evaluated and have never been linked to comorbidities potentially affecting ILT growth.

However, the relative changes rather than total independent parameters could have the potential to enable better timing of therapy and disease monitoring in the future and thus incorporate the TBR into the decision-making processes of clinically active surgeons.

The present study investigated the TBR and its progression in non-treated AAAs by analyzing sequential contrast-enhanced computed tomography angiography (CTA) scans and subsequently calculating the TBR for these patients. Then, CT morphological and clinical characteristics were investigated regarding their potential correlation to TBR progression.

2. Methods

2.1. Data Collection

This retrospective study investigated 35 patients with an AAA (32 male; 3 female) treated at the Clinic for Vascular and Endovascular Surgery at the University Hospital of Düsseldorf, Germany, with two sequential CTA scans available prior to any kind of surgical treatment. Patient data were collected from 1 January 2009 to 31 December 2018 from archived medical records. Information regarding comorbidities and medication was retrieved from the patient's medical records at the time of the first CTA scan. Out of the 707 patients treated for aortic pathologies, only 35 patients were included for ultimate analysis after applying all of the inclusion criteria (Figure 1). The study was approved by the local ethics committee at the Heinrich Heine University Düsseldorf (approval ID: 2018-2, approval date: 28 May 2018), and it followed the standards of good scientific practice and conformed to the provisions of the Declaration of Helsinki.

2.2. Enhanced Computed Tomography Angiography (CTA) Scan Analysis

CTA studies were acquired helically using state-of-the-art CT scanners and standard institutional protocols for CTA. Images were reconstructed at a 1–5 mm thickness. The average overall slice thickness was 2.56 ± 1.52 mm. Scans were uploaded to Osirix DICOM Viewer (Pixmeo SARL, Geneva, Switzerland) and the open-source analysis tool Horos (https://horosproject.org/) for subsequent measurements and analysis. For each patient, the following parameters were collected at both the baseline and follow-up CTA: maximum AAA diameter, total ILT and AAA volume, volume of perfused lumen, AAA wall thickness, ILT surface measured perpendicular to the centerline axis at the maximum AAA diameter, maximum ILT thickness, and AAA wall thickness at maximum ILT diameter. The region of interest (ROI) for volume measurements was defined by setting upper and lower threshold limits. Limits were defined proximally by the loss of parallelism of both aortic walls, until distally, parallelism was regained or until the aortic bifurcation occurred. AAA volume was measured with ROI-based semiautomatic segmentation.

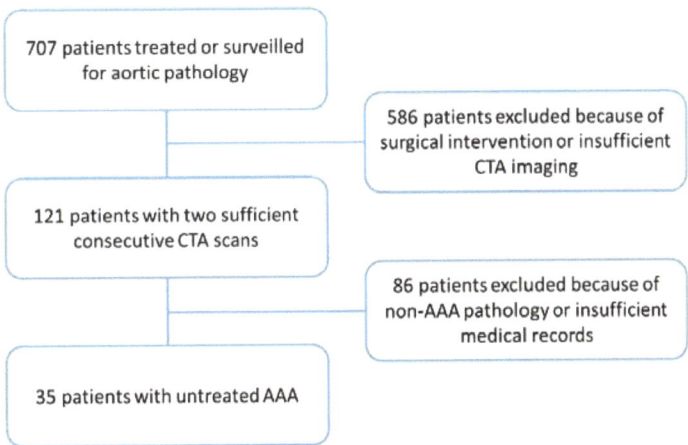

Figure 1. Study population. A total of 707 patients were identified with aortic pathologies between 1 January 2009 and 31 December 2018. Of those, 121 patients had two sequential enhanced computed tomography angiography (CTA) scans available. Ultimately, 35 patients were included for further measurements and analysis as study cohort based on availability of additional clinical data and sufficient CTA quality.

2.3. Definition of TBR

ILT and AAA volume were measured using CTA scans at baseline and follow-up as mentioned above. The ratio of both measurements was defined as the TBR:

$$TBR = ILTvolume/AAAvolume$$

TBR progression was calculated as the difference between the TBR at baseline (BL) and at follow-up (FU) normalized to the baseline TBR and the time between the two sequential CTA scans:

$$((TBR\ FU - TBR\ BL)/TBR\ BL)/time\ period\ [months]$$

2.4. Spearman's Correlation/Multivariate Logistic Regression

Spearman's correlation was applied to analyze the relationship between morphologic parameters and TBR progression. As a next step, multivariate linear regression analysis was performed to evaluate the association of patients' comorbidities, hemostasis-related blood parameters, and changes in AAA and ILT morphology with relative TBR progression. Here, TBR progression was set as the dependent variable, and all parameters collected were set as influencing variables.

2.5. Subgroup Analysis

To explore whether the TBR is different in patients with a large and/or fast-growing AAA, patients were assigned based on either their maximum AAA diameter at baseline CTA or their AAA volume increase between the sequential CTA scans. Threshold values for both were defined as follows: maximum baseline AAA diameter > 50 mm and AAA diameter progression > 1 mm^3/month.

2.6. Statistical Analysis

Where applicable, testing for normality was applied as indicated in the Figure legends, as well as testing for statistical outliers. All continuous data are reported as the mean and standard error of the mean (SEM) with 95% confidence intervals (CI). Categorical data are presented as absolute frequencies with percentages. Statistical analysis was performed using SPSS Statistics Version 27 (IBM, Armonk, NY, USA) and GraphPad Software Version 9 (GraphPad Software, San Diego, CA, USA). Graphs were created with GraphPad Software Version 9 (GraphPad Software, San Diego, CA, USA).

3. Results

3.1. Patient Demographics

The study cohort consisted of 35 patients, comprising 32 males (91.4%) and 3 females (8.6%). The mean age was 68.9 ± 1.4 years (66.1–71.9) at the time of the baseline CTA scan. The time period between the two sequential CTA scans was 16 ± 15.9 months (10.4–21.3). A total of 24 (68.6%) patients had reported arterial hypertension (aHT), 9 (25.7%) patients had hyperlipidemia (HPL), 20 (57.1%) patients had a history of smoking, and 9 (25.7%) patients had a body mass index (BMI) > 30. In addition, 3 (8.6%) patients suffered from type 2 diabetes mellitus (T2D), of whom all were males. Hemostasis-related blood parameters were collected at the time of the second CTA and were within the expected norm thresholds (Table 1).

Table 1. Patient characteristics. Data are shown as mean ± standard error of the mean (SEM) with 95% confidence interval (95% CI) or absolute frequency with percentages (%) (n = 35).

Parameter	Absolute Frequencies (%) Mean ± SEM
Demographics and Comorbidities	n = 35 total
Male gender	69.4 ± 1.4
Age	32 (91.4)
aHT	3 (8.6)
HLP	24 (68.6)
DMTII	9 (25.7)
BMI > 30	20 (57.1)
History of smoking	9 (25.7)
Blood parameters at second CTA	
HCT	39.44 ± 1.31
Hb	13.10 ± 0.44
RBC	4.36 ± 0.18
PLC	219.60 ± 12.89
WBC	10.09 ± 1.00
Quick	90.71 ± 2.92
INR	1.10 ± 0.03

DMTII: type II diabetes mellitus, aHT: arterial hypertension, HLP: hyperlipoproteinemia, BMI: body mass index, HCT: hematocrit, Hb: hemoglobin, RBC: red blood cell count, PLC: platelet count, WBC: white blood cell count, INR: international normalized ratio.

3.2. Morphological Parameters

Morphological parameters were analyzed on two sequential CTA scans. At baseline, the mean AAA diameter was 49.1 ± 1.7 mm (45.6–52.4), ILT volume was 67.9 ± 9.9 cm^3 (27.9–81.0), and the AAA volume was 126.3 ±13.6 cm^3 (98.8–153.9). Within the mean time period between the two sequential CTA scans of 16 months, there was a relative increase in AAA diameter of 12 ± 3% (4–17), in ILT volume of 36 ± 13% (11–62), and in AAA volume of 18 ± 4% (10–27), indicating an accelerated relative ILT growth when compared to AAA growth. Of interest, changes in the aortic wall thickness at the maximum ILT diameter were negligible (Table 2).

Table 2. Morphological parameters on enhanced computed tomography angiography (CTA)-based analysis. Various image-based morphologic parameters for abdominal aortic aneurysm (AAA) and intraluminal thrombus (ILT) were measured from two sequential CTA scans at baseline and at follow-up. Data are shown as mean ± standard error of the mean (SEM) and 95% confidence interval (95% CI). Relative changes between the two time points are reported by normalizing to baseline (n = 35).

Parameter	All (n = 35)		Relative Change vs. Baseline
	Baseline CTA Scan	Follow-Up CTA Scan	
ILT volume (cm^3)	67.9 ± 9.9 (27.9–81.0)	80.6 ± 9.4 (61.6–99.6)	0.36 ± 0.13 (0.11–0.62)
AAA volume (cm^3)	126.3 ± 13.6 (98.8–153.9)	145.3 ± 14.1 (116.6–173.9)	0.18 ± 0.04 (0.10–0.27)
Thrombus burden ratio (TBR)	0.5 ± 0.03 (0.44–0.55)	0.53 ± 0–02 (0.48–0.58)	0.11 ± 0.04 (0.02–0.20)
AAA diameter (mm)	49.1 ± 1.7 (45.6–52.4)	53.5 ± 1.6 (50.2–56.8)	0.12 ± 0.03 (0.04–0.17)
ILT surface at max. aortic diameter (cm^2)	9.6 ± 1.0 (7.5–11.6)	11.7 ± 1.0 (9.6–13.8)	0.51 ± 0.22 (0.05–0.96)
ILT thickness (mm)	17.2 ± 1.5 (14.1–20.3)	21.3 ± 1.7 (17.9–24.7)	0.55 ± 0.28 (−0.01–0.11)
Aortic wall thickness at max. ILT diameter (mm)	1.9 ± 0.06 (1.7–2.0)	1.9 ± 0.05 (1.8–2.0)	0.05 ± 0.03 (−0.01–0.01)

ILT: intraluminal thrombus, AAA: abdominal aortic aneurysm, max.: maximum.

Next, we investigated the TBR by calculating the ratio of ILT and AAA volume at baseline and at follow-up. Here, we observed a significant increase in TBR between the two time points (Figure 2A). The TBR increased by 11 ± 4% (1.8–20), and TBR progression was 0.8 ± 0.0.8% per month (0.8–2.4). To further evaluate whether this significant increase was due to the AAA volume or the ILT volume increase, we compared the relative changes in both parameters between the two time points. We found that the relative ILT volume change was accelerated when compared to the relative AAA volume change, suggesting an overproportioned ILT growth (Figure 2B). This finding was then confirmed by applying Spearman's correlation. Here, ILT volume progression (R = 0.51, p = 0.004) correlated with TBR progression to a greater extent and this was statistically significantly when compared to AAA volume progression (R = 0.29, p = 0.42) (Figure 2C,D).

The Spearman's correlation was then added for other morphologic parameters. Here, we found that the ILT thickness also correlated with TBR progression, which did not apply for AAA diameter progression (Table 3), overall, suggesting a higher relevance of the ILT for TBR progression.

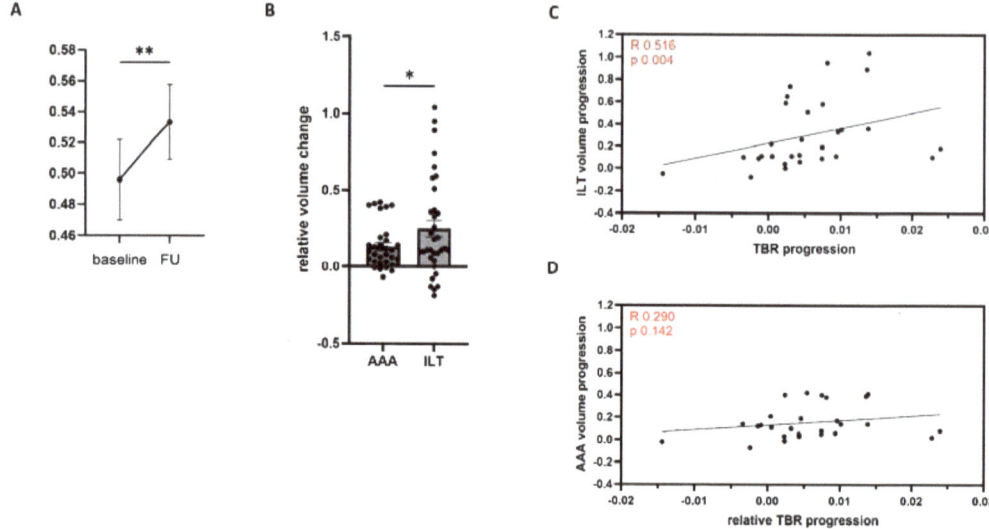

Figure 2. Thrombus burden ratio (TBR) and its progression. The volume of the intraluminal thrombus (ILT) and the abdominal aortic aneurysm (AAA) were measured from enhanced computed tomography angiography (CTA) scans at baseline and follow-up (FU). The ratio between ILT and AAA volume, so-called TBR, increased significantly between two sequential CTA scans (**A**). Analyzing AAA and ILT volume changes normalized to baseline (ILT/AAA volume progression) identified an overproportioned ILT volume progression suggesting ILT volume increase to be more relevant for TBR progression (**B**). Spearman's correlation was applied to assess correlation between TBR progression and ILT (**C**) and AAA (**D**) volume progression following testing for normal distribution using Shapiro–Wilk test. R- and p-values are displayed in the graph. Line is simple linear regression with 95% CI indicated as dotted lines. Wilcoxon matched-pairs signed-rank test. Outliers were identified using GROUT method (Q = 5%), slightly reducing the total of $n = 35$ for some groups. Graphs are mean with SEM. * = $p < 0.05$; ** = $p < 0.01$ (**A**,**B**) or p indicated in graph (**C**,**D**).

Table 3. Spearman's correlation. Spearman's correlation was applied to analyze various morphological parameters and their relative progression on two sequential enhanced computed tomography angiography (CTA) scans on whether they are associated with the thrombus burden ratio (TBR) progression. R- and p-values are displayed together with the 95% confidence interval (95% CI). Calculations were performed after identifying statistical outliers using the ROUT method (Q = 5%), reducing the overall numbers from $n = 35$ for some parameters.

Parameter	R	95% CI	p-Value
ILT volume change	0.51	V0.17–0.74	0.004
AAA volume change	0.29	−0.11–0.61	0.142
AAA diameter change	0.11	−0.28–0.47	0.577
ILT surface at max. aortic diameter change	0.31	−0.09–0.63	0.114
Aortic wall thickness at max. ILT diameter change (mm)	−0.15	−0.50–0.23	0.410
ILT thickness change	0.44	0.05–0.71	0.024

ILT: intraluminal thrombus, AAA: abdominal aortic aneurysm, max.: maximum.

3.3. TBR Progression in a Large and Fast-Growing AAA

We conducted a subgroup analysis to explore whether TBR progression was different in patients with a large or fast-growing AAA. Patients were assigned based on their baseline AAA maximum diameter or their volume increase between baseline and follow-up. We did not observe differences in TBR progression for a large vs. small AAA or fast- vs. slow-growing AAA (Figure 3).

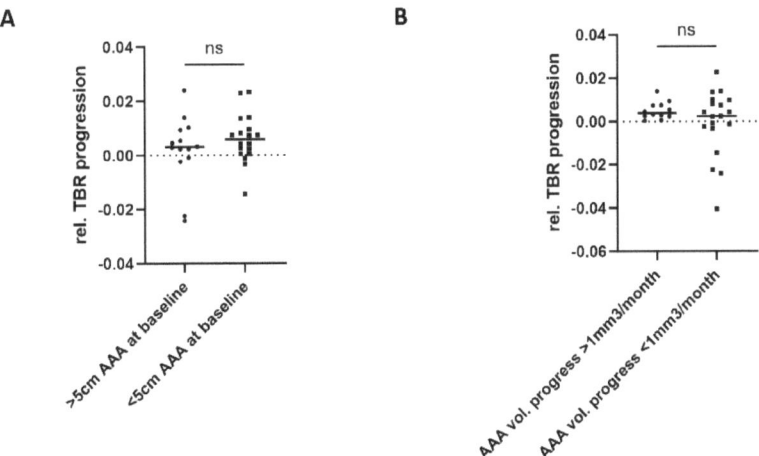

Figure 3. Thrombus burden ration (TBR) in large and fast-growing AAA. Patients of the study cohort were assigned either based on their maximum AAA diameter at baseline (**A**) or their AAA volume increase between the sequential CTA scans (**B**). Threshold values for both were set to AAA baseline diameter > 50 mm and AAA volume progression > 1 mm3/month. TBR progression was compared for both subgroups. There were no significant differences in TBR progression between both subgroups within the study cohort. Mann–Whitney U test was applied after identification of outliers using ROUT method (Q = 5%), slightly reducing the original total number of n = 35; ns: not significant.

3.4. TBR Progression and Potential Correlating Factors

As a next step, we performed a multivariate linear regression analysis to determine whether age, gender, cardiovascular risk factors/comorbidities, hemostasis-related blood parameters, or changes over time in morphologic AAA or ILT parameters were associated with relative TBR progression (Table 4). Among the studied characteristics, we could not identify a statistically significant association. Yet, of all the cardiovascular risk factors, T2D showed the highest regression beta coefficients (unstandardized B 0.122; standardized B 0.735). For the AAA-related morphologic parameters, AAA diameter change over time showed the highest chance of predicting TBR progression (unstandardized B 0.594; standardized B 2.356), though this was not statistically significant.

Table 4. Multivariate logistic regression analysis for comorbidities and blood parameters. Multivariate logistic regression analysis was applied to test the association of co morbidities, blood parameters at baseline, and CTA morphologic parameters with TBR progression. Data are reported with coefficient, standard error, p-value, and upper and lower 95% confidence intervals (95% CI) (n = 35).

Model	Unstandardized Coefficient		Standardized Coefficient				
	B	Standard Error	Beta	t	p-Value	Upper 95% CI	Lower 95% CI
Constant	−0.010	0.470		−0.021	0.984	−1.094	1.074
Demographics and Comorbidities							
Gender	0.045	0.091	0.271	0.498	0.632	−0.164	0.254
Age	−0.001	0.003	−0.218	−0.426	0.681	−0.008	0.005

Table 4. Cont.

Model	Unstandardized Coefficient		Standardized Coefficient				
	B	Standard Error	Beta	t	p-Value	Upper 95% CI	Lower 95% CI
aHT	0.007	0.044	0.072	0.163	0.874	−0.095	0.109
HLP	0.005	0.039	0.043	0.117	0.910	−0.086	0.095
T2D	0.122	0.084	0.735	1.460	0.183	−0.071	0.316
BMI > 30	0.030	0.043	0.285	0.710	0.498	−0.068	0.129
History of smoking	−0.011	0.030	−0.110	−0.353	0.733	−0.080	0.059
Blood parameters at second CTA							
HCT	−0.003	0.007	−0.560	−0.468	0.652	−0.020	0.014
Hb	−0.003	0.020	−0.161	−0.143	0.890	−0.050	0.044
RBC	0.032	0.020	0.721	1.612	0.146	−0.014	0.078
PLC	0.000	0.000	−0.341	−0.837	0.427	−0.001	0.000
WBC	-9.076×10^7	0.005	0.000	0.000	1.000	−0.011	0.011
Quick	0.001	0.002	0.223	0.255	0.805	−0.005	0.006
INR	0.035	0.173	0.110	0.199	0.847	−0.365	0.434
AAA and ILT morphology							
Rel. AAA diameter	0.594	2.468	2.356	0.241	0.816	−5.097	6.285
Rel. ILT volume	−0.043	0.117	−0.685	−0.371	0.720	−0.313	0.226
Rel. AAA volume	−0.293	0.331	−1.525	−0.884	0.403	−1.057	0.471
Rel. ILT surface at max. aortic diameter	0.045	0.100	1.253	0.447	0.667	−0.186	0.275
Rel. ILT max. thickness	0.001	0.018	0.048	0.076	0.941	−0.041	0.044
Rel. Aortic wall thickness at max. ILT diameter	0.141	1.939	0.505	0.073	0.944	−4.330	4.611

aHT: arterial hypertension, HLP: hyperlipoproteinemia, T2D: type II diabetes mellitus, HCT: hematocrit, Hb: hemoglobin, RBC: red blood cell count, PLC: platelet count, WBC: white blood cell count, INR: international normalized ratio.

4. Discussion

The role of ILT in AAA has gained significant interest in recent years. Yet, we are still at the beginning of unveiling its detailed role in the disease. This retrospective study focused on the relationship between ILT and AAA volume progression over time, and the ratio between those two parameters was defined as the thrombus burden ratio (TBR). We found that the growth of an ILT contributes to this ratio to a greater extend when compared to changes in AAA volume, indicating a faster ILT growth over time than overall AAA growth. However, there was no difference in the TBR progression with a fast- vs. slow-growing AAA or an initially large- vs. small-sized AAA. Also, due to the small sample size, we were not able to identify clinical or morphological parameters directly associated with TBR changes.

While the correlation between the risk of AAA rupture and the maximum AAA diameter is well established [13], this linear relationship does not seem to apply for the ILT. For example, recent studies have suggested a thin ILT as an individual risk factor for increased AAA growth and risk of rupture with potential implications for the timing of surgical treatment [14,15]. While this suggests a potentially protective role of the ILT, other studies have taken a fundamentally different view of the role of the ILT in an AAA.

Following such a theory, it is implied that as soon as an undefined threshold of thickness is reached, the potentially protective effects of an ILT are at least equalized by its microstructural composition and the associated proteolytic effects. The sum of these proteolytic effects results in a weakening of the AAA wall, which in turn, may contribute to accelerated AAA growth [4]. Interestingly, this mechanistic role of the ILT is supported by the observation that a high ILT burden was linked to decreased aortic wall strength and an elevated risk of a small AAA rupture [16]. This has also been linked to a reduced supply of oxygen to the aneurysmal wall due to the large ILT mass [17]. This is further supported by findings indicating a ruptured AAA to have a larger diameter and larger ILT volume when compared to an intact AAA [18]. Pointing in the same direction, reports indicate that the presence of an ILT is associated with an increased risk of rupture and faster ILT growth, especially in a small-sized AAA of ≤50 mm [19]. In contrast to these observations, the data from this study show disproportionate ILT vs. AAA growth (TBR), although there was no difference in small AAAs (<50 mm) vs. large AAAs (>50 mm).

Of note, most studies available in the literature to date have one important limitation in common. In most cases, ILT and AAA volume and/or diameter are considered separately from each other; a relative relationship between these two parameters is rarely established, although there is a conclusive argument for that. Here, the implementation of the TBR may be useful for future studies, since this parameter describes the relative ILT growth in relation to the AAA growth over a period of time and could therefore be a decisive future predictor for the determination of an individual's rupture risk or AAA growth rate as well as for the quality of care in regard to the complication rate after open or endovascular therapy [20]. This seems particularly likely, since a large ILT deposition was shown to negatively affect long-term results following endovascular therapy [21].

The results of this study could not establish a direct correlation between any clinical or morphological parameters and the TBR, likely due to the limited sample size. A previous study based on Danish registry data also investigated the role the ILT in an untreated AAA based on ultrasound-derived data. Here, the authors found a small, yet statistically significant correlation between the relative ILT maximum area and AAA growth in their multivariate linear regression model, which we were not able to identify. However, this was carried out in a vastly larger cohort study of 400 patients [22]. In the present study, we were able to gather CTA follow-up data of untreated AAAs, which to our knowledge, has never been published to this extent; the cohort size in this monocentric study hardly allows for any strong conclusions to be drawn regarding the identification of factors affecting ILT growth.

Identification of such factors may be tough in other regards as well. As mentioned above, it is unclear if a large ILT is protective or harmful and whether there is a potentially beneficial threshold for AAA development, which further complicates the process of identifying clear associations.

Conclusively, the multifactorial influence of several parameters in their interaction appears to be the most likely contributor to the TBR. However, some parameters may appear more important than others. For example, T2D and the red blood cell (RBC) count showed the most robust correlation with the TBR. Such a correlation seems particularly plausible against the background of a known increased platelet activation in T2D. In this context, hyperglycemia may have direct osmotic effects by activating platelet GP IIb/IIIa and p-selectin, with protein kinase C (PKC) activation contributing to platelet activation [23–25]. Also, the lack of insulin in patients with diabetes may contribute to enhanced platelet activation as insulin binds to the insulin receptor (IR) located on the platelet surface and activates insulin receptor substrate 1 (IRS-1) via tyrosine phosphorylation. This, in turn, mediates its association with Gi protein α (Giα)-subunit [25–27], which ultimately increases intraplatelet cyclic adenosine monophosphate (cAMP), resulting in decreased platelet activity [28].

The roles of RBCs in hemostasis and thrombosis have become increasingly clear in the recent years. Multiple mechanistic studies suggest that RBCs can actively promote thrombus formation and should no longer be considered as a passive bystander [29]. To this end, multiple hemorheological effects, effects on platelet reactivity, and interactions with the vessel wall are described, although their relevance for ILT formation in AAA has not been investigated at this moment in time [30]. Based on the data presented in this study, the authors strongly encourage further mechanistic studies to identify possible relevant pathways that may contribute to the TBR and that are also beneficially targetable.

If an attempt is now made to finally shed more light on the possible clinical relevance of the TBR, the authors consider two scientific questions to be pressing. On the one hand, the extent to which the TBR may serve as a possible predictor of AAA rupture or increased disease-associated complications needs to be evaluated. Here, a prospective, multicentric study design is needed for patients undergoing AAA surveillance on a larger scale, as introduced in this preliminary study involving multiple institutions. Also, patients with an incidental AAA diagnosis during CT scans for other medical reasons should be included and prospectively followed up. On the other hand, it needs to be verified whether the TBR can predict outcomes after AAA treatment, both endovascular and open. In this context, the TBR may prove useful, as there is accumulating evidence that the ILT affects outcomes after EVAR and TEVAR [21,31]. Again, larger-scaled studies are needed to explore this potential.

This study has various limitations. First, the stringent inclusion criteria have limited the cohort size to 35 patients, since follow-up CT is not regularly available in patients with a large AAA. The small sample size needs to be considered when drawing conclusions from the study. Also, the single-center study design and the retrospective setting may have further biased our findings.

5. Conclusions

In summary, we found that the TBR increases during AAA development indicating an overproportioned ILT vs. AAA volume growth with no preference with regard to a small vs. large and a fast- vs. slow-growing AAA. Nevertheless, the TBR may serve as a useful parameter in future studies since it incorporates several factors in one parameter. Factors that contribute to increased ILT growth or the TBR are not yet known but appear mechanistically interesting.

Author Contributions: Conceptualization, J.M., K.-J.K., H.S., M.E. and M.U.W.; Data curation, J.M., J.S. and M.U.W.; Funding acquisition, H.S., M.E. and M.U.W.; Investigation, J.M., A.M., J.S. and A.A.; Methodology, J.M., A.M., J.S. and K.-J.K.; Project administration, M.U.W.; Resources, H.S., M.E. and M.U.W.; Supervision, M.U.W.; Validation, A.A., W.G. and M.U.W.; Visualization, W.G.; Writing—original draft, J.M., A.M. and M.U.W.; Writing—review and editing, J.S., A.A., W.G., K.-J.K., H.S. and M.E. All authors have read and agreed to the published version of the manuscript.

Funding: The study was supported by the Deutsche Forschungsgemeinschaft (DFG), grant number EL651/6-1 to M.E. and WA 3533/3-1 to M.U.W.; Collaborative Research Center TRR259 (Aortic Disease—Grant No. 397484323) to M.E. and H.S., and a local research grant by the research council of the medical faculty at the Heinrich Heine University Düsseldorf to J.M. (grant number 2021-35) and M.U.W. (grant number 2020-06).

Institutional Review Board Statement: The study was conducted in accordance with the Declaration of Helsinki and approved by the local ethics committee at the Heinrich Heine University Düsseldorf (approval ID: 2018-2, approval date: 28 May 2018).

Informed Consent Statement: Informed consent was obtained from all subjects involved in the study.

Data Availability Statement: The underlying data are available from the corresponding author upon reasonable request.

Conflicts of Interest: The authors declare no conflicts of interest.

References

1. Krumholz, H.M.; Keenan, P.S.; Brush, J.E.; Bufalino, V.J.; Chernew, M.E.; Epstein, A.J.; Heidenreich, P.A.; Ho, V.; Masoudi, F.A.; Matchar, D.B.; et al. Standards for Measures Used for Public Reporting of Efficiency in Health Care: A Scientific Statement from the American Heart Association Interdisciplinary Council on Quality of Care and Outcomes Research and the American College of Cardiology Foundation. *J. Am. Coll. Cardiol.* **2008**, *52*, 1518–1526. [CrossRef] [PubMed]
2. Badger, S.; Forster, R.; Blair, P.H.; Ellis, P.; Kee, F.; Harkin, D.W. Endovascular Treatment for Ruptured Abdominal Aortic Aneurysm. *Cochrane Database Syst. Rev.* **2017**, *5*, CD005261. [CrossRef] [PubMed]
3. Ko, K.J.; Yoo, J.H.; Cho, H.J.; Kim, M.H.; Jun, K.W.; Han, K.D.; Hwang, J.K. The Impact of Abdominal Aortic Aneurysm on Cardiovascular Diseases: A Nationwide Dataset Analysis. *Int. Heart J.* **2021**, *62*, 1235–1240. [CrossRef]
4. O'Leary, S.A.; Kavanagh, E.G.; Grace, P.A.; McGloughlin, T.M.; Doyle, B.J. The Biaxial Mechanical Behaviour of Abdominal Aortic Aneurysm Intraluminal Thrombus: Classification of Morphology and the Determination of Layer and Region Specific Properties. *J. Biomech.* **2014**, *47*, 1430–1437. [CrossRef] [PubMed]
5. Vorp, D.; Mandarino, W.; Webster, M.; Iii, J.G. Potential Influence of Intraluminal Thrombus on Abdominal Aortic Aneurysm as Assessed by a New Non-Invasive Method. *Cardiovasc. Surg.* **1996**, *4*, 732–739. [CrossRef]
6. Michel, J.B.; Martin-Ventura, J.L.; Egido, J.; Sakalihasan, N.; Treska, V.; Lindholt, J.; Allaire, E.; Thorsteinsdottir, U.; Cockerill, G.; Swedenborg, J. Novel Aspects of the Pathogenesis of Aneurysms of the Abdominal Aorta in Humans. *Cardiovasc. Res.* **2011**, *90*, 18–27. [CrossRef]
7. Wang, D.H.J.; Makaroun, M.S.; Webster, M.W.; Vorp, D.A. Effect of Intraluminal Thrombus on Wall Stress in Patient-Specific Models of Abdominal Aortic Aneurysm. *J. Vasc. Surg.* **2002**, *36*, 598–604. [CrossRef]
8. Vande Geest, J.P.; Schmidt, D.E.; Sacks, M.S.; Vorp, D.A. The Effects of Anisotropy on the Stress Analyses of Patient-Specific Abdominal Aortic Aneurysms. *Ann. Biomed. Eng.* **2008**, *36*, 921–932. [CrossRef]
9. Kazi, M.; Thyberg, J.; Religa, P.; Roy, J.; Eriksson, P.; Hedin, U.; Swedenborg, J. Influence of Intraluminal Thrombus on Structural and Cellular Composition of Abdominal Aortic Aneurysm Wall. *J. Vasc. Surg.* **2003**, *38*, 1283–1292. [CrossRef]
10. Zhu, C.; Leach, J.R.; Wang, Y.; Gasper, W.; Saloner, D.; Hope, M.D. Intraluminal Thrombus Predicts Rapid Growth of Abdominal Aortic Aneurysms. *Radiology* **2020**, *294*, 707–713. [CrossRef]
11. Singh, T.P.; Wong, S.A.; Moxon, J.V.; Gasser, T.C.; Golledge, J. Systematic Review and Meta-Analysis of the Association between Intraluminal Thrombus Volume and Abdominal Aortic Aneurysm Rupture. *J. Vasc. Surg.* **2019**, *70*, 2065–2073.e10. [CrossRef] [PubMed]
12. Koncar, I.; Nikolic, D.; Milosevic, Z.; Bogavac-Stanojevic, N.; Ilic, N.; Dragas, M.; Sladojevic, M.; Markovic, M.; Vujcic, A.; Filipovic, N.; et al. Abdominal Aortic Aneurysm Volume and Relative Intraluminal Thrombus Volume Might Be Auxiliary Predictors of Rupture-an Observational Cross-Sectional Study. *Front. Surg.* **2023**, *10*, 1095224. [CrossRef] [PubMed]
13. Scott, R.A.P.; Wilson, N.M.; Ashton, H.A.; Kay, D.N. Is Surgery Necessary for Abdominal Aortic Aneurysm Less than 6 Cm in Diameter? *Lancet* **1993**, *342*, 1395–1396. [CrossRef] [PubMed]
14. Wiernicki, I.; Parafiniuk, M.; Kolasa-Wołosiuk, A.; Gutowska, I.; Kazimierczak, A.; Clark, J.; Baranowska-Bosiacka, I.; Szumilowicz, P.; Gutowski, P. Relationship between aortic wall oxidative stress/proteolytic enzyme expression and intraluminal thrombus thickness indicates a novel pathomechanism in the progression of human abdominal aortic aneurysm. *FASEB J.* **2019**, *33*, 885–895. [CrossRef] [PubMed]
15. Domonkos, A.; Staffa, R.; Kubíček, L. Effect of Intraluminal Thrombus on Growth Rate of Abdominal Aortic Aneurysms. *Int. Angiol.* **2019**, *38*, 39–45. [CrossRef]
16. Haller, S.J.; Crawford, J.D.; Courchaine, K.M.; Bohannan, C.J.; Landry, G.J.; Moneta, G.L.; Azarbal, A.F.; Rugonyi, S. Intraluminal Thrombus Is Associated with Early Rupture of Abdominal Aortic Aneurysm. *J. Vasc. Surg.* **2017**, *67*, 1051–1058.e1. [CrossRef] [PubMed]
17. Vorp, D.A.; Lee, P.C.; Wang, D.H.J.; Makaroun, M.S.; Nemoto, E.M.; Ogawa, S.; Webster, M.W. Association of Intraluminal Thrombus in Abdominal Aortic Aneurysm with Local Hypoxia and Wall Weakening. *J. Vasc. Surg.* **2001**, *34*, 291–299. [CrossRef]
18. Hans, S.S.; Jareunpoon, O.; Balasubramaniam, M.; Zelenock, G.B. Size and Location of Thrombus in Intact and Ruptured Abdominal Aortic Aneurysms. *J. Vasc. Surg.* **2005**, *41*, 584–588. [CrossRef]
19. Stenbaek, J.; Kalin, B.; Swedenborg, J. Growth of Thrombus May Be a Better Predictor of Rupture than Diameter in Patients with Abdominal Aortic Aneurysms. *Eur. J. Vasc. Endovasc. Surg.* **2000**, *20*, 466–469. [CrossRef]
20. Boyd, A.J. Intraluminal Thrombus: Innocent Bystander or Factor in Abdominal Aortic Aneurysm Pathogenesis? *JVS-Vasc. Sci.* **2021**, *2*, 159–169. [CrossRef]
21. Ding, Y.; Shan, Y.; Zhou, M.; Cai, L.; Li, X.; Shi, Z.; Fu, W. Amount of Intraluminal Thrombus Correlates with Severe Adverse Events in Abdominal Aortic Aneurysms after Endovascular Aneurysm Repair. *Ann. Vasc. Surg.* **2020**, *67*, 254–264. [CrossRef]
22. Behr-Rasmussen, C.; Grøndal, N.; Bramsen, M.B.; Thomsen, M.D.; Lindholt, J.S. Mural Thrombus and the Progression of Abdominal Aortic Aneurysms: A Large Population-Based Prospective Cohort Study. *Eur. J. Vasc. Endovasc. Surg. Off. J. Eur. Soc. Vasc. Surg.* **2014**, *48*, 301–307. [CrossRef]
23. Keating, F.K.; Sobel, B.E.; Schneider, D.J. Effects of Increased Concentrations of Glucose on Platelet Reactivity in Healthy Subjects and in Patients with and without Diabetes Mellitus. *Am. J. Cardiol.* **2003**, *92*, 1362–1365. [CrossRef]
24. Assert, R.; Scherk, G.; Bumbure, A.; Pirags, V.; Schatz, H.; Pfeiffer, A.F. Regulation of Protein Kinase C by Short Term Hyperglycaemia in Human Platelets in Vivo and in Vitro. *Diabetologia* **2001**, *44*, 188–195. [CrossRef]

25. Kaur, R.; Kaur, M.; Singh, J. Endothelial Dysfunction and Platelet Hyperactivity in Type 2 Diabetes Mellitus: Molecular Insights and Therapeutic Strategies. *Cardiovasc. Diabetol.* **2018**, *17*, 121. [CrossRef] [PubMed]
26. Trovati, M.; Anfossi, G.; Massucco, P.; Mattiello, L.; Costamagna, C.; Piretto, V.; Mularoni, E.; Cavalot, F.; Bosia, A.; Ghigo, D. Insulin Stimulates Nitric Oxide Synthesis in Human Platelets and, through Nitric Oxide, Increases Platelet Concentrations of Both Guanosine-3′, 5′-Cyclic Monophosphate and Adenosine-3′, 5′-Cyclic Monophosphate. *Diabetes* **1997**, *46*, 742–749. [CrossRef] [PubMed]
27. Ferreira, I.A.; Eybrechts, K.L.; Mocking, A.I.M.; Kroner, C.; Akkerman, J.-W.N. IRS-1 Mediates Inhibition of Ca2+ Mobilization by Insulin via the Inhibitory G-Protein Gi. *J. Biol. Chem.* **2004**, *279*, 3254–3264. [CrossRef] [PubMed]
28. Kakouros, N.; Rade, J.J.; Kourliouros, A.; Resar, J.R. Platelet Function in Patients with Diabetes Mellitus: From a Theoretical to a Practical Perspective. *Int. J. Endocrinol.* **2011**, *2011*, 742719. [CrossRef] [PubMed]
29. Byrnes, J.R.; Wolberg, A.S. Red Blood Cells in Thrombosis. *Blood* **2017**, *130*, 1795–1799. [CrossRef] [PubMed]
30. Weisel, J.W.; Litvinov, R.I. Red Blood Cells: The Forgotten Player in Hemostasis and Thrombosis. *J. Thromb. Haemost.* **2019**, *17*, 271–282. [CrossRef]
31. Whaley, Z.L.; Cassimjee, I.; Novak, Z.; Rowland, D.; Lapolla, P.; Chandrashekar, A.; Pearce, B.J.; Beck, A.W.; Handa, A.; Lee, R. The Spatial Morphology of Intraluminal Thrombus Influences Type II Endoleak after Endovascular Repair of Abdominal Aortic Aneurysms. *Ann. Vasc. Surg.* **2020**, *66*, 77–84. [CrossRef] [PubMed]

Disclaimer/Publisher's Note: The statements, opinions and data contained in all publications are solely those of the individual author(s) and contributor(s) and not of MDPI and/or the editor(s). MDPI and/or the editor(s) disclaim responsibility for any injury to people or property resulting from any ideas, methods, instructions or products referred to in the content.

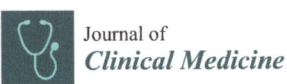

Article

Aortic Vascular Graft and Endograft Infection–Patient Outcome Cannot Be Determined Based on Pre-Operative Characteristics

Ilaria Puttini [1,†], Marvin Kapalla [2,†], Anja Braune [3], Enrico Michler [3], Joselyn Kröger [2], Brigitta Lutz [2], Natzi Sakhalihasan [4], Matthias Trenner [5], Gabor Biro [1], Wolfgang Weber [6], Thomas Rössel [7], Christian Reeps [2], Hans-Henning Eckstein [1], Steffen Wolk [2], Christoph Knappich [1], Susan Notohamiprodjo [6] and Albert Busch [1,2,*]

1. Department for Vascular and Endovascular Surgery, Klinikum Rechts der Isar, Technical University of Munich, 80333 Munich, Germany
2. Division of Vascular and Endovascular Surgery, Department for Visceral, Thoracic and Vascular Surgery, Medical Faculty Carl Gustav Carus, University Hospital, Technical University of Dresden, 01307 Dresden, Germany
3. Nuclear Medicine Department, University Hospital Carl Gustav Carus, Technical University of Dresden, 01307 Dresden, Germany
4. Department of Cardiovascular and Thoracic Surgery, University of Liège, 4000 Liège, Belgium
5. Division of Vascular Medicine, St. Josefs-Hospital Wiesbaden, 65189 Wiesbaden, Germany
6. Department of Nuclear Medicine, Klinikum Rechts der Isar, Technical University of Munich, 81675 Munich, Germany
7. Department of Anaesthesiology and Critical Care Medicine, University Hospital Carl Gustav Carus Dresden, Technical University of Dresden, 01307 Dresden, Germany
* Correspondence: albert.busch@uniklinikum-dresden.de; Tel.: +49-351-458-3072
† These authors contributed equally to this work.

Abstract: Vascular graft/endograft infection (VGEI) is a serious complication after aortic surgery. This study investigates VGEI and patient characteristics, PET/CT quantification before surgical or conservative management of VGEI and post-intervention outcomes in order to identify patients who might benefit from such a procedure. PET standard uptake values (SUV) were quantitatively assessed and compared to a non-VGEI cohort. The primary endpoints were in-hospital mortality and aortic reintervention-free survival at six months. Ninety-three patients (75% male, 65 ± 10 years, 82% operated) were included. The initial operation was mainly for aneurysm (67.7%: 31% EVAR, 12% TEVAR, 57% open aortic repair). Thirty-two patients presented with fistulae. PET SUV_{TLR} (target-to-liver ratio) showed 94% sensitivity and 89% specificity. Replacement included silver-coated Dacron (21.3%), pericardium (61.3%) and femoral vein (17.3%), yet the material did not influence the overall survival ($p = 0.745$). In-hospital mortality did not differ between operative and conservative treatment (19.7% vs. 17.6%, $p = 0.84$). At six months, 50% of the operated cohort survived without aortic reintervention. Short- and midterm morbidity and mortality remained high after aortic graft removal. Neither preoperative characteristics nor the material used for reconstruction influenced the overall survival, and, with limitations, both the in-hospital and midterm survival were similar between the surgically and conservatively managed patients.

Keywords: aortic graft infection; vascular graft endograft infection; pericardial prosthesis; silver graft

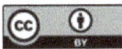

Citation: Puttini, I.; Kapalla, M.; Braune, A.; Michler, E.; Kröger, J.; Lutz, B.; Sakhalihasan, N.; Trenner, M.; Biro, G.; Weber, W.; et al. Aortic Vascular Graft and Endograft Infection–Patient Outcome Cannot Be Determined Based on Pre-Operative Characteristics. *J. Clin. Med.* **2024**, *13*, 269. https://doi.org/10.3390/jcm13010269

Academic Editor: Reinhard Kopp

Received: 29 October 2023
Revised: 1 December 2023
Accepted: 31 December 2023
Published: 3 January 2024

Copyright: © 2024 by the authors. Licensee MDPI, Basel, Switzerland. This article is an open access article distributed under the terms and conditions of the Creative Commons Attribution (CC BY) license (https://creativecommons.org/licenses/by/4.0/).

1. Introduction

Aortic vascular graft and endograft infections (VGEIs) are among the most challenging cases in vascular surgery for both clinicians and patients. Despite the more frequent use of endovascular aortic repair for aortic occlusive disease (AOD) as well as aortic aneurysm (EVAR/TEVAR) over traditional open repair (OR), the incidence of VGEI is on the rise and estimated to affect 1.5–4% of the respective population [1,2].

Typical symptoms range from unspecific fever and pain to impaired wound healing to catastrophic bleeding events in the case of aorto-enteric fistula and might occur early or late (>4 months) after implantation [3]. In order to facilitate VGEI diagnosis, criteria based on clinical/surgical, radiologic and laboratory findings have been defined, providing excellent sensitivity (up to 99%) and high specificity (up to 61%) [2,4]. Recently, ^{18}F-fluordeoxyglucose (FDG) positron emission tomography (PET) is being used more frequently and was demonstrated to increase diagnostic specificity over computed tomography angiography (CTA) [5,6]. Yet, uncertainty remains about a possible diagnostic cut-off regarding a pathologic maximum standard uptake value (SUV$_{max}$) [3,7].

Treatment and specific outcomes for aortic VGEI are reported in a few retrospective cohort studies of 20–80 patients, mostly focusing on the abdominal aorta and a specific replacement material or technique after a follow-up of six months to five years [8–10]. Here, upon graft removal, early and late mortality have been summarized to vary between 4.3–48% and 9–85%, respectively [3,11]. Conservative treatment with or without eventual drainage, irrigation and lifelong anti-infectives is palliative and only scarcely reported [12]. If no bleeding or fistulas occurred, singular cases were shown to have good life expectancy [13,14]. In approximately one-third of cases, blood cultures or intraoperative swabs remain negative. Missing reporting standards on sample acquisition, time-to-infection, antibiotic regimen or infectious specificity make identification of the responsible (poly)microbial flora impossible [2,15]. Hence, various meta-analyses and one European guideline agree on the lack of robust evidence and the continuous need for primary data in this ever-evolving clinical problem [3,16,17].

In this dual-center retrospective cohort study, we report the clinical presentation, procedural and outcome details of VGEI patients treated operatively and conservatively. Additionally, we aim to identify a possible benefit of preoperative risk stratification regarding outcomes involving a quantitative and qualitative PET/CT analysis based on patient and diagnostic characteristics.

2. Patients and Methods

<u>Study design, patient identification and ethical approval</u>: A dual-center retrospective cohort study was conducted. Patients with VGEI were identified at two university centers retrospectively from the electronic information system, operative charts and prospective case registration for the purpose of VGEI cohort analysis from 1 January 2013 (Munich) or 2015 (Dresden) to 31 December 2021. Baseline data were retrieved from electronic patient records and follow-up visits.

Patient data were pseudonymized for further analyses. The study was performed in accordance with the Declaration of Helsinki and approved by the local ethics committees (Medical Faculty, Technical University of Munich: 2022-428-S-NP and Technical University Dresden BO-EK-205042022). The STROBE checklist (v4) for cohort studies was followed as far as possible [18].

<u>Inclusion/exclusion criteria</u>: All patients operated on or diagnosed with their first thoracic or abdominal aortic VGEI were included. Diagnosis was established using MAGIC (Management of Aortic Graft Infection Collaboration) criteria positivity (s. below) from Lyons et al. [2].

Patients <18 years old and patients with isolated iliac graft infections were excluded.

<u>Conservative treatment group</u>: All patients who refused definitive operative treatment after informed consent (ideally including relatives) and patients who were considered unfit for surgery after thorough evaluation including complete cardiac and pulmonary workup and vascular board decision did not undergo graft removal or replacement but may have undergone drainage and/or irrigation. Here, all patients were dismissed on calculated (if available) or empiric (individual case discussion with infectiologist) anti-infective therapy.

<u>Stepwise analysis and definitions</u>: *Patient baseline characteristics* included age, sex, hypertension, diabetes, smoking status, chronic obstructive pulmonary disease (COPD), ethanol consumption, renal insufficiency (any Kidney Disease: Improving Global Outcomes [KDIGO] $\geq$ 2), permanent dialysis, active/previous malignancy, hyperlipidemia, coronary artery disease (CAD) and peripheral arterial occlusive disease (PAOD).

Initial aortic operation was classified as EVAR (including fenestrated and scalloped grafts (n = 2) and iliac branch devices (n = 1) as well as monoiliac reconstruction in combination with extra-anatomic crossover bypass (n = 2)). Furthermore, TEVAR or open aortic repair (OAR) (including tube or aorto-bi/mono-femoral/iliac grafts) for aneurysm (or penetrating aortic ulcers (PAU)), occlusive disease or dissection was noted. Additionally, initial operation due to aortic rupture and in/ex domo procedure was recorded.

A Diagnostic protocol was followed in all cases with suspicion of VGEI. This included blood cultures/swabs (fistula) before antibiotics, CT and, in case of GI bleeding or suspicion of fistula, diagnostic endoscopy. PET/CT was indicated in case of doubt after initial assessment or for confirmation in selected cases. No bacterial DNA was assessed.

VGEI characteristics included time-to-VGEI defined by the date difference between initial operation and established VGEI diagnosis. According to MAGIC criteria, diagnosis was established when at least a single major criterion and any other criterion from another category was fulfilled [2,3]. MAGIC criteria (radiologic) were based on the last CT and/or PET/CT or PET/MR before established diagnosis and the corresponding sampling (microbiologic) via (1) blood culture, (2) CT-guided aspiration and/or (3) direct swab (i.e., cutaneous fistula). Cut-off between late and early VGEI was >4 months [3].

Preoperative CT-guided drainage (or drain only in the conservative treatment group) was for diagnostic purposes, and fluid drainage and eventual temporary irrigation were at the surgeon's discretion. No other procedures were carried out in conservatively managed patients.

Operative handling and definitions: Indication for graft replacement was made via a vascular board decision with patients' (and ideally relatives') informed consent. Emergency surgery was performed due to life-threatening bleeding. Urgent surgery was performed due to suspected aorta-related symptoms (n = 2 summarized with elective procedures). Gastrointestinal fistula involved esophagus and duodenum. The material and type of reconstruction was left to the surgeon's discretion, with the goal of removing all graft material (bare springs eventually left in situ), and extensive debridement of the surrounding infectious tissue was performed as far as possible. Generally, anatomical reconstruction and primary abdominal closure were aims. Eventual additional procedures, including omentum plasty, renal cold perfusion or preemptive temporary left-heart bypass, and especially intestinal reconstruction or discontinuation, were at the treating surgeon's discretion and shown as direct suture (no anastomosis) or resection (including anastomosis and resection).

Additional CT-guided drainage during the postoperative course was performed when necessary. Postoperative complications were aortic (bleeding, rupture), neurologic (stroke, critical illness neuropathy, procedure related nerve injury, delirium), medical (acute kidney failure (any worsening of initial KDIGO stage), temporary dialysis, respiratory problems (longtime respirator treatment, pneumonia, edema), pulmonary embolism, myocardial infarction) and surgical (surgical site infection [SSI], limb ischemia, visceral complication [intestinal ischemia, insufficiency]). Complications were additionally classified according to the Clavien–Dindo classification [19].

Reinfection or persistent infection of the aorta (replacement graft) or the operative situs was defined as suggested by the ESVS guidelines by either (1) any new signs of sepsis/systemic inflammatory response (SIRS) when other sources were ruled out; (2) newly diagnosed bacteria/fungi from periaortic fluid/abscess drainage; (3) newly diagnosed VGEI after replacement according to MAGIC criteria; or (4) anastomotic rupture due to infected graft [1–3]. Reinfection was diagnosed in-hospital or during follow-up and is summarized in results.

Additional complications during follow-up were aortic/graft-related complications (anastomotic rupture; high-grade limb stenosis) requiring reintervention (i.e., secondary extra-anatomic reconstruction, endovascular lining), other surgical complications requiring operation (ureter stenosis, SSI, limb or mesenteric ischemia) and medical complications remotely related to the previous replacement (kidney failure, subileus, pulmonary embolism). Patients in the conservative treatment group were not followed up for complications. All patients or their family physician were contacted in 2022 to establish last contact if not visible from electronic records.

Endpoints and outcome parameters: Primary endpoints were in-hospital mortality (safety endpoint) and 6-month aortic reintervention-free survival (efficacy endpoint).

Secondary endpoints were mortality (at 30 d, 6, 12 months and overall) and the in-hospital complication rates (aortic, surgical, medical, neurologic).

Additionally, the aortic/surgical complication rates and the overall survival in relation to the graft material for aortic reconstruction were analyzed.

PET image acquisition and quantitative and qualitative analysis:

^{18}F-FDG-PET acquisition: All PET/CT examinations were performed on a Biograph-Vision 600, a Biograph mCT machine, or a Biograph16 Hirez (Siemens Healthineers, Erlangen, Germany). Two patients received a PET/MR examination using a 3 Tesla Ingenuity TOF PET/MRI (Philips Medical Systems, Best, The Netherlands).

Patients fasted for at least 4 h prior to the ^{18}F-FDG tracer injection. Blood glucose levels were required to be less than 140 mg/dL during a period of approximately 60 min before the administration of the ^{18}F-FDG. Diagnostic CT imaging was performed in the portal venous phase 80 s after intravenous injection of contrast agent [Imeron 300] (1.5 mL/kg body weight, max. 120 mL) followed by the PET imaging in continuous bed motion mode ("flow-mode") or vice versa.

PET image acquisition techniques differed slightly between the two centers involved and the three different machines applied over time. Generally (Dresden cohort), a median of 4,73 MBq/kg body weight ^{18}F-FDG (range: 2.88–6.39 MBq/kg) was intravenously injected, and PET image acquisition started after a median of 76 min p.i. (range: 58–113 min). Images were acquired in continuous bed motion mode (Biograph mCT: 1.5 mm/s; Biograph Vision 600; 2.2 mm/s) or in step-and-shoot mode (Biograph16 Hirez PET/CT: 2 to 3 min per bed position, Ingenuity PET/MRI: 2 min per bed position).

All PET/CT examinations were reconstructed using an ordered subset expectation maximization (ODEM) iterative reconstruction algorithm and were corrected for randoms, dead time, scatter and attenuation (Biograph mCT: time-of-flight measurements, 3D reconstruction using point-spread-function modeling, three iterations, twenty-one subsets, 200 × 200 matrix, zoom 1.0, defined voxel size, post-reconstruction smoothing (Gaussian filter) or were acquired in 3D mode with an acquisition time of 1.5 mm/s from 2019.

Image Analysis: All ^{18}F-FDG-PET scans were analyzed with syngo.via (software version VB30A, Siemens Healthineers, Erlangen, Germany) under the supervision of an experienced nuclear medicine physician (SN) on a certified digital workstation who was blinded to the clinical data. Quantitative uptake was analyzed with Osirix (Osirix MD, Pixmeo, Geneva, Switzerland). The following parameters were acquired for quantification:

Intensity uptake: SUV_{max} was assessed for aorta, liver and mediastinal blood pool using region of interest (ROI) analysis, which was manually drawn based on co-registered CT or MR images. In all examinations, 10 cm³ circular regions of interest (ROIs) were drawn. The SUV_{max} in the region of the vascular graft was defined as SUV_{max} for the aorta. The SUV_{max} for liver and mediastinal blood pool were recorded in the 7th segment and in the supravalvular ascending aorta, respectively. Calculated values included the SUV_{TLR} (target-to-liver ratio) and the SUV_{TBR} (target-to-back ratio) for better comparison to exclude individual tracer dosage-dependent effects. (Whole body datasets were analyzed for secondary diagnosis, that is, infectious foci not in the vicinity of a graft, or other malignant findings as part of the routine diagnostic procedure). Additionally, intensity uptake was assessed using a visual grading scale (VGS: Grade 0: no uptake; Grade 1: low ^{18}F-FDG uptake, lower than the mediastinal blood pool; Grade 2: moderate uptake between the mediastinal blood pool and the liver uptake; Grade 3: high uptake, moderately higher than the uptake of the liver; Grade 4: strongest uptake, markedly higher than the uptake of the liver).

Focality uptake: Focal FDG uptake was defined as well-circumscribed areas of increased uptake in connection with the graft. The FDG pattern was classified as "uni- or multisegmental" for focal or diffuse uptake or "circumferent or semicircumferent" for a pattern that was encircling the aortic graft entirely or partially. Additionally, a description of the localisation of the uptake (aneurysm sack, aortic wall, graft) was documented.

Non-VGEI control group: For comparison, 19 patients who had ^{18}F-FDG-PET/CT for other reasons (cancer) and no signs of VGEI or history of graft occlusion related to their previously implanted graft based on the above mentioned criteria were selected consecutively from an institutional study database.

Statistical analysis: Statistical analysis was performed using IBM SPSS for Windows, Version 28.0 (IBM Corp., Armonk, NY). Dichotomous variables were recorded as absolute frequencies (number of cases) and relative frequencies (percentages). Continuous data are presented as mean ± one standard deviation (SD) and non-symmetrical data with median and interquartile range (IQR). Pearson's chi-squared or Fisher's exact test was used to analyze the categorical variables. Differences between means were tested with the t-test or the Mann–Whitney U test. Distribution of normality was assumed using histograms where applicable. Survival and patency data were analyzed using Kaplan–Meier estimates, and differences were analyzed using the log-rank test. Univariate Cox regression was used for analysis of risk factors for aortic reinfection with hazard ratios (HR) and 95% confidence intervals (CI) as measures of association. Univariate binary logistic regression analysis was performed to evaluate risk factors for in-hospital mortality with odds ratios (OR) and 95% CI as measures of association. The calculation of cut-off values of PET parameters was determined using receiver operating characteristics (ROC) curve analysis and Youden Index. Analysis of the area under the curve (AUC) of the ROC curves was performed using Delong's test to compare the performance of PET parameters for a predictive response. A two-sided *p*-value < 0.05 was considered statistically significant in all performed tests.

3. Results

3.1. Study Cohort

Overall, 93 VGEI patients (24.7% female, 65.4 ± 10.6 years old) over a nine-year period were included. Of those patients, 29 (31.2%) initially had EVAR, 11 (11.8%) TEVAR and 53 (57%) OAR for aortic aneurysm, occlusive disease or dissection (Figure 1, Table 1). Detailed patient and VGEI characteristics are shown in Table 1/Supplementary Table S1.

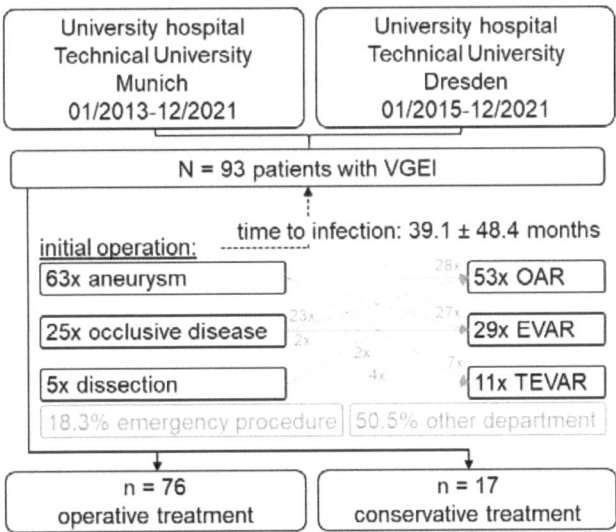

Figure 1. Patient flow chart.

Table 1. Patient characteristics, initial operation and VGEI details.

	Combined N = 93	Operative N = 76	Conservative N = 17
Patient Characteristics			
age (years; mean ± SD)	65.4 ± 10.6	64.5 ± 10.7	69.6 ± 9.17
sex (male: N; %)	70 (75.3)	55 (72.4)	15 (88.2)
hyperlipidemia	68 (73.1)	55 (72.4)	13 (76.5)
diabetes	28 (30.1)	25 (32.9)	3 (17.6)
nicotine abuse (active)	30 (32.3)	30 (39.5)	0
alcohol abuse (active)	8 (8.6)	8 (10.5)	0
COPD	24 (25.8)	19 (25)	5 (29.4)
renal insufficiency	26 (28)	20 (26.3)	6 (35.5)
dialysis	6 (6.5)	6 (7.9)	0
cancer (history)	21 (22.6)	21 (27.6)	0
arterial hypertension	87 (93.5)	71 (93.4)	16 (94.1)
PAOD	43 (46.2)	37 (48.7)	6 (35.3)
CAD	46 (49.5)	31 (40.8)	15 (88.2)
Initial Operation			
EVAR (2xcomplex;1xIBD;1xmono)	29 (31.2)	26 (34.2)	3 (17.6)
TEVAR	11 (11.8)	6 (7.9)	5 (29.4)
OAR	53 (57)	44 (57.9)	9 (52.9)
VGEI Characteristics			
early infection	28 (30.1)	22 (28.9)	6 (35.3)
late infection	65 (69.9)	54 (71.1)	11 (64.7)
fistula — cutaneous	8 (8.6)	7 (9.2)	1 (5.9)
fistula — gastrointestinal	21 (22.6)	17 (22.4)	4 (23.5)
fistula — ureter	3 (3.2)	3 (3.9)	-
B-symptoms	48 (51.6)	37 (48.7)	11 (64.7)
lab — leucocytes (cells/μL)	15.9 ± 6.7	11.2 ± 5.1	10.1 ± 4.5
lab — CRP (mg/dL)	11.9 ± 12.7	11.8 ± 13.2	12.3 ± 10.7
lab — PCT (ng/mL)	2.6 ± 9.0	2.8 ± 9.6	1.2 ± 1.6
preOP CT drain	25 (26.9)	18 (23.7)	7 (41.2)

COPD = chronic obstructive pulmonary disease; PAOD = peripheral arterial occlusive disease; CAD = coronary artery disease; complex = complex EVAR with fenestrations/scallop; IBD = iliac branch device; mono = mono-iliac EVAR with crossover bypass; normal range: leucocytes (3.8–9.8 cells/μL); C-reactive protein (CRP) (<5.0 mg/dL); procalcitonin (PCT) (<0.5 ng/mL).

The median interval between the initial operation and VGEI diagnosis was 24 months (95% CI: 29–49). Twenty-eight cases (30%) were early infections (Table 1). Fistulas were seen in 35.5% and unspecific B symptoms in 51.6% of the patients. Gastrointestinal fistula (n = 21) was most frequent (Table 1, Supplementary Table S1). All patients fulfilled the MAGIC criteria of VGEI, and major radiologic (CT) and laboratory criteria were met by >80% of patients (Supplement Table S2).

Initial laboratory infectious parameters were not altered in general and microbiologic workups, which revealed 49 different bacteria/fungi with no obvious frequency patterns of species or categories in regard to the mode or localization of acquisition (Table 1/Supplementary Table S1). Preoperative blood cultures were taken in 68 patients, yet 67% proved negative. Twenty-five patients had a diagnostic puncture (8% sterile). In twelve patients, the intraoperative swab/graft sonication remained sterile (15.8%) (Supplementary Table S1). Data regarding the pre-/perioperative antibiotic regimen could not be retrieved sufficiently in order to systematically analyze the possible germ selection between infectious diagnostics.

3.2. Quantitative and Qualitative PET/CT Analysis

PET/CT analysis was possible in 53 VGEI patients (60.0%) (Table 2, Figure 2A–C). Subgroup patient details and VGEI characteristics are shown in Supplementary Table S3. The mean aortic SUV_{max} was 12.5 ± 7.3, and the ratios for liver and background were 3.6 ± 2.0 (SUV_{TLR}, target-to-liver SUVmax) and 4.8 ± 3.1 (SUV_{TBR}, target-to-background SUVmax), respectively (Table 2, Supplementary Table S1).

Table 2. Quantitative intensity uptake analysis from PETs comparing VGEI patients with a non-VGEI control cohort.

Quantitative/Qualitative Analysis		VGEI + PET N = 53	Control Group N = 19	p
SUV$_{max}$ aorta		12.5 ± 7.3	4.2 ± 1.7	**<0.001**
		6.45 at 83% sensitivity/89% specificity		
SUV$_{TLR}$ (target-to-liver ratio)		3.6 ± 2.0	1.2 ± 0.4	**<0.001**
		1.35 at 94% sensitivity/89% specificity		
SUV$_{TBR}$ (target-to-back ratio)		4.8 ± 3.1	1.4 ± 0.4	**0.001**
		2.25 at 89% sensitivity/94% specificity		
SUV$_{max}$ liver		3.6 ± 0.9	3.7 ± 0.9	0.63
SUV$_{max}$ blood pool		2.7 ± 0.7	3.0 ± 0.5	0.21
Visual grading scale (VGS)	0	-	1 (5.3)	**<0.001**
	1	-	-	
	2	-	14 (73.7)	
	3	6 (11.3)	4 (21.1)	
	4	47 (88.7)	-	
infection time		early infection 15 (28.3)	late infection 38 (71.7%)	
SUV$_{max}$ aorta		12.27 ± 5.59	12.78 ± 7.95	0.94
SUV$_{TLR}$		3.55 ± 1.76	3.68 ± 2.18	0.9
SUV$_{TBR}$		4.41 ± 2.09	3.5 ± 4.78	0.89
fistula		fistula 19 (36.5%)	no fistula 33 (63.5%)	
SUV$_{max}$ aorta		13.54 ± 8.04	11.06 ± 5.92	0.31
SUV$_{TLR}$		3.79 ± 2.25	3.37 ± 1.68	0.61
SUV$_{TBR}$		5.1 ± 3.67	4.21 ± 1.91	0.54
initial treatment		endovascular 26 (50%)	open 26 (50%)	
SUV$_{max}$ aorta		14.63 ± 8.66	10.64 ± 5.27	0.08
SUV$_{TLR}$		4.25 ± 4.42	3.02 ± 1.38	0.07
SUV$_{TBR}$		5.82 ± 3.95	3.37 ± 1.53	**0.03**
safety EP reached		in-hospital survivor 45 (84.9)	in-hospital death 8 (15.1)	
SUV$_{max}$ aorta		11.90 ± 7.35	16.0 ± 5.77	0.06
SUV$_{TLR}$		3.54 ± 2.14	3.89 ± 1.36	0.24
SUV$_{TBR}$		4.71 ± 3.23	5.13 ± 2.30	0.36

SUV = standard uptake value. Data shown as mean standard deviation (upper line) and cut-off value from Youden analysis with the respective highest sensitivity and specificity (lower line) (Figure 2D). Comparison of SUV values for infection time, presence of fistula, type of initial treatment and safety endpoint reached (Mann–Whitney U test for comparison, $p < 0.05$ is considered significant and highlighted bold).

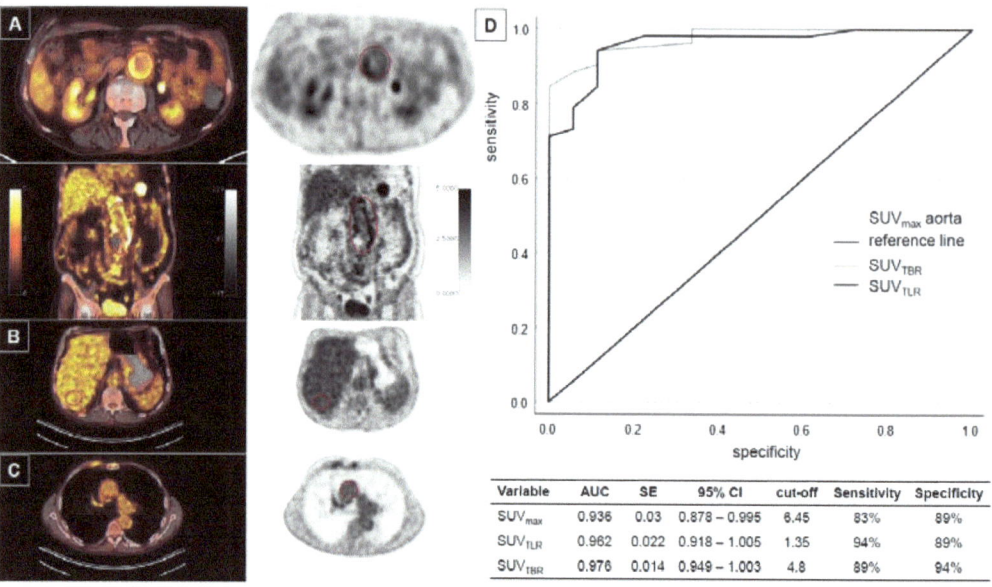

Figure 2. Positron emission tomography (PET)/CT and sensitivity/specificity analysis. (**A**) Axial and coronary depiction of PET/CT overlay and PET scan with correspondingly marked region of interest (ROI; red circle) where mean standard uptake value (SUV) is measured. Additional measurements are made in the liver (**B**) and the ascending aorta (mediastinal blood pool) (**C**). (**D**) Receiver-operator curve (ROC) for sensitivity/specificity based on area under the curve (AUC) measurement for SUV_{max} aorta, SUV_{TBR} and SUV_{TLR}. (SE = standard error; CI = confidence interval; cut-off at maximum sensitivity and specificity).

A control group of 19 patients post EVAR or OAR with no clinical suspicion of VGEI was available for comparison from an institutional PET/CT cancer database (Supplementary Table S3). Here, the aortic SUVmax and the respective dependent ratios were significantly higher for VGEI patients, while liver and blood pool enrichment did not differ between the groups (Table 2). Descriptive intensity uptake based on a VGS was significantly different between patients with graft infections versus controls ($p < 0.001$) (Figure S1, Supplementary Table S1).

In a receiver-operator curve (ROC) analysis for VGEI, a SUV_{TLR} of 1.35 showed 94% sensitivity and 89% specificity (Supplementary Table S1, Figure 2D). However, SUV_{max} aorta and SUV_{TBR} performed almost equally well. Notably, all three values were higher in patients initially treated using endovascular means, whereas the time-to-VGEI and the presence of a fistula did not matter (Table 2).

3.3. Treatment Strategy

Across the entire cohort, 76 patients were treated operatively and 17 were managed conservatively (Table 1). Conservative treatment included long-term anti-infective treatment in all patients and CT-drainage in six patients. Conservatively managed patients were followed up at least once via telephone interview after demission.

For operatively treated patients (all anatomical reconstruction), abdominal replacement was most frequent (84.2%), and 6.5% were emergency procedures (Table 3). The operation time was 502 ± 159 min, and a bifurcated graft (74.7%) and a physician-made pericardium graft (61.3%) were used most frequently. Additional procedures included renal cold perfusion and partial left heart bypass for distal and/or selective perfusion (described previously) [20]. Of 31 additional simultaneous procedures, intestinal resection was most frequent (Table 3).

Table 3. VGEI replacement operative details.

		N = 76
operative setting		
emergency operation		6 (6.5)
extent	thoracic	8 (10.5)
	thoraco-abdominal	4 (5.3)
	abdominal	64 (84.2)
fistula	cutaneous	7 (9.2)
	gastrointestinal	17 (22.4)
	ureter	3 (3.9)
procedural details		
operating time (min)		61.3%
transfusion (# RBC concentrates)		9 (9–12)
reco	tube	19 (25.3)
	bifurcation	56 (74.7)
material	pericardium	46 (61.3)
	silver-coated Dacron	16 (21.3)
	deep vein	13 (17.3)
renal cold perfusion		4 (5.3)
ECMO (partial left heart bypass)		13 (17.1)
omentum plasty		8 (10.5)
gastrointestinal resection		12 (15.8)
gastrointestinal direct suture		4 (5.3)
pulmonary resection/suture		2 (2.6)
other		13 (17.1)
postoperative course (in-hospital)		
scheduled revision		6 (7.9)
additional drainage (CT)		28 (36.8)
complication rates	aortic	18 (23.7)
	bleeding/rupture	16 (21.0)
	neurologic	8 (10.5)
	stroke	3 (3.9)
	surgical	47 (61.8)
	SSI	22 (28.9)
	limb ischemia	10 (13.2)
	visceral complication	9 (11.8)
	medical	50 (65.8)
	acute kidney failure	19 (25)
	dialysis (temp)	10 (13.2)
	respiratory problems	15 (19.7)
	pulmonary embolism	2 (2.6)
	myocardial infarction	4 (5.3)

Two patients were considered urgent (no emergency). One operation was discontinued after laparotomy due to unexpected inoperability. ECMO = extracorporeal membrane oxygenation: used as a partial left heart bypass; RBC = red blood cell; SSI = surgical site infection; other additional procedures included 4× splenectomy; 1× partial vertebral body resection; 2× cholecystectomy, 2× sartorius flap; 1× nephrectomy; 1× sublay mesh augmentation; 1× psoas hitch plasty; and 1× partial ureterectomy.

Postoperatively, an additional CT-guided drainage was necessary in 28 cases. Most notably, aortic complications (rupture, anastomotic bleeding) were noted in 18 cases. Stroke was rare, yet surgical and medical complication rates were considerably high (61.8% and 65.9%, respectively) (Table 3). Hence, surgically treated patients spent 20 ± 37 days in the intensive care unit (ICU) and 51 ± 38 days in the hospital (Table 4).

Table 4. Outcome analysis by treatment.

		Combined N = 93	Operative N = 76	Conservative N = 17
		outcome analysis		
days in hospital		45 ± 37	51 ± 38	21 ± 15
days in ICU		17 ± 34	20 ± 37	3 ± 7
surgical	in-hospital complication (rate)	-	47 (61.8)	-
medical			50 (65.8)	
neurologic			8 (10.5)	
aortic			18 (23.7)	
in-hospital	aortic reintervention (rate)	-	13 (17.1)	-
6 months			14 (18.4)	
12 months			21 (27.6)	
overall			23 (30.3)	
30 d	mortality (rate)	11 (11.8)	8 (10.5)	3 (17.6)
in-hospital		**18 (19.4)**	**15 (19.7)**	**3 (17.6)**
6 months		28 (30.1)	24 (31.5)	4 (23.5)
12 months		32 (34.3)	30 (39.5)	4 (23.5)
overall		40 (43)	35 (46.1)	5 (29.4)
6 months aortic reintervention-free survival		-	38 (50)	-
reinfection (persistent)		-	30 (39.5)	17 (100)
follow-up (months)		22.9 ± 26.4	24.1 ± 24.2	17.9 ± 35

ICU = intensive care unit. The safety and efficiency endpoints are highlighted in bold.

3.4. Outcome Analyses

During 22.9 ± 26.4 months of follow-up, the in-hospital mortality (safety endpoint) was 19.4% (Figure 3A, Table 4). After discharge, ten patients (10.8%) were lost to follow-up. At six months, the mortality rate was 30.1%, and the aortic reintervention free-survival rate (efficacy endpoint) was 50%. Persistent or reinfection was present in 100% of the conservatively treated patients and in 39.5% of the patients in the operative treatment group (Table 4).

While the average time in hospital exceeded one month (45 ± 37 days), the 30-day-, in-hospital-, 6-months-, 12-months and overall mortality gradually increased from 11.8% to 43% (Table 4). Here, no obvious differences were seen between operative and conservative treatments; however, the number at risk decreased rapidly (Figure 3A, Table 4). In addition to the high in-hospital complication rates, the aortic complication and reintervention rates after demission reached up to 30% (Table 4). Analyzing the materials used for abdominal replacement only (n = 64: 38× pericardium, 13× silver-coated Dacron, 13× femoral vein), no significant differences were seen regarding the reinfection or overall survival rate (Figure 3B, Table 5). Higher SUV ratios in PET did not correspond to in-hospital death (Table 2). Specific focality uptake (i.e., aneurysm sac enrichment) analysis was not associated with a specific outcome.

Finally, univariate analysis for in-hospital mortality revealed significantly increased odds ratios (OR) for AAA as an initial indication (OR 4.76, $p = 0.047$), B-symptoms upon clinical presentation (OR 4.22, $p = 0.02$) and tube reconstruction (OR 5.2, $p = 0.007$) (Figure 4, Supplementary Table S5). The reinfection (persistence) rate was significantly associated with emergency replacements (OR 2.41, $p = 0.035$) and mesenteric ischemia during hospital stays (OR 4.5, $p = 0.0002$) (Supplementary Figure S2, Supplementary Table S6).

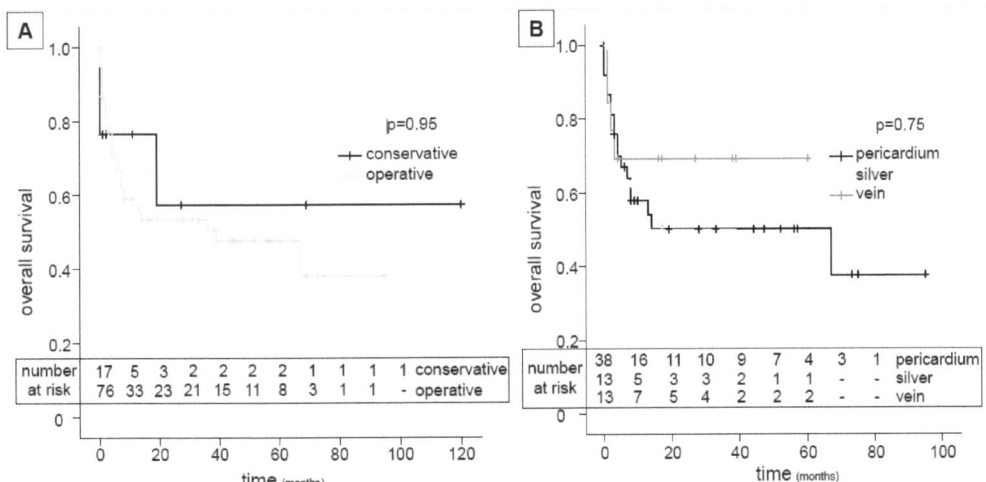

Figure 3. Outcome analysis. (**A**) The overall survival is shown as a Kaplan–Meyer plot comparing operative and conservative treatments for the entire vascular graft and endograft infection (VGEI) cohort (N = 93). (**B**) The overall survival is shown for the three different vascular substitutes used in the abdominal replacement group (N = 64) (log-rank test for comparison; $p < 0.05$ is considered significant).

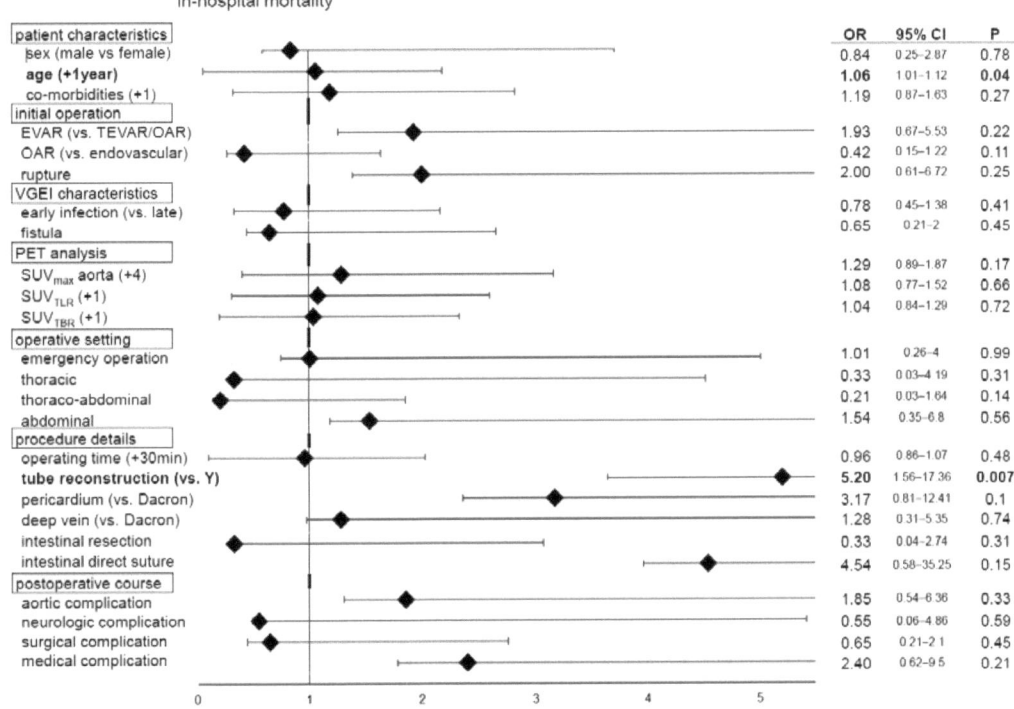

Figure 4. Forest plot shows selected univariate odds ratios for in-hospital mortality, with 95% confidence intervals and p values (logistic regression and Wald test; $p < 0.05$ is considered significant and highlighted bold; all values shown in Supplementary Table S5).

Table 5. Abdominal replacement material analysis.

N = 64 Abdominal Replacement	Pericardium N = 38	Silver-Coated Dacron N = 13	Femoral Vein N = 13	p
aortic complication (in-hospital)	10 (26.3)	1 (7.7)	4 (30.8)	0.31
anastomotic bleeding	7 (18.4)	1 (7.7)	3 (23.1)	0.64
fluid collection (drainage)	2 (5.3)	-	1 (7.7)	-
anastomotic stenosis	1 (2.6)	-	-	
surgical complication	21 (55.3)	10 (76.9)	11 (84.6)	0.09
impaired wound healing	8 (21.1)	5 (38.5)	7 (53.8)	0.07
aortic complication during FU	12 (31.6)	4 (30.8)	5 (38.5)	0.89
death in-hospital	8 (21.1)	0	3 (23.1)	0.18
death during FU	18 (47.4)	6 (46.2)	4 (30.8)	0.57
(persistent) reinfection	17 (44.7)	7 (53.8)	3 (23.1)	0.25

A direct comparison of relevant outcome parameters regarding the replacement material used in the abdominal cohort. Chi-Square test for comparison; <0.05 is considered significant and highlighted bold.

4. Discussion

This study represents one of the largest retrospective cohort studies on VGEI and demonstrates that postoperative morbidity and mortality remain considerable high in this vulnerable patient cohort, but these results were similar to the results obtained in a limited conservative treatment group. While PET is a highly sensitive method to detect VGEI, a qualitative and quantitative approach did not correlate with the clinical endpoints.

Regarding the safety endpoint, we found an overall in-hospital mortality of 19.4%, with no differences between operative vs. conservative treatment (Figure 3A, Table 4). Similarly, the in-hospital complication rates were considerably high and did not change over time. This is in line with the literature overview provided in the 2020 ESVS guidelines, with early mortality ranging from 8–48% and graft-related (aortic) complications from 3–37.2% [3]. One additional systematic review from 2023 found an overall mortality of 14.8–27% in a short-term analysis [16]. Long-term follow-up data (>6 months) are largely missing in these patients, and if provided, the numbers at risk decrease rapidly (Figure 3A, Table 4).

Hence, we found a six-month aortic reintervention-free survival of 50% in the surgical group (efficacy endpoint). Considering the high degree of reinfection (i.e., persistent infection), the aortic complication and reintervention rates described a close monitoring, and frequent follow-up imaging seems mandatory (Table 4). The overall mortality after the two-year mean follow-up was found to be 43% (Figure 3A, Table 4). Regarding the good short- and midterm survival rates of over 90% at six months published lately for both aortic and thoracic VGEIs, surgical graft removal must eventually be considered as "added mortality/morbidity" in this vulnerable cohort [12,13]. Here, the complexity of repair and additional operative procedures had no influence on the in-hospital mortality (Figure 4, Supplementary Table S5). Kahlberg et al. found a trend towards lower 1-year mortality rates when comparing operative and graft-preserving treatments in a systematic review and meta-analysis of 233 cases from 43 studies [17].

The detection of VGEI is most crucial and still a challenge in some cases. Especially regarding the individual operative consequences, sensitivity and specificity must be excellent. Here, the MAGIC criteria showed up to 100% sensitivity, yet were only specific in approx. two-thirds of cases [2,4]. In our cohort, MAGIC positivity was an inclusion criterion; however, most patients "over-fulfilled" the required categories (Supplementary Table S2). ^{18}F-FDG PET/CT has been discussed as a method to increase specificity, especially in cases of clinical doubt [5].

To increase diagnostic accuracy, a quantitative approach using focal uptake SUV_{max} and dependent ratios has been introduced; however, studies evaluating VGEI patients and, specifically, comparisons to studies of non-VGEI patients are scarce [7]. Tsuda et al. have suggested an aortic SUV_{max} = 4.5 as a cut-off to diagnose VGEI, while v. Rijsewijk saw a mean SUV_{max} = 9.5 vs. 5.4 in their VGEI-positive vs. VGEI-negative cohort [7,21]. Our analysis identified the SUV_{TLR} with the highest diagnostic accuracy; however, our results showed an aortic SUV_{max} (cut-off 6.45) and an SUV_{TBR} with almost equally high sensitivity and specificity (Figure 2D, Table 2). Along with previous results, the time-to-infection did not influence basic uptake values; however, the type of initial operation (EVAR vs. OAR) might (Table 2) [7,22]. Similar results have been reported from smaller cohort studies and meta-analyses and also after open ascending aortic repair [23–28]. Yet, quantitative PET analysis could be suggestive of perigraft gas bubbles, but no correlations with eventual bacteria and clinical outcomes of VGEI are reported [6,29]. Further modalities, such as a white blood cell (WBC) scan, could help shed light on this shortcoming [30]. In our study, no differences regarding the in-hospital mortality were seen (Table 2, Supplementary Table S5). The role of follow-up PET to diagnose persistent infection or reinfection in those patients might help to minimize the high rate of aortic complications during follow-up (Table 4) [31].

While individual case reports suggest isolated removal of PET avid segments, complete removal of the allograft material is common sense in eligible patients according to the ESVS guidelines [3,32]. Here, anatomic reconstruction has proven favorable in terms of infection-free survival [33]. However, despite a clear definition bias, the rate of persistent infection and/or reinfection is high after operative treatment and reached 39.5% in our study (Table 4) [34]. Various groups have published their experiences with specific materials used for reconstruction, mostly for the abdominal aorta, with a lack of direct comparisons. The ESVS guidelines, as well as current meta-analyses, have summarized short-term mortality rates and reinfection rates for biological (pericardium, homograft), prosthetic (silver-coated, biosynthetic) and autologous vein vascular substitutes (VS) [3,16,35]. Generally, mortality rates are almost equal, while resistance to infection might be better for biological and venous VS. Here, we found no significant difference between the three materials used regarding overall mortality and immediate or late aortic complications (Figure 3B, Table 5, Supplementary Tables S5 and S6). However, the study was not designed for this analysis.

The identification of the bacterial/fungal etiology and "evolution/selection" considering the antibiotic regimen applied seems key for a potential targeted therapy and a possible improvement of outcomes for both surgical and conservative treatments given the plethora of microorganisms identified (Supplementary Table S1). Standard culturing along with eventual polymerase chain reaction methods can be of help [12]. However, approx. one-third of blood cultures remain negative, and a polymicrobial flora is frequent [12,17,34]. Hence, preoperative classification according to a single microorganism identified might not be justified [36,37]. The additional sonication of explanted grafts increased the microorganism yield by 16% [38]. Either way, the long-term administration of the correct anti-infective agent along with a possible reevaluation during the post-hospital course is crucial for clinical success and might be even more important than surgical success [3,37,39]. The value of other procedures, i.e., partial graft removal or anti-infective graft irrigation, remains unclear [32,40]. Additionally, patients' adherence to therapy and possible outpatient parenteral antimicrobial therapy needs to be assessed on a larger scale [41].

Limitations: As is the case with any other study of this kind, our analysis is limited by the heterogeneity of patients, disease and presentation. Generally, the low number of patients prohibits statistical analysis beyond descriptive methods and thus limits the value of our conclusions, specifically for the comparison of conservatively vs. operatively managed patients. Every surgeon might be subjected to an "intention-to-treat" bias for VGEI, or on the other hand, some conservatively managed patients might be frailer than others. Additionally, the presented PET/CT analysis was only available for 53 patients. The mean follow-up was 22.9 ± 26.4 months only, resulting in a calculated follow-up index of 0.75, allowing only short-/midterm conclusions [42].

5. Conclusions

VGEI is associated with considerably high in-hospital and short-term complication rates and mortality in this cohort. PET shows excellent diagnostic sensitivity and specificity. The material used for reconstruction might not be crucial for clinical outcomes. With a possible selection bias and insufficient group size, we demonstrate that conservatively managed patients might have a similar outcome. However, a more widespread, register-based approach tailored to a thorough infectious diagnosis and treatment is necessary to identify patients who benefit from this type of surgery, especially during longer follow-ups.

Supplementary Materials: The following supporting information can be downloaded at https://www.mdpi.com/article/10.3390/jcm13010269/s1; Figure S1: Visual Grading Scale VGS PET/CT analysis. Figure S2: Univariate analysis re-(persistent)-infection. Table S1: Microbiology data for individual patients. Table S2: MAGIC criteria. Table S3: Comparison PET/CT VGEI and control cohort characteristics. Table S4: Complication rates operative cohort after Clavien-Dindo. Table S5: Univariate analysis of in-hospital mortality. Table S6: Univariate analysis of re-infection (persistent).

Author Contributions: Conceptualization: W.W., C.R., S.N., A.B. (Albert Busch) and N.S.; methodology, I.P., M.K., C.R., H.-H.E., S.W., C.K., S.N., A.B. (Anja Braune), B.L. and M.T.; validation, all authors; formal analysis, all authors; investigation, I.P., M.K., C.R., H.-H.E., S.W., C.K., S.N., A.B. (Anja Braune), E.M., A.B. (Albert Busch), J.K., G.B. and T.R.; resources, A.B. (Albert Busch); data curation, all authors; writing—original draft preparation, S.N. and A.B. (Albert Busch); writing—review and editing, all authors. All authors have read and agreed to the published version of the manuscript.

Funding: This research received no external funding.

Institutional Review Board Statement: This study was performed in accordance with the Declaration of Helsinki and approved by the local ethics committees (Medical Faculty, Technical University of Munich: 2022-428-S-NP and Technical University Dresden BO-EK-205042022, approval date: for Dresden: 6th May 2022, for Munich: 16th August 2022).

Informed Consent Statement: Patient consent was waived due to the retrospective nature of the study.

Data Availability Statement: All original data can be obtained from the corresponding author upon request.

Acknowledgments: We are grateful for a detailed infectiologic assessment and a vivid discussion of our data with K. de With. We are also grateful for statistical advice from B. Bohmann, M.Sc.

Conflicts of Interest: The authors declare no conflicts of interest.

References

1. Wanhainen, A.; Verzini, F.; Van Herzeele, I.; Allaire, E.; Bown, M.; Cohnert, T.; Dick, F.; van Herwaarden, J.; Karkos, C.; Koelemay, M.; et al. Editor's Choice—European Society for Vascular Surgery (ESVS) 2019 Clinical Practice Guidelines on the Management of Abdominal Aorto-iliac Artery Aneurysms. *Eur. J. Vasc. Endovasc. Surg.* **2019**, *57*, 8–93. [CrossRef] [PubMed]
2. Lyons, O.T.; Baguneid, M.; Barwick, T.D.; Bell, R.E.; Foster, N.; Homer-Vanniasinkam, S.; Hopkins, S.; Hussain, A.; Katsanos, K.; Modarai, B.; et al. Diagnosis of Aortic Graft Infection: A Case Definition by the Management of Aortic Graft Infection Collaboration (MAGIC). *Eur. J. Vasc. Endovasc. Surg.* **2016**, *52*, 758–763. [CrossRef] [PubMed]
3. Chakfe, N.; Diener, H.; Lejay, A.; Assadian, O.; Berard, X.; Caillon, J.; Fourneau, I.; Glaudemans, A.; Koncar, I.; Lindholt, J.; et al. Editor's Choice—European Society for Vascular Surgery (ESVS) 2020 Clinical Practice Guidelines on the Management of Vascular Graft and Endograft Infections. *Eur. J. Vasc. Endovasc. Surg.* **2020**, *59*, 339–384. [CrossRef] [PubMed]
4. Anagnostopoulos, A.; Mayer, F.; Ledergerber, B.; Bergada-Pijuan, J.; Husmann, L.; Mestres, C.A.; Rancic, Z.; Hasse, B.; Study, V.C. Editor's Choice—Validation of the Management of Aortic Graft Infection Collaboration (MAGIC) Criteria for the Diagnosis of Vascular Graft/Endograft Infection: Results from the Prospective Vascular Graft Cohort Study. *Eur. J. Vasc. Endovasc. Surg.* **2021**, *62*, 251–257. [CrossRef] [PubMed]
5. Dong, W.; Li, Y.; Zhu, J.; Xia, J.; He, L.; Yun, M.; Jiao, J.; Zhu, G.; Hacker, M.; Wei, Y.; et al. Detection of aortic prosthetic graft infection with ^{18}F-FDG PET/CT imaging, concordance with consensus MAGIC graft infection criteria. *J. Nucl. Cardiol.* **2021**, *28*, 1005–1016. [CrossRef] [PubMed]
6. Mahmoodi, Z.; Salarzaei, M.; Sheikh, M. Prosthetic vascular graft infection: A systematic review and meta-analysis on diagnostic accuracy of 18FDG PET/CT. *Gen. Thorac. Cardiovasc. Surg.* **2022**, *70*, 219–229. [CrossRef]

7. Tsuda, K.; Washiyama, N.; Takahashi, D.; Natsume, K.; Ohashi, Y.; Hirano, M.; Takeuchi, Y.; Shiiya, N. 18-Fluorodeoxyglucose positron emission tomography in the diagnosis of prosthetic aortic graft infection: The difference between open and endovascular repair. *Eur. J. Cardiothorac. Surg.* **2022**, *63*, ezac542. [CrossRef]
8. Cardozo, M.A.; Frankini, A.D.; Bonamigo, T.P. Use of superficial femoral vein in the treatment of infected aortoiliofemoral prosthetic grafts. *Cardiovasc. Surg.* **2002**, *10*, 304–310. [CrossRef]
9. Harlander-Locke, M.P.; Harmon, L.K.; Lawrence, P.F.; Oderich, G.S.; McCready, R.A.; Morasch, M.D.; Feezor, R.J.; Vascular Low-Frequency Disease, C.; Zhou, W.; Bismuth, J.; et al. The use of cryopreserved aortoiliac allograft for aortic reconstruction in the United States. *J. Vasc. Surg.* **2014**, *59*, 669–674. [CrossRef]
10. Oderich, G.S.; Bower, T.C.; Hofer, J.; Kalra, M.; Duncan, A.A.; Wilson, J.W.; Cha, S.; Gloviczki, P. In situ rifampin-soaked grafts with omental coverage and antibiotic suppression are durable with low reinfection rates in patients with aortic graft enteric erosion or fistula. *J. Vasc. Surg.* **2011**, *53*, 99–107.e7. [CrossRef]
11. Caradu, C.; Puges, M.; Cazanave, C.; Martin, G.; Ducasse, E.; Berard, X.; Bicknell, C.; the Imperial Vascular Unit and the University Hospital of Bordeaux Vascular Unit. Outcomes of patients with aortic vascular graft and endograft infections initially contra-indicated for complete graft explantation. *J. Vasc. Surg.* **2022**, *76*, 1364–1373.e3. [CrossRef] [PubMed]
12. Ljungquist, O.; Haidl, S.; Dias, N.; Sonesson, B.; Sorelius, K.; Tragardh, E.; Ahl, J. Conservative Management First Strategy in Aortic Vascular Graft and Endograft Infections. *Eur. J. Vasc. Endovasc. Surg.* **2023**, *65*, 896–904. [CrossRef] [PubMed]
13. Kouijzer, I.J.E.; Baranelli, C.T.; Maat, I.; van den Heuvel, F.M.A.; Aarntzen, E.; Smith, T.; de Mast, Q.; Geuzebroek, G.S.C. Thoracic aortic vascular graft infection: Outcome after conservative treatment without graft removal. *Eur. J. Cardiothorac. Surg.* **2022**, *63*, ezac551. [CrossRef] [PubMed]
14. Akhtar, M.; Meecham, L.; Birkett, R.; Pherwani, A.D.; Fairhead, J.F. Conservative Treatment of an Infected Aortic Graft with Antibiotic Irrigation. *Int. J. Angiol.* **2016**, *25*, e118–e120. [CrossRef] [PubMed]
15. Niaz, O.S.; Rao, A.; Carey, D.; Refson, J.R.; Abidia, A.; Somaiya, P. Systematic Review and Meta: Analysis of Aortic Graft Infections following Abdominal Aortic Aneurysm Repair. *Int. J. Vasc. Med.* **2020**, *2020*, 9574734. [CrossRef] [PubMed]
16. Colacchio, E.C.; D'Oria, M.; Grando, B.; Rinaldi Garofalo, A.; D'Andrea, A.; Bassini, S.; Lepidi, S.; Antonello, M.; Ruaro, B. A Systematic Review of in-Situ Aortic Reconstructions for Abdominal Aortic Graft and Endograft Infections: Outcomes of Currently Available Options for Surgical Replacement. *Ann. Vasc. Surg.* **2023**, *95*, 307–316. [CrossRef] [PubMed]
17. Kahlberg, A.; Grandi, A.; Loschi, D.; Vermassen, F.; Moreels, N.; Chakfe, N.; Melissano, G.; Chiesa, R. A systematic review of infected descending thoracic aortic grafts and endografts. *J. Vasc. Surg.* **2019**, *69*, 1941–1951.e1. [CrossRef]
18. Vandenbroucke, J.P.; von Elm, E.; Altman, D.G.; Gotzsche, P.C.; Mulrow, C.D.; Pocock, S.J.; Poole, C.; Schlesselman, J.J.; Egger, M.; Initiative, S. Strengthening the Reporting of Observational Studies in Epidemiology (STROBE): Explanation and elaboration. *PLoS Med.* **2007**, *4*, e297. [CrossRef]
19. Dindo, D.; Demartines, N.; Clavien, P.A. Classification of surgical complications: A new proposal with evaluation in a cohort of 6336 patients and results of a survey. *Ann Surg* **2004**, *240*, 205–213. [CrossRef]
20. Lutz, B.M.; Schaser, K.-D.; Weitz, J.; Kirchberg, J.; Fritzsche, H.; Disch, A.C.; Busch, A.; Wolk, S.; Reeps, C. Thoracoabdominal Aortic Replacement Together with Curative Oncological Surgery in Retroperitoneal and Spinal Tumours. *Curr. Oncol.* **2023**, *30*, 2555–2568. [CrossRef]
21. van Rijsewijk, N.D.; Helthuis, J.H.G.; Glaudemans, A.; Wouthuyzen-Bakker, M.; Prakken, N.H.J.; Liesker, D.J.; Saleem, B.R.; Slart, R. Added Value of Abnormal Lymph Nodes Detected with FDG-PET/CT in Suspected Vascular Graft Infection. *Biology* **2023**, *12*, 251. [CrossRef] [PubMed]
22. Lauri, C.; Signore, A.; Campagna, G.; Aloisi, F.; Taurino, M.; Sirignano, P. [18F]FDG Uptake in Non-Infected Endovascular Grafts: A Retrospective Study. *Diagnostics* **2023**, *13*, 409. [CrossRef] [PubMed]
23. Rahimi, M.; Adlouni, M.; Ahmed, A.I.; Alnabelsi, T.; Chinnadurai, P.; Al-Mallah, M.H. Diagnostic Accuracy of FDG PET for the Identification of Vascular Graft Infection. *Ann. Vasc. Surg.* **2022**, *87*, 422–429. [CrossRef] [PubMed]
24. Bruls, S.; El Hassani, I.; Hultgren, R.; Hustinx, R.; Courtois, A.; Dumortier, A.; Defraigne, J.O.; Sakalihasan, N. [18F] FDG PET/CT can improve the diagnostic accuracy for aortic endograft infection. *Acta Cardiol.* **2022**, *77*, 399–407. [CrossRef] [PubMed]
25. Husmann, L.; Huellner, M.W.; Eberhard, N.; Ledergerber, B.; Kaelin, M.B.; Anagnostopoulos, A.; Kudura, K.; Burger, I.A.; Mestres, C.A.; Rancic, Z.; et al. PET/CT in therapy control of infective native aortic aneurysms. *Sci. Rep.* **2021**, *11*, 5065. [CrossRef] [PubMed]
26. Martinez-Lopez, D.; Rodriguez Alfonso, B.; Ramos Martinez, A.; Martin Lopez, C.E.; de Villarreal Soto, J.E.; Rios Rosado, E.C.; Villar Garcia, S.; Ospina Mosquera, V.M.; Serrano Fiz, S.; Burgos Lazaro, R.; et al. Are 18F-fluorodeoxyglucose positron emission tomography results reliable in patients with ascending aortic grafts? A prospective study in non-infected patients. *Eur. J. Cardiothorac. Surg.* **2021**, *60*, 148–154. [CrossRef] [PubMed]
27. Mitra, A.; Pencharz, D.; Davis, M.; Wagner, T. Determining the Diagnostic Value of 18F-Fluorodeoxyglucose Positron Emission/Computed Tomography in Detecting Prosthetic Aortic Graft Infection. *Ann. Vasc. Surg.* **2018**, *53*, 78–85. [CrossRef]
28. Reinders Folmer, E.I.; Von Meijenfeldt, G.C.I.; Van der Laan, M.J.; Glaudemans, A.; Slart, R.; Saleem, B.R.; Zeebregts, C.J. Diagnostic Imaging in Vascular Graft Infection: A Systematic Review and Meta-Analysis. *Eur. J. Vasc. Endovasc. Surg.* **2018**, *56*, 719–729. [CrossRef]
29. Chrapko, B.E.; Chrapko, M.; Nocun, A.; Zubilewicz, T.; Stefaniak, B.; Mitura, J.; Wolski, A.; Terelecki, P. Patterns of vascular graft infection in 18F-FDG PET/CT. *Nucl. Med. Rev. Cent. East. Eur.* **2020**, *23*, 63–70. [CrossRef]

30. Puges, M.; Berard, X.; Ruiz, J.B.; Debordeaux, F.; Desclaux, A.; Stecken, L.; Pereyre, S.; Hocquelet, A.; Bordenave, L.; Pinaquy, J.B.; et al. Retrospective Study Comparing WBC scan and ^{18}F-FDG PET/CT in Patients with Suspected Prosthetic Vascular Graft Infection. *Eur. J. Vasc. Endovasc. Surg.* **2019**, *57*, 876–884. [CrossRef]
31. Berchiolli, R.; Torri, L.; Bertagna, G.; Canovaro, F.; Zanca, R.; Bartoli, F.; Mocellin, D.M.; Ferrari, M.; Erba, P.A.; Troisi, N. [^{18}F]-Fludeoxyglucose Positron Emission Tomography/Computed Tomography with Radiomics Analysis in Patients Undergoing Aortic In-Situ Reconstruction with Cryopreserved Allografts. *Diagnostics* **2022**, *12*, 2831. [CrossRef] [PubMed]
32. Goto, T.; Shimamura, K.; Kuratani, T.; Kin, K.; Shijo, T.; Masada, K.; Sawa, Y. Successful surgery localized to the infected lesion as diagnosed by ^{18}F-fluorodeoxyglucose positron emission tomography/computed tomography for extended-aortic prosthetic graft infection. *Int. J. Surg. Case Rep.* **2019**, *59*, 76–79. [CrossRef]
33. Janko, M.R.; Hubbard, G.; Back, M.; Shah, S.K.; Pomozi, E.; Szeberin, Z.; DeMartino, R.; Wang, L.J.; Crofts, S.; Belkin, M.; et al. In-situ bypass is associated with superior infection-free survival compared with extra-anatomic bypass for the management of secondary aortic graft infections without enteric involvement. *J. Vasc. Surg.* **2022**, *76*, 546–555.e3. [CrossRef] [PubMed]
34. Janko, M.; Hubbard, G.; Woo, K.; Kashyap, V.S.; Mitchell, M.; Murugesan, A.; Chen, L.; Gardner, R.; Baril, D.; Hacker, R.I.; et al. Contemporary Outcomes After Partial Resection of Infected Aortic Grafts. *Ann. Vasc. Surg.* **2021**, *76*, 202–210. [CrossRef] [PubMed]
35. El-Diaz, N.; Walker-Jacobs, A.; Althaher, A.; Alalwani, Z.; Borucki, J.; Stather, P.W. A systematic review and meta-analysis of the use of the Omniflow II biosynthetic graft for aortic reconstruction. *J. Vasc. Surg.* **2023**, *77*, 964–970.e4. [CrossRef] [PubMed]
36. Uyttebroek, S.; Chen, B.; Onsea, J.; Ruythooren, F.; Debaveye, Y.; Devolder, D.; Spriet, I.; Depypere, M.; Wagemans, J.; Lavigne, R.; et al. Safety and efficacy of phage therapy in difficult-to-treat infections: A systematic review. *Lancet Infect. Dis.* **2022**, *22*, e208–e220. [CrossRef] [PubMed]
37. Wouthuyzen-Bakker, M.; van Oosten, M.; Bierman, W.; Winter, R.; Glaudemans, A.; Slart, R.; Toren-Wielema, M.; Tielliu, I.; Zeebregts, C.J.; Prakken, N.H.J.; et al. Diagnosis and treatment of vascular graft and endograft infections: A structured clinical approach. *Int. J. Infect. Dis.* **2023**, *126*, 22–27. [CrossRef] [PubMed]
38. Braams, L.; Vlaspolder, G.; Boiten, K.; Salomon, E.; Winter, R.; Saleem, B.; Wouthuyzen-Bakker, M.; van Oosten, M. Sonication of Vascular Grafts and Endografts to Diagnose Vascular Graft Infection: A Head-To-Head Comparison with Conventional Culture and Its Clinical Impact. *Microbiol. Spectr.* **2023**, *11*, e0372222. [CrossRef]
39. Sixt, T.; Aho, S.; Chavanet, P.; Moretto, F.; Denes, E.; Mahy, S.; Blot, M.; Catherine, F.X.; Steinmetz, E.; Piroth, L. Long-term Prognosis Following Vascular Graft Infection: A 10-Year Cohort Study. *Open Forum Infect. Dis.* **2022**, *9*, ofac054. [CrossRef]
40. Morris, G.E.; Friend, P.J.; Vassallo, D.J.; Farrington, M.; Leapman, S.; Quick, C.R. Antibiotic irrigation and conservative surgery for major aortic graft infection. *J. Vasc. Surg.* **1994**, *20*, 88–95. [CrossRef]
41. Allen, N.; Adam, M.; O'Regan, G.; Seery, A.; McNally, C.; McConkey, S.; Brown, A.; de Barra, E. Outpatient parenteral antimicrobial therapy (OPAT) for aortic vascular graft infection; a five-year retrospective evaluation. *BMC Infect. Dis.* **2021**, *21*, 670. [CrossRef] [PubMed]
42. von Allmen, R.S.; Weiss, S.; Tevaearai, H.T.; Kuemmerli, C.; Tinner, C.; Carrel, T.P.; Schmidli, J.; Dick, F. Completeness of Follow-Up Determines Validity of Study Findings: Results of a Prospective Repeated Measures Cohort Study. *PLoS ONE* **2015**, *10*, e0140817. [CrossRef] [PubMed]

Disclaimer/Publisher's Note: The statements, opinions and data contained in all publications are solely those of the individual author(s) and contributor(s) and not of MDPI and/or the editor(s). MDPI and/or the editor(s) disclaim responsibility for any injury to people or property resulting from any ideas, methods, instructions or products referred to in the content.

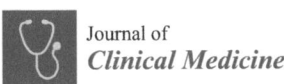

Article

Preoperative Imaging Signs of Cerebral Malperfusion in Acute Type A Aortic Dissection: Influence on Outcomes and Prognostic Implications—A 20-Year Experience

Mohammed Al-Tawil *,†, Mohamed Salem †, Christine Friedrich, Shirin Diraz, Alexandra Broll, Najma Rezahie, Jan Schoettler, Nora de Silva, Thomas Puehler, Jochen Cremer and Assad Haneya

Department of Cardiovascular Surgery, University Hospital of Schleswig-Holstein, 24118 Kiel, Germany; christine.friedrich@uksh.de (C.F.); shirin.diraz@uksh.de (S.D.)
* Correspondence: mo.altawil98@gmail.com
† These authors contributed equally to this work.

Abstract: Background: Acute type A aortic dissection (ATAAD) continues to be a subject of active research due to its high mortality rates and associated complications. Cerebral malperfusion in ATAAD can have a devastating impact on patients' neurological function and overall quality of life. We aimed to explore the risk profile and prognosis in ATAAD patients presenting with preoperative imaging signs of cerebral malperfusion (PSCM). Methods: We obtained patient data from our Aortic Dissection Registry, which included 480 consecutive ATAAD cases who underwent surgical repair between 2001 and 2021. Primary endpoint outcomes included the in-hospital and 30-day mortality, postoperative new neurological deficit, mechanical ventilation hours, and intensive care unit (ICU) length of stay. Results: Of the total cohort, 82 patients (17.1%) had PSCM. Both groups had similar distributions in terms of age, sex, and body mass index. The patients in the PSCM group presented with a higher logistic EuroSCORE (47, IQR [31, 64] vs. 24, IQR [15, 39]; $p < 0.001$) and a higher portion of patients with a previous cardiac surgery (7.3% vs. 2.0%; $p = 0.020$). Intraoperatively, the bypass, cardioplegia, and aortic cross-clamp times were similar between both groups. However, the patients in the PSCM group received significantly more intraoperative packed red blood cells, fresh frozen plasma, and platelets transfusions ($p < 0.05$). Following the surgery, the patients who presented with PSCM had markedly longer ventilation hours (108.5 h, IQR [44, 277] vs. 43 h, IQR [16, 158], $p < 0.001$) and a significantly longer ICU length of stay (7 days, IQR [4, 13] vs. 5 days, IQR [2, 11]; $p = 0.013$). Additionally, the patients with PSCM had significantly higher rates of postoperative new neurological deficits (35.4% vs. 19.4%; $p = 0.002$). In the Cox regression analysis, PSCM was associated with significantly poorer long-term survival (hazard ratio (HR) 1.75, 95%CI [1.20–2.53], $p = 0.003$). Surprisingly, hypertension was shown as a protective factor against long-term mortality (HR: 0.59, 95%CI [0.43–0.82], $p = 0.001$). Conclusion: PSCM in ATAAD patients is linked to worse postoperative outcomes and poorer long-term survival, emphasizing the need for early recognition and tailored management.

Keywords: type A aortic dissection; cerebral malperfusion; stroke

1. Introduction

Acute type A aortic dissection (ATAAD) continues to be a subject of active research due to its high mortality rates and associated perioperative complications. Despite the ongoing advancements in the diagnosis and expedited management of ATAAD, the early mortality rates remain alarmingly high. In contemporary practice, the in-hospital mortality rate for ATAAD patients who undergo surgery ranges between 10 and 18% with considerable between-hospital variations [1–5].

Still, the preoperative ATAAD profile is a major moderator of outcomes in those patients. A critical aspect that necessitates careful attention is when the dissection involves one of the vital organs' perfusing vessels, causing malperfusion. The presence of preoperative malperfusion affecting cerebral, myocardial, mesenteric, spinal, renal, or lower limb regions significantly increases the risk of mortality and perioperative adverse events [6–10].

Among the various forms of malperfusion, cerebral malperfusion (CM) holds particular significance. CM can be indicated by preoperative imaging signs (PSCM) or intraoperatively, and can have a devastating impact on a patient's neurological function, cognitive abilities, and overall quality of life. A recent systematic review estimated that CM occurs in approximately 16% of patients presenting with ATAAD and is associated with an in-hospital mortality rate of around 20% [11]. However, advancements in the early surgical intervention and expedited management of patients with CM have contributed to a substantial decrease in mortality rates in recent years [4,11].

The main objective of this study was to analyze the outcomes and investigate the impact of CM indicated by PSCM on the patient prognosis. Furthermore, we aimed to examine the differences in the various preoperative, intraoperative, and postoperative factors associated with prognosis.

2. Materials and Methods

2.1. Study Design and Patient Population

We obtained patient data from our Aortic Dissection Registry, which included 480 consecutive ATAAD cases who underwent surgical repair under moderate hypothermic circulatory arrest between 2001 and 2021. ATAAD was defined as the dissection of the ascending aorta with extension to the arch or to the descending aorta, regardless of the site of the primary intimal tear. Diagnosis was generally established with emergent computed tomographic (CT) angiography of the chest, abdomen, and pelvis. Bedside transthoracic echocardiography assessed pericardial effusion and left ventricular function. Patients also underwent transesophageal echocardiography in the operating room to evaluate heart valves and the potential need for concomitant procedures. The presence of PSCM was identified using CT scan or equivalent and was evaluated for the presence of signs of stroke or cerebral ischemia. Primary endpoint outcomes were the following: (1) in-hospital and 30-day mortality, (2) postoperative new neurological deficit, (3) mechanical ventilation hours, and (4) intensive care unit (ICU) length of stay.

2.2. Surgical Technique and Postoperative Management

The surgical technique and the protocol followed in our university hospital has been previously described [12]. Experienced senior surgeons performed all cases under general anesthesia with standard hemodynamic monitoring. After cross-clamping of the aorta, myocardial protection involved retrograde cold blood cardioplegia. To provide bilateral antegrade cerebral perfusion, oxygenated cold blood (18 °C) was delivered through a balloon catheter inserted into the arch vessels, ensuring controlled flow pressure at 50–60 mmHg. The extent of the intimal tear determined the surgical approach, including supracoronary ascending aortic replacement, total vs. hemi- arch replacement, frozen elephant trunk, and reimplantation of supra-aortic arteries. The need for associated coronary artery bypass grafting or a Conduit/Bentall procedure with reimplantation of coronary arteries versus a David operation was also determined according to assessment of disease extent. After anastomosis, intracardiac air was ruled out using transesophageal echocardiography. Once primary hemostasis was achieved, the chest was closed, and the patient was subsequently transferred to the cardiac intensive care unit (ICU) to receive standard postoperative care.

Neurological deficits were routinely assessed in patients every hour during their stay in the ICU and every eight hours after being transferred to the floor. If a new deficit was detected, a CT scan of the head was performed, followed by formal neurological evaluation and magnetic resonance imaging to confirm the diagnosis. Mechanical ventilation was gradually discontinued following a standard postoperative protocol, with the aim of achieving liberation as soon as possible. Tracheostomy was considered if weaning from mechanical ventilation and extubation were not achievable within 10–12 days after the surgery.

2.3. Statistical Analysis

Descriptive statistics were used to present the baseline characteristics, operative details, and postoperative outcomes of patients in both groups. The normality of continuous variables was assessed using the Kolmogorov–Smirnov and the Shapiro–Wilk tests. For normally distributed data, group differences were assessed using the T-test, while for non-normally distributed data, the Mann–Whitney U-test was employed. The results were reported as the median and interquartile range (IQR). Categorical data were summarized as absolute (n) and relative (%) frequencies and compared by Chi^2-test or Fisher's exact test. Survival was estimated using the Kaplan–Meier curves for right censored data and analyzed for differences between the PSCM and the non-CM groups by the log rank test. Cox regression analysis was employed to examine the risk factors associated with long-term survival. Variable selection was based on clinical relevance and forward selection. All tests were conducted 2-sided and a p-value of ≤ 0.05 was considered statistically significant. IBM SPSS Statistics for Windows (Version 27.0) was used for statistical analysis.

3. Results

3.1. Preoperative and Baseline Patients' Characteristics

Of the total cohort, 82 patients (17.1%) had PSCM. The age, sex, and body mass index showed no significant differences between the groups. The patients with PSCM exhibited a higher logistic EuroSCORE I (median: 47, IQR [31, 64] vs. 24, IQR [15, 39]; $p < 0.001$) and had a higher prevalence of arterial hypertension (74.4% vs. 63.1%; $p = 0.05$). Although the EuroSCORE II was numerically higher in the PSCM group, the difference did not reach statistical significance (9.42 vs. 6.62; $p = 0.44$).

Interestingly, the patients in the PSCM group had a smaller aneurysmal diameter (48 mm, IQR [45, 53] vs. 52 mm, IQR [49, 60]; $p = 0.048$) compared to those without PSCM. Furthermore, the patients in the PSCM group were more likely to have undergone a previous cardiac surgery (7.3% vs. 2%; $p = 0.02$). Table 1 provides a summary of the baseline characteristics of the included patients. In terms of the laboratory data, we observed that the C-reactive protein levels were significantly higher in the PSCM group prior to surgery (6.5 mg/dL, IQR [2.1, 52.6] vs. 4.25 mg/dL, IQR [1.2, 21.5]; $p = 0.01$).

Table 1. Summary of the baseline characteristics and preoperative data of the included patients.

Variable	Total (n = 480)	No PSCM (n = 398/82.9%)	PSCM (n = 82/17.1%)	p-Value
Age (years)	63 (53; 73)	62 (53; 73)	66 (56; 73)	0.077
Female gender	170 (35.4%)	139 (34.9%)	31 (37.8%)	0.619
Body mass index [kg/m^2]	26.3 (24; 29.3)	26.3 (24; 29.3)	26.3 (23.4; 28.6)	0.530
Logistic EuroScore I	27 (16; 42)	24 (15; 39)	47 (31; 64)	**<0.001**
EuroScore II	6.86 (4.07; 14.14)	6.62 (3.92; 13.27)	9.42 (4.96; 14.66)	0.44
LVEF [%]	60 (55; 70)	60 (55; 70)	60 (55; 70)	0.804
Aneurysm Diameter [mm]	52 (47; 60)	52 (49; 60)	48 (45; 53)	**0.048**
DeBakey I	380 (79.3%)	314 (79.1%)	66 (80.5%)	0.776
DeBakey II	100 (20.7%)	84 (20.9%)	16 (19.5%)	0.776
Arterial hypertension	312 (65%)	251 (63.1%)	61 (74.4%)	0.050
IDDM	6 (1.3%)	4 (1%)	2 (2.4%)	0.275
Acute kidney failure	9 (1.9%)	8 (2%)	1 (1.2%)	1.000
Chronic kidney failure	51 (10.6%)	43 (10.8%)	8 (9.8%)	0.774

Table 1. Cont.

Variable	Total (n = 480)	No PSCM (n = 398/82.9%)	PSCM (n = 82/17.1%)	p-Value
COPD	33 (6.9%)	30 (7.5%)	3 (3.7%)	0.206
PAD	15 (3.1%)	12 (3%)	3 (3.7%)	0.729
CAD	75 (15.6%)	62 (15.6%)	13 (15.8%)	0.537
Bicuspid aortic valve	23 (4.8%)	22 (5.6%)	1 (1.2%)	0.297
Marfan syndrome	13 (2.7%)	10 (2.5%)	3 (3.7%)	0.473
Previous PCI	33 (6.9%)	30 (7.6%)	3 (3.7%)	0.213
Previous thoracic intervention	41 (8.5%)	30 (7.5%)	11 (13.4%)	0.083
Previous cardiac surgery	14 (2.9%)	8 (2%)	6 (7.3%)	**0.020**
Pericardial tamponade	78 (16.3%)	65 (16.4%)	13 (15.9%)	0.901
Acute MI (≤48 h)	15 (3.1%)	13 (3.3%)	2 (2.4%)	1.000
Cardiogenic shock	33 (6.9%)	29 (7.3%)	4 (4.9%)	0.430
CPR (≤48 h)	40 (8.3%)	37 (9.3%)	3 (3.7%)	0.093
ICU transfer	71 (14.8%)	62 (15.6%)	9 (11%)	0.282
Ventilated on admission	52 (10.9%)	44 (11.1%)	8 (9.8%)	0.725
Atrial fibrillation	56 (11.7%)	43 (10.8%)	13 (15.9%)	0.195
Aortic valve regurgitation	157 (33.7%)	131 (33.8%)	26 (33.3%)	0.302
C-reactive protein (mg/dL)	4.75 (1.28; 23.7)	4.25 (1.2; 21.5)	6.5 (2.1; 52.6)	**0.014**

PSCM: preoperative signs of cerebral malperfusion, EuroScore: European System for Cardiac Operative Risk Evaluation; COPD: chronic obstructive pulmonary disease; LVEF: left ventricular ejection fraction; IDDM: insulin dependent diabetes mellitus; PAD: peripheral arterial disease; CAD: coronary artery disease; PCI: percutaneous coronary intervention; MI: myocardial infarction; CPR: cardiopulmonary resuscitation; ICU: intensive care unit; Bold: Statistically significant.

3.2. Intraoperative Details

The operative, bypass, cardioplegia, and aortic cross clamp times were similar between both groups, as shown in Table 2. The patients without PSCM underwent more Bentall surgeries (8.5% vs. 22.4%; $p = 0.004$) and had more aortic valve replacements (6.1% vs. 21.6%; $p = 0.001$). The patients presenting with PSCM received more intraoperative packed red blood cells (4 units, IQR [2, 6] vs. 2 units, IQR [0, 5]; $p < 0.001$), fresh frozen plasma (3 units, IQR [0, 6] vs. 0 units, IQR [0, 4]; $p = 0.003$), and platelets (2 units, IQR [1, 2] vs. 2 units, IQR [1, 2]; $p = 0.035$). There were no significant differences observed in the choice of arterial or venous cannulation sites between both groups.

3.3. Postoperative Outcomes

Following the surgery, the patients who presented with PSCM had markedly longer ventilation hours (108.5 h, IQR [44, 277] vs. 43 h, IQR [16, 158], $p < 0.001$) and a significantly longer ICU length of stay (7 days, IQR [4, 13] vs. 5 days, IQR [2, 11]; $p = 0.013$). Additionally, the patients with preoperative PSCM had significantly higher rates of postoperative new neurological deficits (35.4% vs. 19.4%; $p = 0.002$). Moreover, they underwent more tracheotomies (35.4% vs. 20.7%; $p = 0.004$) and experienced more postoperative pneumonia (22% vs. 12.5%; $p = 0.026$). No significant difference was noted in terms of the postoperative inotrope requirement, chest tube drainage, or postoperative delirium between both groups. Table 3.

Table 2. Intraoperative details.

Variable	Total (n = 480)	No PSCM (n = 398/82.9%)	PSCM (n = 82/17.1%)	p-Value
Surgery duration [min]	281 (228; 347)	280 (227; 349)	289 (230; 335)	0.993
CPB [min]	168 (135; 215)	171 (135; 224)	160 (139; 193)	0.132
Cross clamp duration [min]	95 (72; 137)	96 (72; 140)	90 (71; 118)	0.166
Circulatory arrest [min]	35 (26; 51)	34 (26; 51)	39 (28; 55)	0.199
RBC [unit]	2 (0; 6)	2 (0; 5)	4 (2; 6)	**<0.001**
FFP [unit]	0 (0; 6)	0 (0; 4)	3 (0; 6)	**0.003**
Platelets [unit]	2 (1; 2)	2 (1; 2)	2 (1; 2)	**0.035**
Supracoronary aortic replacement ONLY	202 (42.1%)	163 (41%)	39 (47.6%)	0.270
Hemi-arch	119 (24.8%)	96 (24.1%)	23 (28%)	0.453
Total-arch	72 (15%)	61 (15.3%)	11 (13.4%)	0.659
Conduit/Bentall	96 (20%)	89 (22.4%)	7 (8.5%)	**0.004**
David	29 (6%)	26 (6.5%)	3 (3.7%)	0.447
Elephant-trunk	13 (2.7%)	11 (2.8%)	2 (2.4%)	1.000
Aortic valve replacement	91 (19%)	86 (21.6%)	5 (6.1%)	**0.001**
CABG	37 (7.7%)	34 (8.5%)	3 (3.7%)	0.131
Arterial cannulation site				
Femoral artery	81 (17.3%)	62 (16%)	19 (23.5%)	0.283
Ascending aorta	93 (19.9%)	74 (19.1%)	19 (23.5%)	0.283
Aortic arch	13 (2.8%)	10 (2.6%)	3 (3.7%)	0.283
Subclavian artery	2 (0.4%)	2 (0.5%)	0 (0%)	0.283
Apex	5 (1.1%)	4 (1%)	1 (1.2%)	0.283
Pulmonary vein	274 (58.5%)	235 (60.7%)	39 (48.1%)	0.283
Venous cannulation site				
Right Atrium	455 (97.2%)	378 (97.7%)	77 (95.1%)	0.086
bicaval	4 (0.9%)	4 (1%)	0 (0%)	0.086
Femoral vein	9 (1.9%)	5 (1.3%)	4 (4.9%)	0.086

PSCM: preoperative signs of cerebral malperfusion; CPB: cardiopulmonary bypass; RBC: red blood cells; FFP: fresh frozen plasma; CABG: coronary artery bypass grafting. Bold: Statistically significant.

In terms of the laboratory data, we observed that patients in the PSCM group had higher levels of plasma potassium (5 mmol/L, IQR [4.7, 5.31]) compared to the patients without PSCM (4.8 mmol/L, IQR [4.5, 5.1]; p = 0.002) on the first postoperative day. Additionally, the PSCM group had higher levels of C-reactive protein (141.6 mg/dL, IQR [92, 194] vs. 102 mg/dL, IQR [42.5, 161.3]; p = 0.005) and a lower platelet count (111 × 10^9/L IQR [90, 141] vs. 130 [104, 161]; p = 0.004) on the first postoperative day.

The PSCM group tended to have higher in-hospital mortality rates; however, the results were not statistically significant (19.8% vs. 15.3%; p = 0.32). Furthermore, no significant difference was observed in the 30-day mortality between both groups (22% vs. 17.2%; p = 0.31). Table 4 illustrates the differences in the cause-specific mortality between both groups.

Table 3. Postoperative outcomes.

Variable	Total (n = 480)	No PSCM (n = 398/82.9%)	PSCM (n = 82/17.1%)	p-Value
Postoperative inotropic therapy	64 (14%)	54 (14.3%)	10 (12.7%)	0.213
48 h chest tube output [mL]	910 (500; 1650)	950 (500; 1700)	900 (500; 1600)	0.987
24 h RBC [unit]	0 (0; 2)	0 (0; 2)	1 (0; 2)	0.525
24 h FFP [unit]	0 (0; 4)	0 (0; 4)	0 (0; 4)	0.894
24 h Platelets [unit]	0 (0; 0)	0 (0; 0)	0 (0; 1)	0.424
Total RBC given [unit]	3 (0; 8)	2 (0; 8)	4 (0; 8)	0.314
Total FFP [unit]	1.5 (0; 6)	2 (0; 6)	0 (0; 4)	0.189
Total platelets [unit]	0 (0; 2)	0 (0; 2)	0 (0; 1)	**0.042**
Ventilation [h]	17 (60; 189)	43 (16; 158)	108.5 (44; 277)	**<0.001**
ICU stay [d]	5 (2; 11)	5 (2; 11)	7 (4; 13)	**0.013**
ICU re-admission	39 (8.2%)	33 (8.4%)	6 (7.3%)	0.737
Reintubation	77 (16.3%)	63 (16.1%)	14 (17.1%)	0.830
Tracheotomy	110 (23.2%)	81 (20.7%)	29 (35.4%)	**0.004**
Delirium	93 (19.8%)	81 (20.9%)	12 (14.6%)	0.197
MI	6 (1.3%)	6 (1.5%)	0 (0%)	0.596
New neurological deficits	105 (22.2%)	76 (19.4%)	29 (35.4%)	**0.002**
CPR	29 (6.1%)	25 (6.4%)	4 (4.9%)	0.603
Pneumonia	67 (14.2%)	49 (12.5%)	18 (22%)	**0.026**
Sepsis	21 (4.4%)	16 (4.1%)	5 (6.1%)	0.385
TEVAR(EVAR)	31 (6.5%)	27 (6.9%)	4 (4.9%)	0.522
Re-thoracotomy	89 (18.7%)	78 (19.7%)	11 (13.4%)	0.180
Wound healing deficits	7 (1.5%)	6 (1.5%)	1 (1.2%)	1.000
AKI KDIGO	102 (21.7%)	85 (21.9%)	17 (20.7%)	0.815
Postoperative AF	46 (9.8%)	37 (9.5%)	9 (11.1%)	0.654
New pacer	23 (4.9%)	20 (5.1%)	3 (3.7%)	0.780
Postoperative C-reactive protein (mg/dL)	110.5 (47; 173.1)	102 (42.55; 161.38)	141.6 (91.8; 193.65)	**0.005**
Postoperative platelets count	127.5 (101.25; 157)	130 (104; 161)	111 (90; 141)	**0.004**

PSCM: preoperative signs of cerebral malperfusion; RBC: red blood cells; FFP: fresh frozen plasma; ICU: intensive care unit; MI: myocardial infarction; CPR: cardiopulmonary resuscitation; TEVAR: thoracic endovascular aortic repair; AKI: acute kidney injury; AF: atrial fibrillation. Bold: Statistically significant.

Table 4. Early overall and cause-specific mortality.

Variable	Total (n = 480)	No Cerebral Malperfusion (n = 398/82.9%)	Cerebral Malperfusion (n = 82/17.1%)	p-Value
In-hospital mortality	77 (16.1%)	61 (15.3%)	16 (19.8%)	0.323
Cause of death				
Cardiac	44 (50%)	34 (49.3%)	10 (52.6%)	0.064
Cerebrovascular	8 (9.1%)	4 (5.8%)	4 (21.1%)	0.064
Sepsis	4 (4.5%)	2 (2.9%)	2 (10.5%)	0.064
Multi-organ failure	28 (31.8%)	25 (36.2%)	3 (15.8%)	0.064
Unknown	4 (4.5%)	4 (5.8%)	0 (0%)	0.064
Surgery till death [d]	3 (1; 12)	3 (1; 11)	6 (1; 16)	0.223
7-day mortality	56 (11.8%)	46 (11.7%)	10 (12.2%)	0.900
30-day mortality	86 (18%)	68 (17.2%)	18 (22%)	0.310

In the long term, there was a significant decline in survival in the PSCM group, as indicated by the KM curve ($p = 0.007$). Figure 1 shows the Kaplan–Meier analysis.

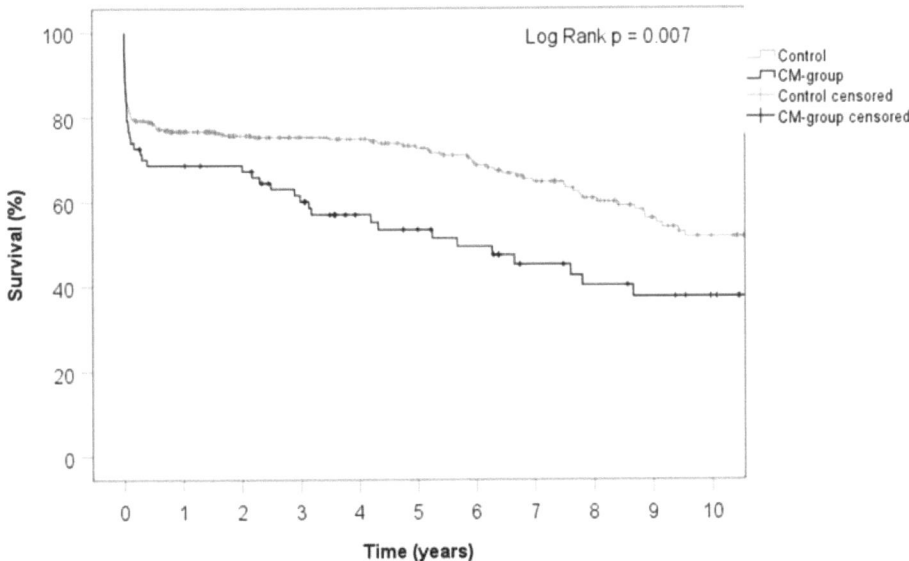

Figure 1. Kaplan–Meier curve illustrating long-term survival throughout follow-up. There is a significantly lower survival rate in patients who had PSCM after ten years of follow-up (38% vs. 52%, log-rank test p value = 0.007).

3.4. Risk Factors for Long-Term Mortality

In our multivariate Cox regression analysis, several significant risk factors associated with long-term mortality were identified. PSCM emerged as a significant risk factor (hazard ratio (HR) 1.75, 95%CI [1.20–2.53], $p = 0.003$). Additionally, factors such as ventilation upon admission and cardiopulmonary resuscitation within 48 h of admission were also found to be associated with a lower survival. Surprisingly, hypertension was shown as a protective factor against long-term mortality. (HR: 0.59, 95%CI [0.43–0.82], $p = 0.001$). Table 5 presents a summary of the variables that were tested in the Cox regression analysis, along with their respective hazard ratios.

Table 5. Cox regression analysis on risk factors for long-term survival.

Risk Factor	Hazard Ratio	95% Confidence Interval	p-Value
Age (years)	1.041	[1.026–1.057]	**<0.001**
Female gender	0.949	[0.682–1.321]	0.758
PSCM	1.747	[1.204–2.534]	**0.003**
Arterial hypertension	0.595	[0.433–0.817]	**0.001**
PAD	1.890	[0.917–3.896]	0.085
Ventilated on admission	1.677	[1.050–2.679]	**0.031**
CPR (<48 h)	2.610	[1.622–4.202]	**<0.001**
CPB (min)	1.007	[1.004–1.009]	**<0.001**
RBC (unit)	1.043	[1.000–1.088]	**0.048**

PSCM: preoperative signs of cerebral malperfusion, PAD: peripheral artery disease, CPR: cardiopulmonary resuscitation, CPB: cardiopulmonary bypass time, RBC: red blood cell transfusion. Bold: Statistically significant.

4. Discussion

ATAAD is a complex and life-threatening condition characterized by high mortality rates and perioperative complications. The presence of malperfusion syndromes further aggravates these challenges and contributes to the poorer outcomes. Our study aimed to investigate the characteristics and outcomes of ATAAD patients who presented with CM.

In our large center experience, we observed that 17.1% of the patients diagnosed with ATAAD also presented with CM. This finding is consistent with previous estimates, which have reported CM occurring in approximately one sixth of ATAAD cases [11].

Furthermore, our results showed a trend indicating an association between PSCM and increased in-hospital mortality rates. Wang and colleagues [11] reported an average in-hospital mortality rate of around 20% in ATAAD patients presenting with CM. Our findings, showing an in-hospital mortality of 19.8% and a 30-day mortality of 22%, align with these previous studies. Although we did not observe a statistically significant difference compared to the patients without PSCM, the observed trends suggest a potential link between PSCM and a poorer prognosis. Interestingly, we found that the impact of PSCM on the patient survival becomes more evident in the long term, with significantly lower survival rates in the PSCM group.

Importantly, our findings highlight the significant impact of PSCM on the postoperative outcomes. For example, the patients with PSCM had significantly longer ventilation hours and intensive care unit stays compared to those without PSCM. This highlights the complex impact leading to respiratory insufficiency. Previous reports have also highlighted the intricate nature of postoperative respiratory complications in patients with CM, showing consistently prolonged durations of mechanical ventilation in patients with CM [13–15]. Furthermore, the prolonged ventilation can be mirrored by the higher rate of tracheotomies and the increased incidence of postoperative pneumonia in the CM group, indicating the severity of respiratory compromise in patients with CM and the challenges in weaning them off mechanical ventilation.

Several reports have emphasized the risk imposed by preoperative CM and the influence on the incidence of postoperative new neurological deficits [11,15–19]. Our results showed that 35.4% of the patients with PSCM experienced new postoperative neurological deficits. Wang and colleagues also showed that postoperative new neurological deficits can occur in up to 45.5% of patients who have PSCM [11]. Nonetheless, it is important to note that the preoperative CM can be difficult to categorize at admission and the accurate assessment of neurological symptoms is difficult, especially when patients are admitted intubated. Gomibuchi et al. [17] demonstrated that the presence of supra-aortic branch occlusion or stenosis is a significant risk factor for permanent neurological deficit (odds ratio: 7.66; $p < 0.001$), regardless of the preoperative neurological symptoms. On the other hand, Vendramin et al. [15] noted in their series that patients presenting with coma had the highest in-hospital mortality, regardless of the brain protection.

Despite the earlier debate on whether patients with preoperative CM should undergo prompt surgery [18], the current guidelines encourage no delay in surgery for those patients [6,7]. The systematic review by Wang showed that 54.3% of patients with preoperative CM experienced complete recovery or improvement in their neurological symptoms, while the symptoms remained the same in 27.1% of patients and worsened in 8.5% of patients. Similarly, Di Eusanio et al. [18] demonstrated an improved late survival and frequent reversal of neurologic deficits.

The extent of supra-aortic vessel involvement was reported as a significant moderator of poor neurological outcomes. Fukuhara and colleagues [16] showed that the extension of the dissection to the internal carotid artery was the worst predictor of poor outcomes when compared to common carotid involvement. In their experience, all patients with internal carotid artery occlusion developed cerebral edema and herniation syndromes, and died regardless of the management.

Several management strategies have been proposed to manage ATAAD patients presenting with PSCM and reduce the risk of neurological complications. Those include early aggressive direct carotid reperfusion before surgical repair [19], percutaneous stenting or endovascular repair [20], and extra-anatomic revascularization [17]. Moreover, a hemi-arch replacement was proposed as a strategy to manage patients with supra-aortic vessel dissection but no PSCM, still, such a strategy carried a higher risk of reoperation [21]. The optimal management approach for CM in ATAAD remains uncertain. Fukuhara et al. [16] emphasized the importance of performing neck computed tomography prior to surgery, as it can provide valuable information about the extent of dissection involving the supra-aortic vessels and guide the intraoperative management decisions for these cases.

Recent evidence has provided insights into the potential value of serum biomarkers in ATAAD patients. Besides elevated C-reactive protein, the lymphocyte-to-neutrophil ratio and lymphocyte-to-platelet ratio (LPR) have emerged as predictive markers of mortality [22,23]. Interestingly, a study conducted by Yuan et al. [4] identified a plasma potassium of >4.4 mmol/L as an independent predictor of mortality in ATAAD patients. Consistent with these findings, our study revealed that patients with PSCM exhibited elevated postoperative serum potassium levels, increased levels of C-reactive protein, and lower platelet counts. The exact role and clinical significance of these biomarkers in ATAAD warrant further investigation for a better understanding of their diagnostic and prognostic implications.

In our multivariate Cox regression analysis, we identified PSCM as a significant risk factor for long-term mortality, emphasizing its significant impact posed on patients' long-term survival. Additionally, factors such as ventilation upon admission and cardiopulmonary resuscitation within 48 h of admission were associated with lower survival rates, which could be rationally attributed to the critical baseline morbidity in those patients. Intriguingly, our study revealed that hypertension has a protective effect against long-term mortality. Previous studies have suggested that a known history of hypertension may contribute to the earlier diagnosis and management of patients with ATAAD, potentially leading to lower mortality rates [24,25]. This earlier recognition and management may also mitigate the impact of CM on brain tissue viability in patients with PSCM. Moreover, hypertension could theoretically enhance the collateral circulation and reduce the damage to the penumbral tissue [26], potentially reducing the overall impact of CM on patients' long-term survival. Nevertheless, this theory warrants further investigation to better understand its potential role in this specific subgroup of ATAAD patients.

Further research is also warranted to explore the optimal approaches for addressing CM in patients with ATAAD and minimizing its impact on patient outcomes.

5. Strengths, Limitations, and Future Recommendations

Our study provides valuable real-world data that reflect the clinical practice and patient populations encountered in daily practice. It is important to acknowledge several limitations that should be considered when interpreting the results. Firstly, being a retrospective observational study, there is the potential for an inherent confounding bias that may impact the generalizability of our findings. Secondly, the complex nature of the patient pathology in ATAAD makes it challenging to draw definitive conclusions regarding the specific impact of CM on outcomes, particularly considering the potential influence of other malperfusion syndromes. Moreover, CT scans were employed to detect the presence of PSCM; therefore, our data do not provide a clear cause of CM whether due to a dissection-related artery obstruction or severe hemodynamic changes that resulted in a stroke. Future research may benefit from performing a preoperative perfusion CT or an intraoperative transcranial Doppler to obtain more conclusive evidence on the presence of PSCM.

It is important to mention that the postoperative parameters discussed may not be solely attributed to CM but could reflect the overall complexity of cases. It is crucial to exercise caution and to consider these limitations when interpreting the results. Further research, including prospective studies with larger sample sizes and more comprehensive assessments, is warranted to better elucidate the association between CM and outcomes in ATAAD patients.

6. Conclusions

PSCM in patients with ATAAD were associated with longer ventilation hours, the ICU length of stay, and a higher incidence of postoperative new neurological deficits. Moreover, the long-term survival outcomes were significantly poorer in patients presenting with PSCM. These results highlight the need for early recognition and appropriate management of neurologic deficits in ATAAD to improve the postoperative outcomes and long-term survival.

Author Contributions: Conceptualization, A.H.; methodology, C.F.; formal analysis, C.F.; investigation, M.A.-T., M.S., S.D., A.B., N.R., T.P. and J.C.; data curation, C.F. and A.B.; writing—original draft, M.A.-T., M.S., S.D., A.B., N.R., J.S. and N.d.S.; writing—review and editing, J.S., T.P. and J.C.; supervision, A.H. All authors have read and agreed to the published version of the manuscript.

Funding: This research received no external funding.

Institutional Review Board Statement: Ethical review and approval were waived for this study due to its retrospective nature.

Informed Consent Statement: Patient consent was waived due to the retrospective nature of the study.

Data Availability Statement: The data presented in this study are available on request from the corresponding author. The data are not publicly available due to institutional policies.

Conflicts of Interest: The authors declare no conflict of interest.

References

1. Biancari, F.; Dell'aquila, A.M.; Gatti, G.; Perrotti, A.; Hervé, A.; Touma, J.; Pettinari, M.; Peterss, S.; Buech, J.; Wisniewski, K.; et al. Interinstitutional analysis of the outcome after surgery for type A aortic dissection. *Eur. J. Trauma Emerg. Surg.* **2023**, *49*, 1791–1801. [CrossRef]
2. Gemelli, M.; Di Tommaso, E.; Natali, R.; Dixon, L.K.; Mohamed Ahmed, E.; Rajakaruna, C.; Bruno, V.D. Validation of the German Registry for Acute Aortic Dissection Type A Score in predicting 30-day mortality after type A aortic dissection surgery. *Eur. J. Cardio-Thorac. Surg.* **2023**, *63*, ezad141. [CrossRef]
3. Lee, T.C.; Kon, Z.; Cheema, F.H.; Grau-Sepulveda, M.V.; Englum, B.; Kim, S.; Chaudhuri, P.S.; Thourani, V.H.; Ailawadi, G.; Hughes, G.C.; et al. Contemporary management and outcomes of acute type A aortic dissection: An analysis of the STS adult cardiac surgery database. *J. Card. Surg.* **2018**, *33*, 7–18. [CrossRef] [PubMed]
4. Yuan, H.; Sun, Z.; Zhang, Y.; Wu, W.; Liu, M.; Yang, Y.; Wang, J.; Lv, Q.; Zhang, L.; Li, Y.; et al. Clinical Analysis of Risk Factors for Mortality in Type A Acute Aortic Dissection: A Single Study From China. *Front. Cardiovasc. Med.* **2021**, *8*, 728568. [CrossRef] [PubMed]
5. Pape, L.A.; Awais, M.; Woznicki, E.M.; Suzuki, T.; Trimarchi, S.; Evangelista, A.; Myrmel, T.; Larsen, M.; Harris, K.M.; Greason, K.; et al. Presentation, Diagnosis, and Outcomes of Acute Aortic Dissection: 17-Year Trends From the International Registry of Acute Aortic Dissection. *J. Am. Coll. Cardiol.* **2015**, *66*, 350–358. [CrossRef]
6. Erbel, R.; Aboyans, V.; Boileau, C.; Bossone, E.; Di Bartolomeo, R.; Eggebrecht, H.; Evangelista, A.; Falk, V.; Frank, H.; Gaemperli, O.; et al. 2014 ESC Guidelines on the diagnosis and treatment of aortic diseases: Document covering acute and chronic aortic diseases of the thoracic and abdominal aorta of the adult. The Task Force for the Diagnosis and Treatment of Aortic Diseases of the European Society of Cardiology (ESC). *Eur. Heart J.* **2014**, *35*, 2873–2926. [PubMed]
7. Isselbacher, E.M.; Preventza, O.; Black, J.H.; Augoustides, J.G.; Beck, A.W.; Bolen, M.A.; Braverman, A.C.; Bray, B.E.; Brown-Zimmerman, M.M.; Chen, E.P.; et al. 2022 ACC/AHA Guideline for the Diagnosis and Management of Aortic Disease: A Report of the American Heart Association/American College of Cardiology Joint Committee on Clinical Practice Guidelines. *Circulation* **2022**, *146*, E334–E482. [CrossRef] [PubMed]
8. Jaffar-Karballai, M.; Tran, T.T.; Oremakinde, O.; Zafar, S.; Harky, A. Malperfusion in Acute Type A Aortic Dissection: Management Strategies. *Vasc. Endovasc. Surg.* **2021**, *55*, 721–729. [CrossRef] [PubMed]
9. Kayali, F.; Jubouri, M.; Al-Tawil, M.; Tan, S.Z.C.P.; Williams, I.M.; Mohammed, I.; Velayudhan, B.; Bashir, M. Coronary artery involvement in type A aortic dissection: Fate of the coronaries. *J. Card. Surg.* **2022**, *37*, 5233–5242. [CrossRef]
10. Pacini, D.; Murana, G.; Di Marco, L.; Berardi, M.; Mariani, C.; Coppola, G.; Fiorentino, M.; Leone, A.; Di Bartolomeo, R. Cerebral perfusion issues in type A aortic dissection. *J. Vis. Surg.* **2018**, *4*, 77. [CrossRef]
11. Wang, C.; Zhang, L.; Li, T.; Xi, Z.; Wu, H.; Li, D. Surgical treatment of type A acute aortic dissection with cerebral malperfusion: A systematic review. *J. Cardiothorac. Surg.* **2022**, *17*, 140. [CrossRef] [PubMed]
12. Salem, M.; Friedrich, C.; Rusch, R.; Frank, D.; Hoffmann, G.; Lutter, G.; Berndt, R.; Cremer, J.; Haneya, A.; Puehler, T. Is total arch replacement associated with an increased risk after acute type A dissection? *J. Thorac. Dis.* **2020**, *12*, 5517–5531. [CrossRef] [PubMed]

13. Pacini, D.; Leone, A.; Belotti, L.M.B.; Fortuna, D.; Gabbieri, D.; Zussa, C.; Contini, A.; Di Bartolomeo, R.; on behalf of RERIC (Emilia Romagna Cardiac Surgery Registry) Investigators. Acute type A aortic dissection: Significance of multiorgan malperfusion. *Eur. J. Cardio-Thoracic Surg.* **2013**, *43*, 820–826. [CrossRef] [PubMed]
14. Sultan, I.; Bianco, V.; Patel, H.J.; Arnaoutakis, G.J.; Di Eusanio, M.; Chen, E.P.; Leshnower, B.; Sundt, T.M.; Sechtem, U.; Montgomery, D.G.; et al. Surgery for type A aortic dissection in patients with cerebral malperfusion: Results from the International Registry of Acute Aortic Dissection. *J. Thorac. Cardiovasc. Surg.* **2021**, *161*, 1713–1720.e1. [CrossRef]
15. Vendramin, I.; Isola, M.; Piani, D.; Onorati, F.; Salizzoni, S.; D'Onofrio, A.; Di Marco, L.; Gatti, G.; De Martino, M.; Faggian, G.; et al. Surgical management and outcomes in patients with acute type A aortic dissection and cerebral malperfusion. *JTCVS Open* **2022**, *10*, 22–33. [CrossRef]
16. Fukuhara, S.; Norton, E.L.; Chaudhary, N.; Burris, N.; Shiomi, S.; Kim, K.M.; Patel, H.J.; Deeb, G.M.; Yang, B. Type A Aortic Dissection with Cerebral Malperfusion: New Insights. *Ann. Thorac. Surg.* **2021**, *112*, 501–509. [CrossRef]
17. Gomibuchi, T.; Seto, T.; Naito, K.; Chino, S.; Mikoshiba, T.; Komatsu, M.; Tanaka, H.; Ichimura, H.; Yamamoto, T.; Nakahara, K.; et al. Strategies to improve outcomes for acute type A aortic dissection with cerebral malperfusion. *Eur. J. Cardio-Thorac. Surg.* **2021**, *59*, 666–673. [CrossRef]
18. Di Eusanio, M.; Patel, H.J.; Nienaber, C.A.; Montgomery, D.M.; Korach, A.; Sundt, T.M.; DeVincentiis, C.; Voehringer, M.; Peterson, M.D.; Myrmel, T.; et al. Patients with type A acute aortic dissection presenting with major brain injury: Should we operate on them? *J. Thorac. Cardiovasc. Surg.* **2013**, *145* (Suppl. S3), S213–S221.e1. [CrossRef]
19. Okita, Y.; Ikeno, Y.; Yokawa, K.; Koda, Y.; Henmi, S.; Gotake, Y.; Nakai, H.; Matsueda, T.; Inoue, T.; Tanaka, H. Direct perfusion of the carotid artery in patients with brain malperfusion secondary to acute aortic dissection. *Gen. Thorac. Cardiovasc. Surg.* **2019**, *67*, 161–167. [CrossRef]
20. Heran, M.K.; Balaji, N.; Cook, R.C. Novel Percutaneous Treatment of Cerebral Malperfusion Before Surgery for Acute Type A Dissection. *Ann. Thorac. Surg.* **2019**, *108*, e15–e17. [CrossRef]
21. Norton, E.L.; Wu, X.; Kim, K.M.; Fukuhara, S.; Patel, H.J.; Deeb, G.M.; Yang, B. Is hemiarch replacement adequate in acute type A aortic dissection repair in patients with arch branch vessel dissection without cerebral malperfusion? *J. Thorac. Cardiovasc. Surg.* **2021**, *161*, 873–884.e2. [CrossRef] [PubMed]
22. Guvenc, O.; Engin, M. The role of neutrophil-lymphocyte platelet ratio in predicting in-hospital mortality after acute Type A aortic dissection operations. *Eur. Rev. Med. Pharmacol. Sci.* **2023**, *27*, 1534–1539. [CrossRef] [PubMed]
23. Erdolu, B.; As, A.K. C-Reactive Protein and Neutrophil to Lymphocyte Ratio Values in Predicting Inhospital Death in Patients with Stanford Type A Acute Aortic Dissection. *Heart Surg. Forum* **2020**, *23*, E488–E492. [CrossRef] [PubMed]
24. Trimarchi, S.; Eagle, K.A.; Nienaber, C.A.; Rampoldi, V.; Jonker, F.H.; De Vincentiis, C.; Frigiola, A.; Menicanti, L.; Tsai, T.; Froehlich, J.; et al. Role of age in acute type A aortic dissection outcome: Report from the International Registry of Acute Aortic Dissection (IRAD). *J. Thorac. Cardiovasc. Surg.* **2010**, *140*, 784–789. [CrossRef] [PubMed]
25. Friedrich, C.; Salem, M.A.; Puehler, T.; Hoffmann, G.; Lutter, G.; Cremer, J.; Haneya, A. Sex-specific risk factors for early mortality and survival after surgery of acute aortic dissection type a: A retrospective observational study. *J. Cardiothorac. Surg.* **2020**, *15*, 145. [CrossRef]
26. Regenhardt, R.W.; Das, A.S.; Stapleton, C.J.; Chandra, R.V.; Rabinov, J.D.; Patel, A.B.; Hirsch, J.A.; Leslie-Mazwi, T.M. Blood Pressure and Penumbral Sustenance in Stroke from Large Vessel Occlusion. *Front. Neurol.* **2017**, *8*, 317. [CrossRef]

Disclaimer/Publisher's Note: The statements, opinions and data contained in all publications are solely those of the individual author(s) and contributor(s) and not of MDPI and/or the editor(s). MDPI and/or the editor(s) disclaim responsibility for any injury to people or property resulting from any ideas, methods, instructions or products referred to in the content.

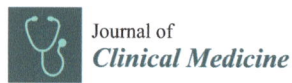 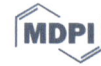

Article

Paracolic Gutter Routing: A Novel Retroperitoneal Extra-Anatomical Repair for Infected Aorto-Iliac Axis†

Hazem El Beyrouti [1,*], Mohamed Omar [1], Cristi-Teodor Calimanescu [2], Hendrik Treede [1] and Nancy Halloum [1]

[1] Department of Cardiac and Vascular Surgery, University Medical Center, Johannes Gutenberg University, 55131 Mainz, Germany
[2] Division of Vascular Surgery, Ameos Clinic Center Bremerhaven, 27568 Bremerhaven, Germany
* Correspondence: hbeyrouti@gmail.com; Tel.: +49-6131-170
† Presented at the ESVS 2022 Annual Meeting, Rome, Italy, 20–23 September 2022, and at the 2022 Three-Country Meeting of the Austrian, German and Swiss Society for Vascular Surgery, Vienna, Austria, 19–22 October 2022.

Abstract: Objective: We describe and analyze outcomes of a novel extra-anatomical paracolic gutter routing technique for surgical repair of aorto-iliac infections. Methods: A double-center, observational, cohort study of all consecutive patients with aorto-iliac infections treated using extra-anatomical paracolic gutter technique. Between May 2015 and December 2022, six patients with aorto-iliac infections were treated with the paracolic gutter routing technique. Cases were identified retrospectively in an institutional database, and data were retrieved from surgical records, imaging studies, and follow-up records. Results: Aorto-bifemoral vascular reconstructions were performed using this technique in six patients. During mean follow-up of 52 ± 44 months, there was one case of graft thrombosis (17%) with subsequent successful thrombectomy. Primary and secondary graft patency rates were 83% and 100%, respectively. There was one mortality (17%) due to candida sepsis. All graft prostheses were patent at last follow-up. Conclusions: The paracolic gutter technique is a useful technique in patients with extensive aorto-iliac infections, arteriovenous and iliac-ureteric fistulas, or at a high risk of vascular graft infection and is associated with favorable reinfection and patency rates.

Keywords: aorta; infection; graft; prosthesis; vascular; endovascular; VGEI; INAA

Citation: El Beyrouti, H.; Omar, M.; Calimanescu, C.-T.; Treede, H.; Halloum, N. Paracolic Gutter Routing: A Novel Retroperitoneal Extra-Anatomical Repair for Infected Aorto-Iliac Axis. *J. Clin. Med.* **2023**, *12*, 5765. https://doi.org/10.3390/jcm12175765

Academic Editors: Benedikt Reutersberg, Matthias Trenner and Dmitriy Atochin

Received: 24 July 2023
Revised: 24 August 2023
Accepted: 29 August 2023
Published: 4 September 2023

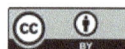

Copyright: © 2023 by the authors. Licensee MDPI, Basel, Switzerland. This article is an open access article distributed under the terms and conditions of the Creative Commons Attribution (CC BY) license (https://creativecommons.org/licenses/by/4.0/).

1. Introduction

Graft infections are infrequent (incidence 0.6–5%) but serious complications of vascular surgery. Aorto-iliac graft infections can threaten limb viability and are associated with high morbidity and mortality rates. A conservative treatment is associated with high mortality rates of 25–88% and limb loss in 5–25% [1–3]. The mortality and morbidity of aortic infection depend on several factors, including the presence of concomitant comorbidities, the causative agent, the invasivity of the infection, the timing of diagnosis, and the operative management [4,5].

In one study of 72 vascular graft infections (VGI) with positive graft cultures in 65 patients, infection-related mortality was 11%; of the 65 patients, 14 had undergone aorto-bifemoral bypass, 13 axillo-femoral bypass, 5 femoro-femoral bypass, 27 femoro-popliteal bypass, and 4 femoral endarterectomy with synthetic patch angioplasty [6]. Surgical debridement and replacement of infected segments is necessary, but the close proximity of synthetic grafts to the infected field may lead to high rates of reinfection. Several graft materials for in situ reconstruction (using an antibiotic soaked or rifampicin-bounded graft, cryopreserved allograft, autogenous femoral vein, tube graft made of bovine pericardium, silver-coated prostheses, Omniflow or cryopreserved allograft) have been studied to prevent infection recurrence with variable results [7–16]. Extra-anatomical bypass techniques (axillo-femoral bypass) have also been proposed but with increased morbidity: low patency (40–73% at 5 years), limb amputation (up to 24%), aortic stump blow-out (2–30%), and mortality (up to 27%) [11]. None of these approaches is universally applicable due to sometimes there being longer graft preparation times, the limited availability of certain prostheses, and increased risk of reinfection. We describe here a novel extra-anatomical para-colic technique to manage aorto-iliac infections and clinical outcomes of patients treated to date with this technique.

2. Methods

This is a retrospective review of all consecutive patients who received extra-anatomical paracolic gutter technique as aorto-bifemoral grafts. Cases were identified retrospectively in our institutional database, and data were retrieved from surgical records, imaging studies, and follow-up records. Medical records of all patients with confirmed infection between May 2015 and December 2022 were screened for inclusion in the study. Patients treated using other surgical techniques, with incomplete medical records or who did not meet the diagnostic criteria for VGI were excluded from the analysis. Demographic, clinical, and laboratory data were collected from electronic medical records. Variables of interest included age, sex, and underlying medical conditions.

The choice of technique was based mainly on the preference of the operating surgeon. In general, this technique was used in patients with aorto-iliac infections. Infection diagnosis was established by computed tomography (CT) supported by clinical, microbiological, and laboratory findings, and was confirmed by intraoperative findings.

Ethical approval was obtained from the institutional ethical committee, and informed consents were waived due to the retrospective and observational nature of this study.

The outcomes analyzed distinguished between early ($\leq$30 days after graft placement) and late (>30 days) surgical revision, primary and secondary patency and early and late mortality, reinfection, and freedom from formation of aorto-enteric or aorto-ureteral fistulation during the follow-up after vascular reconstruction using the novel extra-anatomical paracolic gutter routing technique in aorto-iliac infection.

2.1. Surgical Technique

Prior to surgery, all patients undergo a thorough preoperative evaluation, which includes a detailed medical history, physical examination, and infectious disease consultation. Typical imaging studies such as CT angiography are performed to assess the extent of infection, anatomical considerations, and the feasibility of the extra-anatomical repair approach. In cases of sepsis and hemodynamic instability, patients are admitted to intensive care for stabilization prior to surgery.

Bilateral ureteral splints are inserted 1–2 days before surgery. The extra-anatomical aorto-bifemoral graft procedure is carried out under general anesthesia and through a midline laparotomy with the patient in the supine position. The abdomen is explored to assess the extent of infection and to identify any intra-abdominal involvement.

To facilitate exposure, we use a self-retaining retractor to retract the omentum and transverse colon cephalad. The small bowel is removed laterally. We irrigate the infected area with an antibiotic solution, which is chosen on the basis of the pre-operative cultures. Our routine intraoperative anticoagulation regimen includes unfractionated heparin prior to arterial clamping (5000 IE).

The infected aorto-iliac axis is exposed by meticulous dissection and isolation of the vascular structures. Proximal vascular control is achieved using vascular clamps and the iliac vessels are occluded with Foley catheters. After cross clamping the aorta and the iliac vessels, all infected native and synthetic materials are removed (Figure 1B,C), and surrounding tissues are radically debrided. The proximal segment of the aorta is anastomosed in an end-to-end fashion with 4–0 Prolene running sutures to either an antibiotic-soaked Dacron Y-graft or a silver-triclosan collagen-coated polyester graft selected based on anatomical considerations and availability. A new channel is created behind the ureter (which can be easily palpated using the ureteral splint) and the colon on either side using blind separation. The extra-anatomical bypass is performed by creating tunnels through the retroperitoneal space, carefully dissected to avoid injury to vital structures. The branch vascular graft on each side is then passed retroperitoneally through the channel and laterally into the paracolic gutter (Figure 2), and then extended along the lateral abdomen wall to the groin, where it is anastomosed to the femoral artery using 4–0 Prolene running sutures (Figures 3 and 4A). Complete retro-peritonealization of the graft is thus ensured. The proximal and distal ends of the graft are anastomosed to the uninfected portions of the aorta and femoral vessels using standard vascular techniques. An omental flap is added unless the omentum is too small to cover the reconstruction. Care should be taken to ensure that the graft is not subjected to excessive tension or kinking. The retroperitoneal tunnels are closed using absorbable sutures (Video S1).

Postoperatively, we recommend prophylactic heparin and aspirin 100 mg once daily during hospital stay if there are no other indications. All patients are closely monitored in intensive care.

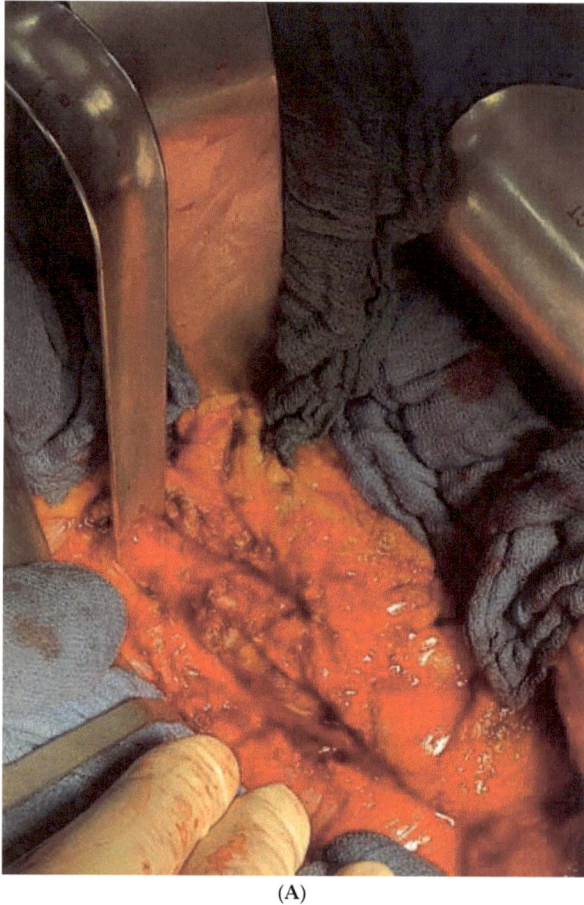

(A)

Figure 1. *Cont.*

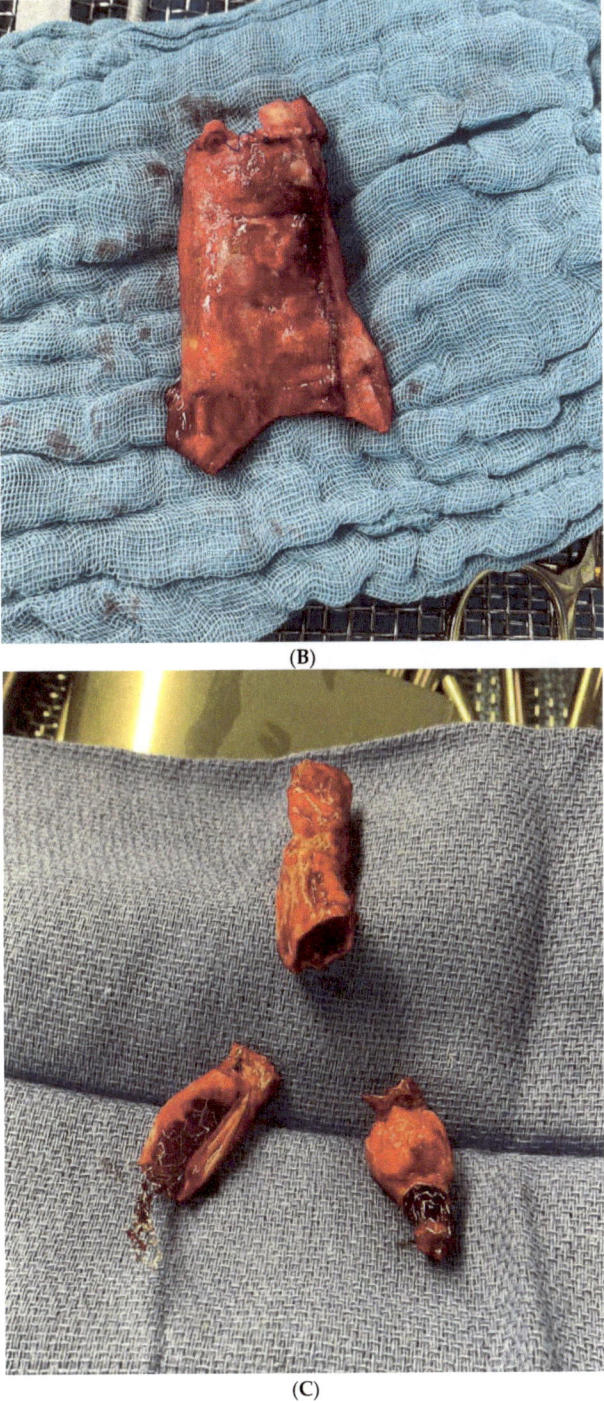

Figure 1. (**A**) Infection of bovine pericardial reconstruction and stents in the aorto-iliac axis by redo aorto-axis reconstruction in a patient operated four times previously. (**B**) The infected pericardial tube is resected. (**C**) Removal of infected implanted stents in the aorto-iliac axis.

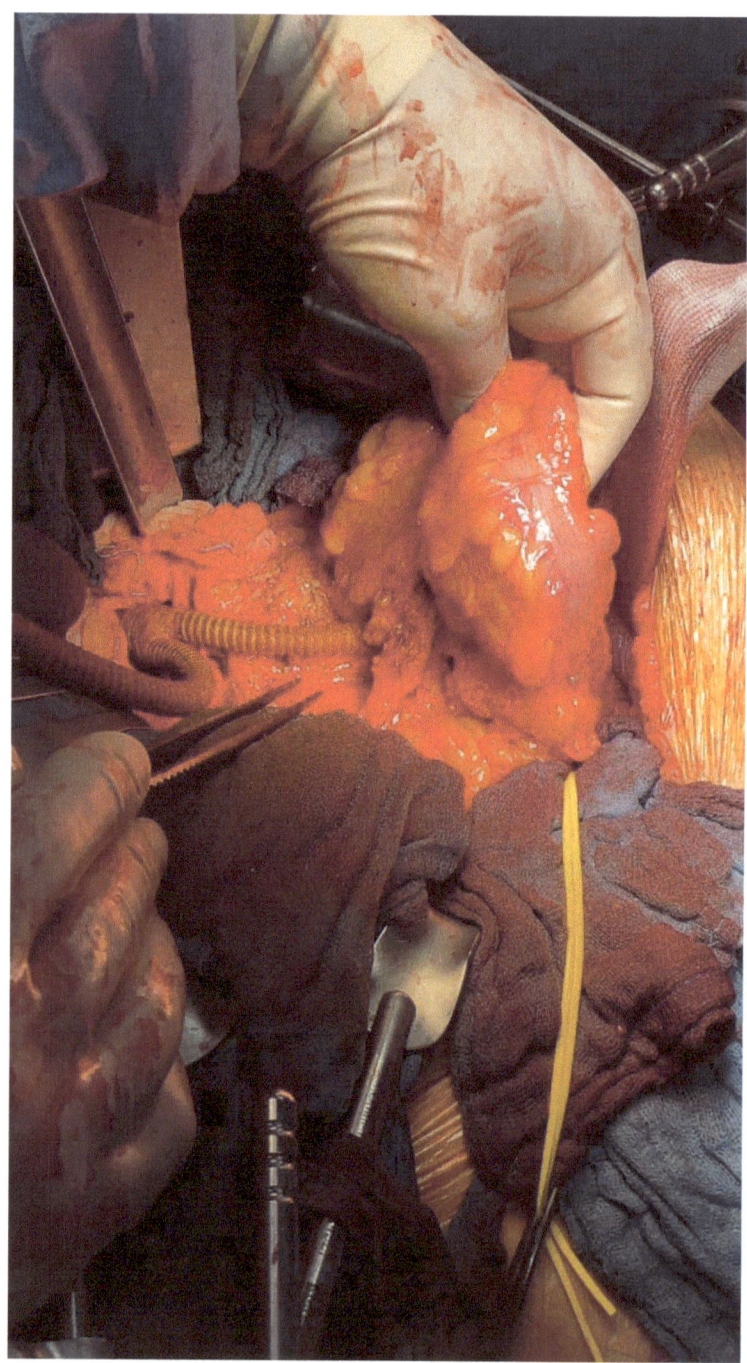

Figure 2. The branch of the vascular graft on each side is passed retrocolon and retro-peritoneally through the channel and laterally into the paracolic gutter.

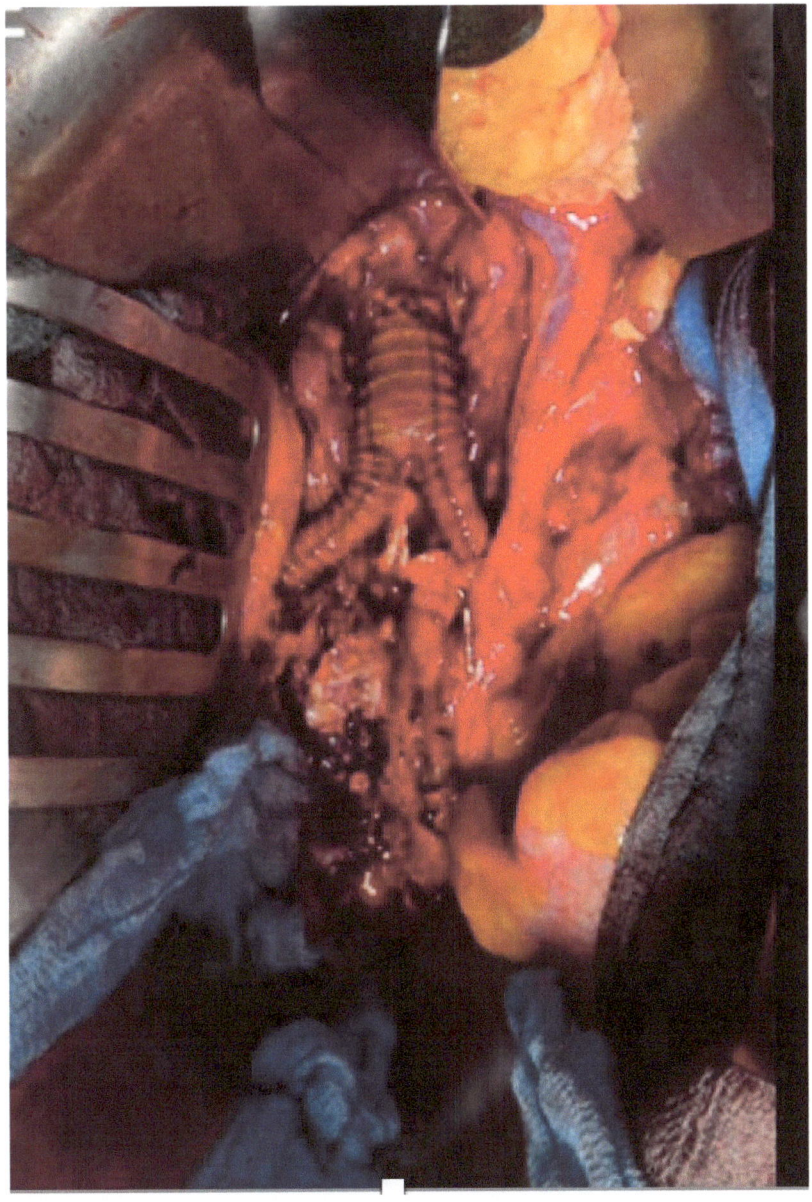

Figure 3. Intraoperative replacement of infrarenal aorta with a silver–triclosan collagen-coated polyester vascular graft.

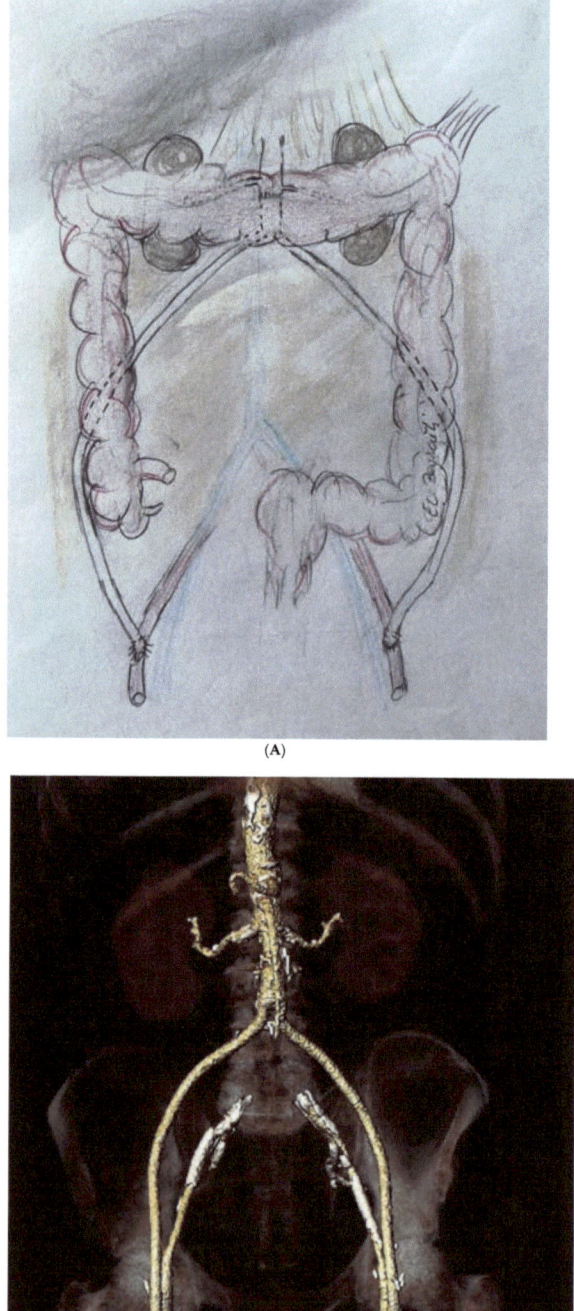

Figure 4. (**A**) Artistic representation of the technique. (**B**) Postoperative, volume-rendering three-dimensional computed tomographic reconstruction of the aorto-iliac grafts with para-colic routing.

2.2. Intraoperative Microbiological Cultures and Antimicrobial Therapy

Accurate diagnosis of VGI can involve several radiological and nuclear medicine modalities with white blood cell scintigraphy or PET recommended to improve diagnostic accuracy [17]. Our standard practice is to request for PET-CT unless the patient is considered at risk of a severe complication like sepsis. Specimens collected intraoperatively are routinely sent for culture; in the case of prosthetic graft infections; a piece of the removed graft is also sent for microbiological testing. Infection is classification according to the Management of Aortic Graft Infection Collaboration (MAGIC) criteria [18]. All patients receive antifungal or wide-spectrum antibiotic intravenous therapy upon diagnosis—subsequently adapted according to the pathogens identified from intraoperative microbiological cultures—and is continued for a minimum of six weeks after discharge and as per laboratory markers and microbiological findings of infection. In the cases of candida infection, we typically advise antibiotic medication for at least one year. Graft-related outcomes such as patency are evaluated during follow-up using ultrasonography and/or CT.

2.3. Statistical Analyses

Descriptive statistics are used to summarize patient demographics, intraoperative variables, and postoperative outcomes. Statistical Package of Social Sciences for Windows, version 20 (SPSS Inc., Chicago, IL, USA) was used for statistical analysis. Continuous numerical variables are presented as median ± standard deviation and were compared with the Student's *t*-test. Categorical variables are presented as numbers and percentages and were compared with a chi-square test.

3. Results

Six patients with aorto-iliac infections were treated using the paracolic gutter technique (Table 1, Figure 1A). At the time of presentation, the average age was 69 ± 12 years. The cohort included three men and three women. Mean BMI was 27 ± 4 kg/m^2. Comorbidities included the following: six (100%) had chronic obstructive pulmonary disease (COPD) and hypertension, five (83%) had hyperlipidemia and were smokers at the time of surgery, four (67%) had diabetes mellitus, malignancy, and peripheral artery disease, and three (50%) had coronary artery disease. One (17%) patient had undergone prior endovascular repair, two (33%) patients had recurrent reinfections, three (50%) patients had undergone at least one redo procedure, and four (67%) had contained rupture at the aorto-iliac axis. Infective native aortic aneurysms were present in two (33%) patients, and an aorto-ureteric fistula was present in one (17%) patient. (Table 2).

Table 1. Summary of patient data.

	n = 6
Male	3 (50%)
Age (years)	69 ± 12
Peripheral artery disease	4 (67%)
BMI (kg/m^2)	27 ± 4
Coronary artery disease	3 (50%)
Hypertension	6 (100%)
Hyperlipidemia	5 (83%)
Diabetes	4 (67%)
Smoking	5 (83%)
COPD	6 (100%)
Malignancy	4 (67%)
Prior endovascular repair	1 (17%)
Aorto-iliac rupture	4 (67%)
Recurrent infections	2 (33%)
Prior tumor resection	3 (50%)
Infective native aortic aneurysm	2 (33%)
Aorto-ureteric fistula	1 (17%)
ASA ≥ 4	5 (83%)

Data are *n* (%) or (median ± SD). ASA, American Society of Anesthesiologists; BMI, body mass index; COPD, chronic obstructive pulmonary disease; SD, standard deviation.

Table 2. Indication and operative data.

	n = 6
Infective native aortic aneurysm (INAA)	2 (33%)
Vascular graft/endograft infection (VGEI)	4 (67%)
Major infection (MAGIC classification)	6 (100%)
Antibiotic-soaked Y-graft (Dacron)	3 (50%)
Silver–triclosan collagen-coated (polyester)	3 (50%)
Omental flap	3 (50%)
Procedure time (min)	322 ± 44
Technical success	6 (100%)
Procedural complications	0
Perioperative mortality	0
Intensive care (days)	2.2 ± 1
Hospitalization (days)	17 ± 6
Positive cultures/Infection (Intraoperative microbiological cultures)	
Staphyolococcus	2 (34%)
Enterococcus	2 (34%)
Pseudomonas	1 (17%)
Candida	1 (17%)

Data are n (%) or (median ± SD). MAGIC, Management of Aortic Graft Infection; SD, standard deviation; INAA, Infective native aortic aneurysm; VGEI Vascular graft/endograft infection.

Operative and procedural details are given in Table 2. All patients were confirmed with a major infection according to the MAGIC classification: four with VGI and two with infective native aortic aneurysm. The following bacteria were detected microbiologically from positive intraoperative cultures in all six (100%) patients: Staphylococcus and Enterococcus (34% each); Pseudomonas and Candida (17% each).

All procedures were technical successes and there were no major intraoperative or early postoperative complications. No intraoperative deaths occurred. Median procedure time was 322 ± 44 min. The median length of intensive care stay was 2.2 ± 1 days and total hospitalization was 17 ± 6 days.

Graft patency was assessed through regular postoperative imaging. There was no early surgical revision and one late (>30 days) due to graft thrombosis (treated with thrombectomy). Primary and secondary graft patency rates were 83% and 100%, respectively. Postoperative infection control was evaluated based on clinical and radiological parameters. All six patients demonstrated complete resolution of infection as evidenced by the absence of fever, wound discharge, and negative imaging findings for infection at discharge. There were no signs of aortic infection with formation of aorto-enteric or aorto-ureteral fistulation (Figure 4B). No complications were observed. Patients were followed for median 52 ± 44 months. One late mortality occurred due to candida reinfection with sepsis and respiratory failure, and to multiorgan failure. This patient had been advised to continue long-term antimycotic therapy but was subsequently discovered to have discontinued medication eight months previously of his own accord.

During the first six postoperative months, all patients received dual antiplatelet therapy (aspirin, clopidogrel). Three (50%) continued with dual antiplatelet therapy due to coronary artery stenting for coronary artery disease or atrial fibrillation. Three (50%) switched to aspirin alone.

4. Discussion

Infections of the aorto-iliac bifurcation—especially fungal infections and those involving arteriovenous and iliac-ureteric (IUF) and iliac-duodenal (IDF) fistulas—are rare but very challenging surgical problems to address. Aorto-iliac infection has a mortality rate between 9% and 75% and associated morbidity can include amputation (up to 30%) depending on the severity of the infection and type of treatment [19–21]. Those that occur after previous aortic surgery are often more difficult to treat and have a higher mortality rate due to the presence of scar tissue from the previous surgery. Reinfection in the aortoiliac arteries can cause graft occlusion, sepsis, limb ischemia, internal organ ischemia, sepsis, and aortic rupture.

Several techniques have been described for the treatment of aortic graft infections, ranging from isolated anti-infection therapy to graft explantation with extensive debridement of all infected tissue followed by revascularization using extra-anatomic bypass or in situ reconstruction [9,11–16]. All these approaches remain challenging because of prolonged operating times, sufficient length of the autologous graft, limited availability of certain prostheses, patency (especially through extra-anatomical bypass), and the risk of re-infection [9,22]. In a study of 122 VGI patients with various surgical approaches—semiconservative (21%) with infection drainage and preservation of the vascular prosthesis; resection (38%) with extra-anatomic bypass; and in situ reconstruction (32%)—the semi-conservative approach was associated with the poorest long-term outcomes [23].

The proximity of the graft to the infected area is associated with a high rate of infection, which is why many surgeons tend to perform an extra-anatomic bypass [24]. But disappointing results of the extra-anatomic bypass due to high mortality (up to 27%), poor patency rates (40–73% at 5 years), high amputation rates (up to 24%), and risk of aortic stump rupture (2–30%) [11] have encouraged many to resort to in situ reconstruction with autogenous grafts. However, the results of autologous reconstruction with femoral vein (FV) were not encouraging due to operative mortality (up to 10%) and low survival (45% at five years); in addition the venous morbidity after FV harvest was up to 14% of deep venous thrombosis [25].

Fistulas between aortic graft and the adjacent ureter or duodenum can lead to severe morbidity and mortality if untreated. Endovascular treatment of IUF and IDF has emerged as a promising alternative to open surgical repair, offering a less invasive and potentially safer option by placing a stent-graft over the fistula, effectively sealing the abnormal junction between the aortic graft and the adjacent ureter or duodenum [26]. The literature includes several case reports with high rates of technical success and favorable outcomes with endovascular repair of IUF and IDF [26–28].

However, the endovascular option for IDF remains technically challenging and requires careful stent-graft selection, prudent deployment, and close postoperative monitoring for stent-graft-related complications. In addition to these technical challenges, endovascular repair is associated with several potential complications, including stent-graft migration, endoleaks, infection, bleeding, puncture site complications, and thrombosis and thromboembolic events [29,30]. Furthermore, long-term outcomes have not been established.

A methodological review of 245 reports (445 patients with arterio-ureteral fistula) showed that the predominant location of the fistula was the common iliac artery and that mortality ranged from 7–19% [31]. In recent years, the treatment of aorto-iliac infection has shifted from open surgical repair to minimally invasive endovascular stenting. Because most surgeons have treated only isolated cases, treatment algorithms are often ill-defined, especially in the case of arterio-ureteral or arterio-duodenal fistula. This is because these patients usually have a challenging environment due to previous extensive pelvic surgery and radiation therapy causing adhesions and fibrosis. Endovascular surgery is preferred over open surgery because of improved arterio-ureteral fistula related mortality (4% vs. 11%) [26,31].

Our experience indicates that the paracolic gutter course is an excellent alternative. This approach avoids the proximity of graft materials to the infected area and permits intra-abdominal and juxta-anatomic implantation, which is preferable to the extra-anatomical subcutaneous course of the axillo-bifemoral bypass. Moreover, the channel-in-channel course permits omental flap covering and complete retro-peritonealization. Another advantage of this approach is that it is feasible in patients with large aortas where mismatch between the aorta and certain prostheses (such as femoral venous or biosynthetic graft prostheses) might be an issue. Ureteral splints implanted pre-operatively facilitate the procedure considerably and ensure recto-colonic and retro-ureteral routing and minimize the risk of iatrogenic injury.

The limitations of this study can be seen in the retrospective nature of the analysis, the small number of patients, and the limited follow-up period. However, such series are necessary to describe experience with these relatively rare cases and to share novel techniques.

5. Conclusions

Creation of a neo-aortofemoral system using the retro-peritoneal paracolic gutter is a safe approach in a heterogeneous cohort of patients with aorto-iliac graft infections and presents an alternative to other methods that can be associated with a high risk of re-infection. Long-term follow-up with imaging and to ensure medication compliance is required.

Supplementary Materials: The following supporting information can be downloaded at: https://www.mdpi.com/article/10.3390/jcm12175765/s1, Video S1: Paracolic gutter routing.

Author Contributions: Data collection, C.-T.C., M.O., N.H.; Conceptualization, H.E.B. and M.O.; writing—original draft preparation, H.E.B., N.H.; writing—review and editing, H.E.B., N.H., H.T.; Supervision, H.E.B., N.H., H.T. All authors have read and agreed to the published version of the manuscript.

Funding: This research received no external funding.

Institutional Review Board Statement: Ethical approval was obtained from the institutional ethical committee, and informed consents were waived due to the retrospective and observational nature of this study.

Informed Consent Statement: Informed consent was obtained from all subjects involved in the study.

Data Availability Statement: The data presented in this study are available on request from the corresponding author.

Conflicts of Interest: The authors declare no conflict of interest.

References

1. Kilic, A.; Arnaoutakis, D.J.; Reifsnyder, T.; Black, J.H., 3rd; Abularrage, C.J.; A Perler, B.; Lum, Y.W. Management of infected vascular grafts. *Vasc. Med.* **2016**, *21*, 53–60. [CrossRef] [PubMed]
2. Wilson, W.R.; Bower, T.C.; Creager, M.A.; Amin-Hanjani, S.; O'gara, P.T.; Lockhart, P.B.; Darouiche, R.O.; Ramlawi, B.; Derdeyn, C.P.; Bolger, A.F.; et al. Vascular Graft Infections, Mycotic Aneurysms, and Endovascular Infections: A Scientific Statement from the American Heart Association. *Circulation* **2016**, *134*, e412–e460. [CrossRef] [PubMed]
3. Bruggink, J.L.; Slart, R.H.; Pol, J.A.; Reijnen, M.M.; Zeebregts, C.J. Current Role of Imaging in Diagnosing Aortic Graft Infections. *Semin. Vasc. Surg.* **2011**, *24*, 182–190. [CrossRef] [PubMed]
4. Lyons, O.; Baguneid, M.; Barwick, T.; Bell, R.; Foster, N.; Homer-Vanniasinkam, S.; Hopkins, S.; Hussain, A.; Katsanos, K.; Modarai, B.; et al. Diagnosis of Aortic Graft Infection: A Case Definition by the Management of Aortic Graft Infection Collaboration (MAGIC). *Eur. J. Vasc. Endovasc. Surg.* **2016**, *52*, 758–763. [CrossRef] [PubMed]
5. Chakfé, N.; Diener, H.; Lejay, A.; Assadian, O.; Berard, X.; Caillon, J.; Fourneau, I.; Glaudemans, A.W.; Koncar, I.; Lindholt, J.; et al. Editor's Choice—European Society for Vascular Surgery (ESVS) 2020 Clinical Practice Guidelines on the Management of Vascular Graft and Endograft Infections. *Eur. J. Vasc. Endovasc. Surg.* **2020**, *59*, 339–384. [CrossRef] [PubMed]
6. Gouveia e Melo, R.; Martins, B.; Pedro, D.M.; Santos, C.M.; Duarte, A.; Fernandes e Fernandes, R.; Garrido, P.; Pedro, L.M. Microbial evolution of vascular graft infections in a tertiary hospital based on positive graft cultures. *J. Vasc. Surg.* **2021**, *74*, 276–284.e4. [CrossRef] [PubMed]
7. Chung, J.; Clagett, G.P. Neoaortoiliac System (NAIS) Procedure for the Treatment of the Infected Aortic Graft. *Semin. Vasc. Surg.* **2011**, *24*, 220–226. [CrossRef]
8. Vogt, P.R. Arterial Allografts in Treating Aortic Graft Infections: Something Old, Something New. *Semin. Vasc. Surg.* **2011**, *24*, 227–233. [CrossRef]
9. El Beyrouti, H.; Izzat, M.B.; Kornberger, A.; Halloum, N.; Dohle, K.; Trinh, T.T.; Vahl, C.-F.; Dorweiler, B. Ovine Biosynthetic Grafts for Aortoiliac Reconstructions in Nonsterile Operative Fields. *Thorac. Cardiovasc. Surg.* **2022**, *70*, 645–651. [CrossRef]
10. Czerny, M.; von Allmen, R.; Opfermann, P.; Sodeck, G.; Dick, F.; Stellmes, A.; Makaloski, V.; Bühlmann, R.; Derungs, U.; Widmer, M.K.; et al. Self-Made Pericardial Tube Graft: A New Surgical Concept for Treatment of Graft Infections After Thoracic and Abdominal Aortic Procedures. *Ann. Thorac. Surg.* **2011**, *92*, 1657–1662. [CrossRef]
11. Berger, P.; Moll, F.L. Aortic Graft Infections: Is There Still a Role for Axillobifemoral Reconstruction? *Semin. Vasc. Surg.* **2011**, *24*, 205–210. [CrossRef]
12. Shiraev, T.; Barrett, S.; Heywood, S.; Mirza, W.; Hunter-Dickson, M.; Bradshaw, C.; Hardman, D.; Neilson, W.; Bradshaw, S. Incidence, Management, and Outcomes of Aortic Graft Infection. *Ann. Vasc. Surg.* **2019**, *59*, 73–83. [CrossRef]

13. Vogel, T.R.; Symons, R.; Flum, D.R. The incidence and factors associated with graft infection after aortic aneurysm repair. *J. Vasc. Surg.* **2008**, *47*, 264–269. [CrossRef]
14. Post, I.C.; Vos, C.G. Systematic Review and Meta-Analysis on the Management of Open Abdominal Aortic Graft Infections. *Eur. J. Vasc. Endovasc. Surg.* **2019**, *58*, 258–281. [CrossRef]
15. O'connor, S.; Andrew, P.; Batt, M.; Becquemin, J.P. A systematic review and meta-analysis of treatments for aortic graft infection. *J. Vasc. Surg.* **2006**, *44*, 38–45.e8. [CrossRef]
16. Oderich, G.S.; Bower, T.C.; Hofer, J.; Kalra, M.; Duncan, A.A.; Wilson, J.W.; Cha, S.; Gloviczki, P. In situ rifampin-soaked grafts with omental coverage and antibiotic suppression are durable with low reinfection rates in patients with aortic graft enteric erosion or fistula. *J. Vasc. Surg.* **2011**, *53*, 99–107.e7. [CrossRef]
17. Lauri, C.; Iezzi, R.; Rossi, M.; Tinelli, G.; Sica, S.; Signore, A.; Posa, A.; Tanzilli, A.; Panzera, C.; Taurino, M.; et al. Imaging Modalities for the Diagnosis of Vascular Graft Infections: A Consensus Paper amongst Different Specialists. *J. Clin. Med.* **2020**, *9*, 1510. [CrossRef]
18. Anagnostopoulos, A.; Mayer, F.; Ledergerber, B.; Bergadà-Pijuan, J.; Husmann, L.; Mestres, C.A.; Rancic, Z.; Hasse, B. Editor's Choice—Validation of the Management of Aortic Graft Infection Collaboration (MAGIC) Criteria for the Diagnosis of Vascular Graft/Endograft Infection: Results from the Prospective Vascular Graft Cohort Study. *Eur. J. Vasc. Endovasc. Surg.* **2021**, *62*, 251–257. [CrossRef]
19. Sugimoto, M.; Banno, H.; Idetsu, A.; Matsushita, M.; Ikezawa, T.; Komori, K. Surgical experience of 13 infected infrarenal aortoiliac aneurysms: Preoperative control of septic condition determines early outcome. *Surgery* **2011**, *149*, 699–704. [CrossRef]
20. Bunt, T.J.; Haynes, J.L. Synthetic vascular graft infection. The continuing headache. *Am. Surg.* **1984**, *50*, 43–48.
21. O'Hara, P.J.; Hertzer, N.R.; Beven, E.G.; Krajewski, L.P. Surgical management of infected abdominal aortic grafts: Review of a 25-year experience. *J. Vasc. Surg.* **1986**, *3*, 725–731. [CrossRef]
22. Harlander-Locke, M.P.; Harmon, L.K.; Lawrence, P.F.; Oderich, G.S.; McCready, R.A.; Morasch, M.D.; Feezor, R.J. The use of cryopreserved aortoiliac allograft for aortic reconstruction in the United States. *J. Vasc. Surg.* **2014**, *59*, 669–674. [CrossRef] [PubMed]
23. Gavali, H.; Furebring, M.; Mani, K.; Wanhainen, A. Aortic Graft Infections—A Nationwide Study. *Eur. J. Vasc. Endovasc. Surg.* **2019**, *58*, e602–e603. [CrossRef]
24. Kuestner, L.M.; Reilly, L.M.; Jicha, D.L.; Ehrenfeld, W.K.; Goldstone, J.; Stoney, R.J. Secondary aortoenteric fistula: Contemporary outcome with use of extraanatomic bypass and infected graft excision. *J. Vasc. Surg.* **1995**, *21*, 184–196. [CrossRef] [PubMed]
25. Dorweiler, B.; Neufang, A.; Chaban, R.; Reinstadler, J.; Duenschede, F.; Vahl, C.-F. Use and durability of femoral vein for autologous reconstruction with infection of the aortoiliofemoral axis. *J. Vasc. Surg.* **2014**, *59*, 675–683. [CrossRef] [PubMed]
26. Malgor, R.D.; Oderich, G.S.; Andrews, J.C.; McKusick, M.; Kalra, M.; Misra, S.; Gloviczki, P.; Bower, T.C. Evolution from open surgical to endovascular treatment of ureteral-iliac artery fistula. *J. Vasc. Surg.* **2012**, *55*, 1072–1080. [CrossRef] [PubMed]
27. Muraoka, N.; Sakai, T.; Kimura, H.; Kosaka, N.; Itoh, H.; Tanase, K.; Yokoyama, O. Endovascular Treatment for an Iliac Artery–Ureteral Fistula with a Covered Stent. *J. Vasc. Interv. Radiol.* **2006**, *17*, 1681–1685. [CrossRef]
28. Kerns, D.B.; Darcy, M.D.; Baumann, D.S.; Allen, B.T. Autologous vein–covered stent for the endovascular management of an iliac artery–ureteral fistula: Case report and review of the literature. *J. Vasc. Surg.* **1996**, *24*, 680–686. [CrossRef]
29. Zaki, M.; Tawfick, W.; Alawy, M.; ElKassaby, M.; Hynes, N.; Sultan, S. Secondary aortoduodenal fistula following endovascular repair of inflammatory abdominal aortic aneurysm due to Streptococcus anginosus infection: A case report and literature review. *Int. J. Surg. Case Rep.* **2014**, *5*, 710–713. [CrossRef]
30. Antoniou, G.A.; Koutsias, S.; Antoniou, S.A.; Georgiakakis, A.; Lazarides, M.K.; Giannoukas, A.D. Outcome after endovascular stent graft repair of aortoenteric fistula: A systematic review. *J. Vasc. Surg.* **2009**, *49*, 782–789. [CrossRef]
31. Kamphorst, K.; Lock, T.M.T.W.; Bergh, R.C.N.v.D.; Moll, F.L.; de Vries, J.-P.P.M.; Lo, R.T.H.; de Kort, G.A.P.; Bruijnen, R.C.G.; Dik, P.; Horenblas, S.; et al. Arterio-Ureteral Fistula: Systematic Review of 445 Patients. *J. Urol.* **2022**, *207*, 35–43. [CrossRef] [PubMed]

Disclaimer/Publisher's Note: The statements, opinions and data contained in all publications are solely those of the individual author(s) and contributor(s) and not of MDPI and/or the editor(s). MDPI and/or the editor(s) disclaim responsibility for any injury to people or property resulting from any ideas, methods, instructions or products referred to in the content.

MDPI AG
Grosspeteranlage 5
4052 Basel
Switzerland
Tel.: +41 61 683 77 34

Journal of Clinical Medicine Editorial Office
E-mail: jcm@mdpi.com
www.mdpi.com/journal/jcm

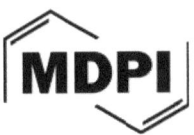

Disclaimer/Publisher's Note: The title and front matter of this reprint are at the discretion of the Guest Editors. The publisher is not responsible for their content or any associated concerns. The statements, opinions and data contained in all individual articles are solely those of the individual Editors and contributors and not of MDPI. MDPI disclaims responsibility for any injury to people or property resulting from any ideas, methods, instructions or products referred to in the content.

www.ingramcontent.com/pod-product-compliance
Lightning Source LLC
LaVergne TN
LVHW070000100526
838202LV00019B/2591